BILIARY LITHOTRIPSY

BILIARY LITHOTRIPSY

Adapted from the
Proceedings of The First International Symposium
On Biliary Lithotripsy
Boston, Massachusetts
July 11-13, 1988

Department of Radiology
Massachusetts General Hospital
Division of Continuing Medical Education
Harvard Medical School

Editors

Joseph T. Ferrucci, M.D.
Professor of Radiology
Massachusetts General Hospital
Harvard Medical School

Michael Delius, M.D.
Institute For Surgical Research
Munich, West Germany

H. Joachim Burhenne, M.D.
Head, Department of Radiology
University of British Columbia
Vancouver General Hospital
Vancouver, British Columbia

Assistant Editor
Gregory Freiherr

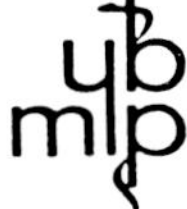

YEAR BOOK MEDICAL PUBLISHERS, INC.
Chicago • London • Boca Raton

1 2 3 4 5 6 7 8 9 0 P 93 92 91 90 89

Library of Congress Cataloging-in-Publication Data

Biliary lithotripsy / edited by Joseph T. Ferrucci, Michael Delius, H. Joachim Burhenne with over 20 international contributors.
p. cm.
Based on the First International Symposium on Biliary Lithotripsy held July 1988 in Boston, Mass.
Includes bibliographies and index.
ISBN 0-8151-3202-6
1. Gallstones--Treatment--Congresses. 2. Ultrasonic lithotripsy--Congresses. I. Ferrucci, Joseph T., 1937- . II. Delius, Michael. III. Burhenne, H. Joachim (Hans Joachim), 1925- IV. International Symposium on Biliary Lithotripsy (1st : 1988 : Boston, Mass.)
[DNLM: 1. Biliary Tract Diseases--therapy--congresses. 2. Lithotripsy--congresses. WI 750 B5955 1988]
RD547.655 1989
617'.556--dc19
DNLM/DLC
for Library of Congress 88-39925
CIP

Sponsoring Editor: James D. Ryan/James F. Shanahan

Assistant Director, Manuscript Services: Frances M. Perveiler

Production Project Manager: Nancy Baker

Contributors

HENRY C. ALDER
Director, Division of Clinical Services and Technology
American Hospital Association
Chicago, Illinois

MUMTAZ AHMED, M.D.
Ciba-Geigy Corporation
Pharmaceuticals Division
Summit, New Jersey

CHRISTOPH D. BECKER, M.D.
Department of Radiology
University of British Columbia
Vancouver General Hospital
Vancouver, British Columbia, Canada

W. BRENDEL, M.D.
Institute for Surgical Research
Ludwig Maximillians Universitat
Munich, West Germany

HALYNA P. BRESLAYWEC, PHD
Chief, Division of Gastroenterology and Urology
General Use Devices
Food and Drug Administration
Silver Springs, Maryland

ROBERT G. BRITAIN
Manager, Diagnostic Imaging and Therapy Systems Division
National Association of Electrical Manufacturers
Washington, D.C.

H. JOACHIM BURHENNE, M.D.
Department of Radiology
University of British Columbia
Vancouver, British Columbia, Canada

LEONARD R. CAPUANO
Ciba-Geigy Corporation
Pharmaceuticals Division
Summit, New Jersey

ANDREW COLEMAN, PHD
Department of Medical Physics
St. Thomas' Hospital
London, England

MICHAEL DELIUS, M.D.
Institute for Surgical Research
Ludwig Maximillians Universitat
Munich, West Germany

JEAN DELMONT, M.D.
Hepato-Gastroenterology Service
Hopital De Cimiez
University of Nice
Nice, France

RICHARD DIMONDA
Director, Medical Research Foundation
Dornier Medical Systems, Inc.
Marietta, Georgia

R. HERMON DOWLING, M.D.
Guy's Hospital
Gastroenterology Unit
London, England

PHILIP DREW, Ph.D
Drew Consultants, Inc
Carlisle, Massachusetts

CHRISTIAN ELL, M.D.
Medical Clinic
University of Erlangen-Nurnberg
Erlangen, West Germany

JOSEPH T. FERRUCCI, M.D.
Department of Radiology
Massachusetts General Hospital
Harvard Medical School
Boston, Massachusetts

ALAN HOFMANN, M.D.
Division of Gastroenterology
Department of Medicine
University of California, San Diego
La Jolla, California

A. G. JOHNSON, M.D.
Surgical Unit
University of Sheffield
Royal Hallamshire Hospital
Sheffield, England

RONALD A. MALT, M.D.
Surgical Service
Massachusetts General Hospital
Harvard Medical School
Boston, Massachusetts

GERALD MAY, M.D.
Department of Radiology
Virginnia Mason Clinic
Seattle, Washington

BRUCE L. MCCLENNAN, M.D.
Department of Radiology
Washington University Medical Center
St. Louis, Missouri

PETER R. MUELLER, M.D.
Department of Radiology
Massachusetts General Hospital
Harvard Medical School
Boston, Massachusetts

GUSTAV PAUMGARTNER, M.D.
Department of Gastroenterology
Ludwig Maxmillians-Universitat
Klinikum Grosshadern
Munich, West Germany

THIERY PONCHON, M.D.
Division of Gastroenterology
Hospital Edward Herriot
Lyon, France

EDWIN L. PRIEN, M.D.
Department of Medicine
Massachusetts General Hospital
Harvard Medical School
Boston, Massachusetts

JAMES M. RICHTER, M.D.
Department of Medicine
Massachusetts General Hospital
Harvard Medical School
Boston, Massachusetts

ENRICO RODA, M.D.
Department of Gastroenterology
University of Bologna
Bologna, Italy

GERALD SALEN, M.D.
Gastroenterology Section
Department of Medicine
V.A. Medical Center
University of New Jersey Medical Center
East Orange, New Jersey

TILMAN SAUERBRUCH, M.D.
Department of Gastroenterology
Klinikum Grosshadern
Ludwig Maximillians-Universitat
Munich, West Germany

JOHN E. SAUNDERS, PHD
Department of Medical Physics
St. Thomas Hospital
London, England

ROBERT H. SCHAPIRO, M.D.
Department of Medicine
Massachusetts General Hospital
Harvard Medical School
Boston, Massachusetts

JOSEPH F. SIMEONE, M.D.
Department of Radiology
Massachusetts General Hospital
Harvard Medical School
Boston, Massachusetts

MARTIN STARITZ, M.D.
Medical Clinic
Johannes Gutenberg University
Mainz, West Germany

HARVEY V. STEINBERG, M.D.
Department of Radiology
Crawford Long Hospital
Atlanta, Georgia

JOHNSON L. THISTLE, M.D.
Gastroenterology and Internal Medicine
Mayo Clinic
Rochester, Minnesota

WILLIAM E. TORRES, M.D.
Department of Radiology
Crawford Long Hospital
Atlanta, Georgia

ERIC VANSONNENBERG, M.D.
Department of Radiology
University of California, San Diego
San Diego, California

DAVID VANDERPOOL, M.D.
Department of Surgery
Baylor University
Dallas, Texas

Foreword

Biliary lithotripsy is a rapidly evolving new modality for nonsurgical treatment of gallstones. Only 3 years after the first treatment of a patient with a gallbladder stone by extracorporeal shock wave lithotripsy in 1985 at the Klinikum Grosshadern in Munich, the First International Symposium on Biliary Lithotripsy was called by Joseph T. Ferrucci. Its purpose was to bring together researchers, engineers, and clinicians from various disciplines pioneering and pursuing new therapeutic modalities for the nonsurgical treatment of cholelithiasis, be it extracorporeal shock wave lithotripsy itself or methods that are employed as adjuvant or complementary measures to this novel technique. The contributions to this symposium comprise this volume. They clearly show the interest and input that extracorporeal shock wave lithotripsy of gallstones is receiving from different specialists such as gastroenterologists, surgeons, and radiologists.

Obviously, the interdisciplinary approach will be very productive in the further development of this young but evolving new technology. Hopefully, it will not lead to new specialists, the lithotriptists, or a new discipline, knowing all about the shattering of stones but little about the disease and the patient. Thus, it is important not to overemphasize the single procedure, be it surgical, radiologic, endoscopic, or lithotriptic, but to approach the patient as a physician who is treating the patient and not only the stone. The better the technology is perfected and the better the interdisciplinary dialogue is cultivated, the easier it will be to attain this goal. It was impressive to see at this symposium how much one discipline had to offer the other and how the different manufacturers are striving to exceed each other in technical innovations. This development will continue and we shall see more of this in the future.

It can be concluded from the presentations and from the discussions of this symposium that for selected patients with cholelithiasis, extracorporeal shockwave lithotripsy is evolving as a safe and effective alternative to open abdominal surgery. At present, it should be restricted to symptomatic patients with radiolucent stones in a functioning gallbladder that are well suited for targeting and fragmentation. Since cholelithiasis is one of the most prevalent diseases, affecting approximately 10% of the adult population in the United States and in Europe, these results attract much attention. Caution, however, is prudent not to nourish hopes that are difficult to fullfill, such as to make open abdominal surgery obsolete. Even if the above requirements are fullfilled, cholecystectomy will remain the therapy of choice for patients with a pathologically altered gallbladder and for those with complicated disease.

Gustav Paumgartner, M.D.
Tilman Sauerbruch, M.D.

Preface

The convergence of several events in early 1988 have sparked a rapidly evolving transformation in the clinical management of gallstone disease, i.e., the emergence of safe, effective alternatives to cholecystectomy. First was the initiation of FDA approved clinical trials of gallstone lithotripsy by several lithotripter manufacturers. Second was the receipt of FDA approval to market the bile acid, ursodeoxycholic acid, an effective, nontoxic oral agent for dissolving cholesterol gallstones and presumably their fragments. Third was the publication in the *New England Journal of Medicine,* by German researchers from Munich, of highly favorable results with negligible complications in their first 175 gallstone lithotripsy patients. Fourth was the widening interest in the use of direct percutaneous contact dissolution of gallstones by the potent cholesterol solvent methyl tert-butyl-ether (MTBE). For the one in eight adults over 50 years of age in the civilized Western world who may harbor gallstones, these techniques alone or in various combinations promise as fundamental a change in therapy as the performance of the first cholecystectomy in Germany over 100 years ago.

This volume has been assembled in connection with the first worldwide meeting whose explicit focus is biliary lithotripsy, the technologic center of this new field of nonsurgical therapy of gallstone disease. The First International Symposium on Biliary Lithotripsy was held in early July of 1988 in Boston under the auspices of the Department of Radiology, Massachusetts General Hospital, and the Division of Continuing Medical Education of the Harvard Medical School. During the 3-day meeting, over 500 registrants received presentations from more than 30 invited speakers, heard 20 original proferred scientific papers, and viewed technical exhibits by nearly two dozen commercial firms.

The flavor of this symposium and of the entire field at this early stage has several different elements. These include the number and complexity of technical and clinical issues, the early dominance of European gastroenterologists and their interactions with the American commercial and medical communities, and the rivalry between different lithotripter manufacturers with vastly different shock wave systems and early clinical results. In combination, these elements are creating a rapidly expanding body of scientific knowledge and new professional relationships.

At the moment it is unclear whether the early European data will be reproducible in the United States and what the different commercial systems operating either alone or in combination with drugs will ultimately achieve. It is also uncertain how the highly competitive, rapidly evolving medical marketplace will influence dissemination of these technologies. As of this writing, only a few United States centers have clinical experience with any of these techniques.

It is fully recognized that the information exchanged in the symposium and presented within this volume will have a limited useful life. Nevertheless, in view of the intensity of interest among so many diverse parties, the challenge to transform the material into a permanent and hopefully useful volume was inescapable.

In order to produce a volume of timely interest, most of the material contained herein was obtained as finished manuscripts from the speakers at the time of the meeting. In a few cases, edited transcript of verbal presentations are included and several additional manuscripts not presented at the time of the meeting have been obtained from distinguished members of the faculty to supplement basic research knowledge and newer clinical experience.

Finally, the senior editors wish to acknowledge the unique spirit of collegiality that has characterized the transatlantic dissemination of information from the initial European workers. The hospitality and patience with visitors, especially that shown by Professors Paumgartner and Sauerbruch to American physicians, has been remarkable. It is hoped that this international spirit will evolve and be reciprocated, at the very least, at subsequent multinational-multidisciplinary symposia now being planned.

Joseph T. Ferrucci, M.D.
Michael Delius, M.D.
H. Joachim Burhenne, M.D.

Acknowledgments

We wish to acknowledge with thanks the able and enthusiastic direction of James Ryan of Year Book Medical Publishers, Inc., and the special patient support and professionalism of our secretaries, Ms. Lynda Bessette and Ms. Diane McMahon.

Joseph T. Ferrucci, M.D.
Michael Delius, M.D.
H. Joachim Burhenne, M.D.

Editor's Note

The Greco-Latin derivation of the word *lithotripsy* is well known: lithos (stone) and tript (crush or fragment). The literature to date contains descriptions of both lithotrip*tors* and lithotrip*ters*, a source of some consternation to purists. We therefore consulted the Classics Departments of Harvard University and the University of British Columbia to obtain a concensus as to the preferred usage. *Lithotripter* shall refer to the machine. *Lithotriptor* shall refer to the operator. And. . . . for those who insist, *Lithotriptee* shall refer to the patient, *Lithotriptress* to female patients, etc. . . .

Contents

Section V. Urinary Versus Biliary Lithotripsy

Section VI. Gallstones—Natural History

Section VII. Gallstone Chemolysis With Oral Bile Acids

Section VIII. Direct Mechanical and Solvent Dissolution Techniques

Section IX. Gallstone Recurrence and Prophylaxis

Section X. Lithotripsy of Bile Duct Stones

Section XI. The New Gallstone Therapies: Ramifications for Medical Practice

Section XII. Assessing the Technology, the Market, the Future: A Panel Discussion

BILIARY LITHOTRIPSY

Biliary Lithotripsy: What Will Be the Issues?

Joseph T. Ferrucci

The successful application of extracorporeal shock wave lithotripsy to cholesterol gallstones at the Groshadern Clinic, Munich, West Germany, in 1985 was the flashpoint of an unfolding revolution in the clinical management of gallstone patients.[1] Following the leadership of Dornier engineers, some 10 other firms are now testing various different lithotripter devices in Europe, the United States, and Japan. As of this writing, perhaps 1000 gallstone patients have undergone shockwave lithotripsy worldwide, and prestigious medical journals are gladly publishing the early results.[2]

As visible and dramatic as lithotripsy is, other competing and complementary therapeutic techniques are being introduced almost simultaneously to further accelerate the trend to nonsurgical management. These include both pharmacological and mechanical interventional methods. For example, direct contact dissolution of cholesterol gallstones by the potent solvent methyl tert-butyl ether (MTBE) has given highly successful results in early series.[3] Chemolysis of cholesterol gallstones using oral bile acids has had a long and successful clinical experience in Europe,[4–6] and the widely preferred agent ursodeoxycholic acid has recently been approved by the FDA for clinical use in the United States Various interventional techniques using direct mechanical basket or laser destructive techniques are also being widely applied under endoscopic and fluoroscopic guidance, especially for common bile duct stones. It is also highly likely that all these various techniques—lithotripsy, solvent dissolution, and mechanical intervention—can be used to advantage in a variety of yet unforeseen combinations.

It is therefore apparent that a new threshold of medical scientific knowledge is in view. For the one in ten adults worldwide who harbors cholesterol gallstones, a new range of therapeutic options is emerging, which ultimately promises to eclipse surgical cholecystectomy as the gold standard treatment of gallstone disease.

The field of nonsurgical management of gallstones is complex and, at present, somewhat immature. However, with the proliferation of equipment, metabolic information, and technical knowhow, new opportunities for research and scientific advancement are clear. A great deal of information has already been accumulated; and without minimizing the validity or importance of these data, it is likely that much of the information will prove to be preliminary and undergo refinement over the next several years. The major technical and clinical questions are becoming apparent, and some of the major issues that this Symposium will address are described below.

THE SHOCK WAVE: PHYSICAL PRINCIPLES

MECHANISMS OF SHOCK WAVE FORMATION

The Symposium will cover the *mechanisms of shock wave* formation and distinction of shock waves from acoustic waves, the significance of the ability to focus shock waves, and the interrelation of the parameters affecting the focus (e.g., focal distance, aperture diameter, and focal zone size and shape). Mechanisms of transmission of shock waves in tissue and nature of energy deposition will also be discussed.

CHARACTERISTICS OF SHOCK WAVES

What are the pertinent physical characteristics of shock waves, and how are they measured? These include significance and techniques of measurement of peak pressure, rise times, focal zone, isodose fall-off, and wave form. What are the best parameters to characterize the shock wave field? What are the best measures of efficacy of stone disintegration?

BIOEFFECTS

What are the mechanisms and determinants of tissue injury during shock wave therapy? The phenomenon of cavitation requires more elucidation. What are the interactions between shock frequency, total number of shocks, and initial pressure on tissue damage and repair processes? On pain perception? How are shock waves transmitted in water versus air versus tissues, and what effects do they display as they cross tissue-skin-air interfaces?

THE LITHOTRIPTER: DESIGN FEATURES

FUNCTIONAL COMPONENTS OF A LITHOTRIPTER SYSTEM

These include:

The energy source or type of shock wave generator
The focusing or reflecting device
The coupling medium
The image localization technique (i.e., ultrasound, fluoroscopy).

What are the advantages, disadvantages, and tradeoffs?

CATEGORIES OF SHOCK WAVE GENERATORS

These categories include the basic concept and design of an immersion spark-gap generator, electromagnetic acoustic generator, piezoelectric generator, micro-explosive generator. What are the unique properties of each, their strengths, their problems?

METHODS FOR MEASUREMENT, COMPARISON, AND STANDARDIZATION

At present, clinical in vivo quality assurance of shock wave production is relatively primitive. Physical measurement observations are relied upon rather than internal electronic or computer generated fail-safe controls. Attempts at standardization are thwarted by company-specific measuring techniques, disclosure, patent, and country of origin issues. On-line quality assurance to ascertain the pressure front output for clinical site operations is the bottom line. Industry wide standardization of operating parameters would be of value.

THE STONE

MECHANISMS OF STONE FRAGMENTATION

What are the differences between kidney stones and gallstones, relative to their susceptibility to lithotripsy (hardness or crystallinity in the matrix)? How are these measured, and how are they modeled in the research laboratory? What is the physical mechanism by which the tensile and shock forces interact within a stone? What is the relationship between the front wall and back wall reverberation effects? What is meant by spallation as a mechanism of stone disintegration? What is cavitation; and how do bubbles form, enlarge, and collapse? How real is the piezo-electric disruption effect in terms of its surface active erosion rather than pure fragmentation? What about the ability to predict susceptibility of a stone or stones to fragmentation?

CLINICAL DISTINCTIONS BETWEEN GALLSTONE AND KIDNEY STONE LITHOTRIPSY

These distinctions include the need for ultrasonic rather than fluoroscopic localization; the probable necessity of adjuvant solvent therapy to dissolve gallstone fragments, even though no solvent therapy is generally required for kidney stone fragments; and at the present time, the much more rapid elimination of kidney fragments (3 months) versus gallstone fragments (6 to 18 months).

THE TREATMENT

ANESTHESIA

Although early lithotripsies were done with patients under general or epidural anesthesia, the industrywide standard has moved to the concept of anesthesia-free lithotripsy. Introduced by the piezoelectric companies, this concept has now been adopted by manufacturers of spark-gap systems. Principal physical factors controlling pain perception include lower total shock wave energy and a wider reflector aperture, which distributes the energy more diffusely over the somatic pain receptors at the skin surface. Nearly pain-free or anesthesia-free procedures can thus be accomplished, and as a result most patients will be treated on an out-patient basis. What are the down-side issues, if any, of the need for less analgesia?

POSITIONING

What will be the optimum patient position for lithotripsy vis-à-vis ease and reliability of an acoustic window with stones positioned appropriately at the same time? Initially, there has been a general preference for the prone position, but patient tolerance may be limited. How will these considerations fit with existing system design features?

THE GALLBLADDER

FRAGMENT PASSAGE

Early clinical results from Munich indicate that 3 to 18 months may be required for fragment passage, depending on the original stone burden.[2] Factors accounting for this prolonged delay probably include the scant daily volume of bile flow (vis-à-vis urine flow), the higher viscosity of bile, the narrow (2 to 3 mm), tortuous character of the cystic duct, the dependent position of fragments in the gallbladder fundus relative to the cystic duct, and the relative dysmotility of the gallbladder, especially in the weeks and months after lithotripsy. How much of a clinical problem does this create? How important is it to measure and quantitate fragment burden and rate of passage? Can this be accurately achieved?

THE FRAGMENTS

ADJUVANT THERAPY

The prolonged time for elimination of gallstone fragments has prompted interest in adjuvant therapy to speed the process. Adjuvant therapy could include the use of contact dissolution with MTBE and direct transcutaneous suction, among several other methods. However, interventional instrumentation to remove gallstone fragments is a more formidable undertaking than ureteral instrumentation.

ROLE OF ORAL BILE ACIDS

Initial gallstone lithotripsy experience from European centers has generally included oral bile acid adjuvant therapy to speed dissolution and elimination of cholesterol fragments. Based on clinical experience with primary oral bile acid therapy, it is assumed that for stones of a given size, fragmentation will increase the surface area, accelerating the rate of dissolution (Fig 1). The absolute necessity of adjuvant bile

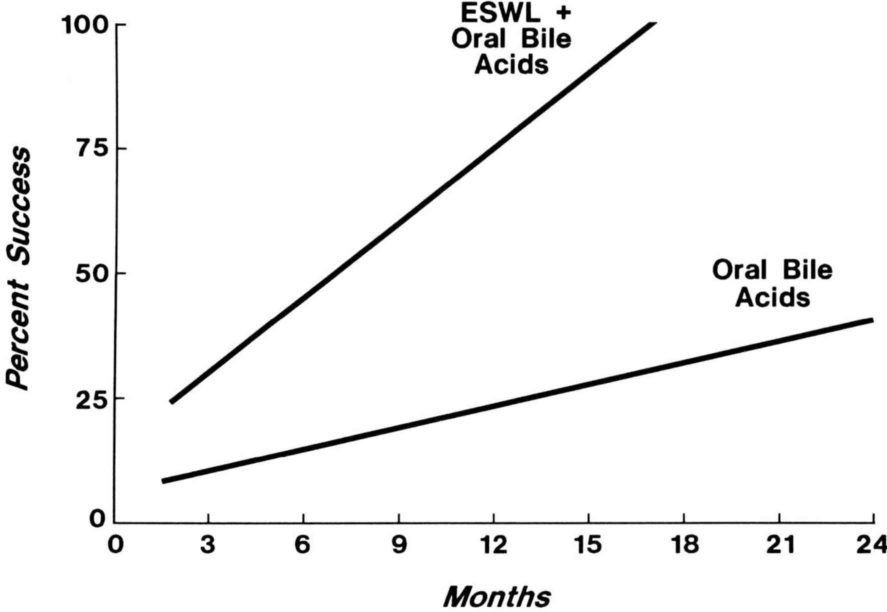

FIG 1.
Idealized plot of the enhanced effect of mechanical fragmentation of cholesterol gallstones versus primary oral bile acid therapy. (Ferrucci, JT: Gallstone ESWL: The first 175 patients. *AJR* 1988; 150:1231. Used by permission.)

acid therapy, while considered likely, has not yet been proven by randomized clinical trials. These are now underway.

RELATION OF MECHANICAL AND CHEMOLYTIC TECHNIQUES

Medically oriented investigators perceive cholesterol gallstone disease as primarily a chemical problem, with mechanical and shock wave techniques as the adjuvants. Commercial lithotripter manufacturers tend to view the fragmentation as the principal beneficial effect. Other investigators believe it highly likely that the best results will be obtained with combinations of mechanical and chemical methods: mechanical methods to increase stone surface area and/or mixing; chemical methods to dissolve the cholesterol.

RESULT REPORTING

What is the measure of efficacy to be used for gallstone lithotripsy: Initial fragmentation rate? Fragmentation to a specific size? Stone-free rate? Stone-free rate at a specified time after treatment? Different manufacturers and groups have used different definitions, most likely to optimally frame their own results.

AFTER LITHOTRIPSY

PROPHYLAXIS

Surgeons' criticism of lithotripsy and other nonsurgical therapies is the compelling argument that a high cholesterol milieu and a diseased gallbladder remain after lithotripsy, and recurrent stone formation is highly likely. Thus, the issue will be prophylaxis against stone recurrence. Diametrically opposed approaches have been taken to address this problem, including direct sclerosis or chemical ablation of the gallbladder mucosa and/or cystic duct and long-term low dose prophylaxis with oral ursodeoxycholic acid. Success rates, costs, and risks of these forms of therapy remain to be elucidated.

THE INDICATIONS

PATIENT ELIGIBILITY

Initial protocol criteria for lithotripsy have been quite restrictive, based on number and size of gallstones, presence of gallbladder function by OCG, and absence of calcification by plain roentgenogram. Various data indicate total eligibility with the present criteria will not greatly exceed about 25 percent.[7] Initially all treated patients have been required to be symptomatic. The speed with which asymptomatic high-risk patients will be accepted for treatment remains an interesting question. Among the first of those with silent gallstones who would not be candidates for surgery but might be treatable by lithotripsy are patients with diabetes and those with cardiac problems.

GALLSTONE IMAGING

Major implications for gallstone imaging arise from the new nonsurgical forms of therapy becoming available. In the past, the only issue for the imaging diagnosis of gallstones was binary, gallstones were either present or not present. Now there is a need to quantitate gallstone number, morphology, and total gallbladder stone burden. Radiologists will be required to relearn the techniques of oral cholecystography.

THE COMPLICATIONS

EARLY

Both cholecystitis and pancreatitis can result from direct shock wave injury or from fragment passage. European centers report only few instances in initial reports. The exact incidence of these problems remains to be ascertained, but likely variables will include fragment burden, total number of shocks, shock wave energy, accuracy in target localization, and precision of follow-up reporting.

DELAYED

Some physicians have expressed concern at the finding of late renal hypertension in 8 percent of patients undergoing renal ESL. Possible late effects of biliary lithotripsy remain to be defined.

THE TRAINING

RENAL PRECEDENT

The rather open-and-shunt arrangement for kidney lithotripsy user certification by the American Urologic Association, Dornier, and individual urologists will not be so easily developed for biliary applications. Multiple manufacturers, multiple involved specialties, and reliance on real-time ultrasonography, a difficult imaging technique to master, promise that a more varied series of training solutions or nonsolutions will emerge. It is worthy of note, however, that the renal ESL precedent for specialty certification in a new modality was the exception, not the rule. In most cases, use of a new technology diffuses into practice by opportunity and linkage, not fiat.

COMPARING LITHOTRIPTERS

MULTIFUNCTIONAL LITHOTRIPTERS

This refers to the concept of treating both kidney and gallstones. Almost all second generation machines will do this without difficulty, using ultrasound for localization. More important, the term *multifunctional* has also been used to refer to the concept of adding x-ray fluoroscopy and radiographic capability. In such designs, a simple lithotripter machine that is streamlined to do only lithotripsy is fitted with add-ons. This increases the size, complexity, and cost of the system but also increases system versatility, revenue-generating potential, and, some hope, marketability. The merits of the streamlined versus the multifunctional concept are presently unclear.

TRADE-OFFS OF PAIN VERSUS EFFICACY

A major issue is the clinical trade-off between

high initial fragmentation efficiency and more perceived pain versus lower initial fragmentation efficiency and nearly painless treatments that may have to be repeated. At present it is unclear whether this is anything more than a matter of preference.

THE MULTI-TIERED MARKET

As noted above, the type of energy generator, the amount of pain, and the efficiency of fragmentation and re-treatment are creating a multitiered market. High cost, high shock power, and high fragmentation are at the top with the various manufacturers distributed down the scale.

SYSTEM OPERATIONS

Comparisons of lithotripters must also include ease of patient handling, complexity of training, number of operating personnel required, operating costs, and expected patient mix (i.e., gallbladder, common bile duct, and genitourinary cases).

ACQUISITION ISSUES

Will all systems eventually be scaled down in size and cost? Will the concept of a mobile lithotripter become outmoded as a result? What about the concept of a transportable system that can be easily moved from site to site and rolled into an existing fixed facility?

FINANCES AND POLITICS

REIMBURSEMENT

How will the precedent of renal lithotripsy performed by a single specialty fit with the competing and/or complementary efforts of multiple specialties interested in gallstone lithotripsy? Is it practical to have only a global fee? Should component fees be established for biliary lithotripsy in addition or instead? These could include surgical plus medical plus radiologic components adding up to the global fee or less.

TURF ISSUES

Obviously, multiple specialty interests exist in the case of biliary lithotripsy (Fig 2). The surgeon views the gallstone in terms of providing a total solution by removing the gallbladder. The gastroenterologist perceives the gallstone as an accumulation of cholesterol, which may or may not trouble the patient. The radiologist considers the gallstone his to detect, characterize, and localize during lithotripsy. The manufacturer considers the gallstone primarily as a target for the machine. In addition to these primary parties to gallstone lithotripsy, a second sphere of interest could be envisioned as shown in Figure 3. The FDA and the National Electrical Manufacturers Association are concerned both with safety of the devices and with uniform standards for performance. The Health Care Financing Administration and the insurance carriers will have considerable influence as to the penetration of this technology through their reimbursement policies. The NIH and charitable foundations will study this field from the standpoint of funding worthy research proposals. Hospital administrators and joint venture groups will actively engage in discussions of financing and marketing strategies. One final group not included in these spheres of interest are the urologists. They certainly will claim some residual interest in the field of biliary lithotripsy by virtue of their familiarity with the technology. It is likely, however, that this claim will have little support and will gradually wane.

ADVANTAGES OF A MULTISPECIALTY APPROACH

Common wisdom suggests that with the new explosion of scientific opportunity and clinical knowledge, a multidisciplinary approach will be in the best interests of the patient and of science. This would include jointly constituted committees or concensus groups to implement this new technology into medical practice.

These are but some of the issues. It is antici-

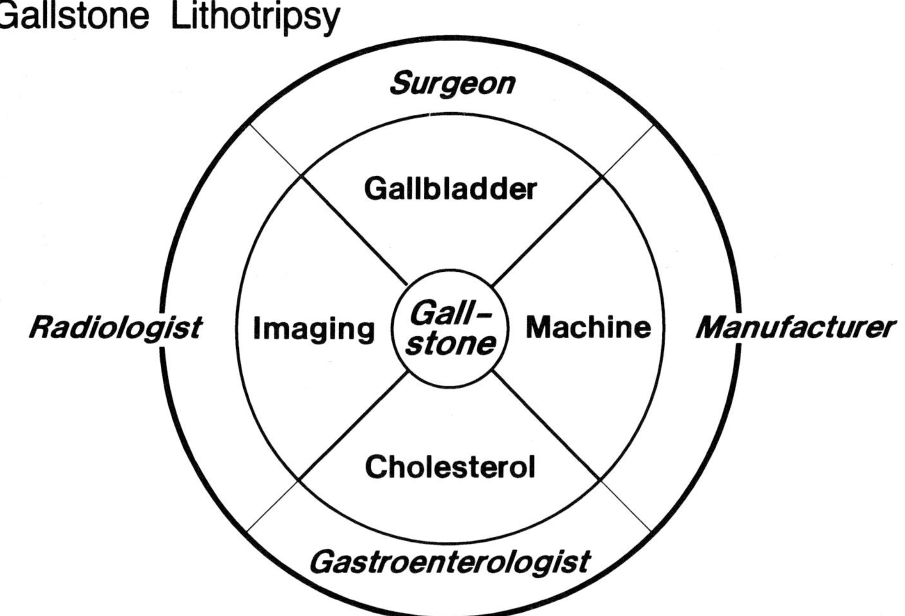

FIG 2.
Primary spheres of interest in gallstone lithotripsy.

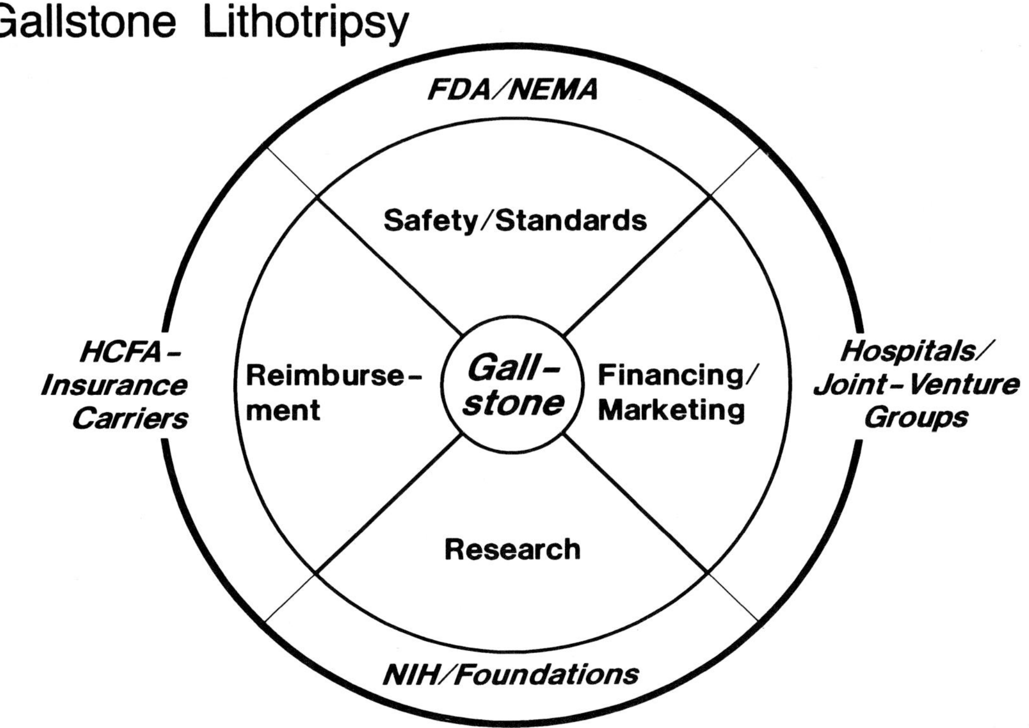

FIG 3.
Secondary spheres of interest in gallstone lithotripsy.

pated that this Symposium will begin the process of providing answers. The once lowly gallbladder has been suddenly raised to a new position of lofty prominence. Much is already known about it. Much more will be and very soon.

REFERENCES

1. Sauerbruch T, Delius M, Paumgartner G, et al: Fragmentation of gallstones by extracorporeal shock waves. *N Engl J Med* 1986; 314:818–822.
2. Sackmann M, Delius M, Sauerbruch T et. al: Shock-wave lithotripsy of gallbladder stones: The first 175 patients. *N Engl J Med* 1988; 318:394–397.
3. Allen MJ, Borody TJ, Bugliosi TF, et al: Rapid dissolution of gallstones by methyl tert-butyl ether: Preliminary observations. *N Eng J Med* 1985; 312:217–220.
4. Schoenfield LJ, Lachin JM, et al: Chenodiol (chenodeoxycholic acid) for dissolution of gallstones. The National Cooperative Gallstones Study: A controlled trial of efficacy and safety. *Ann Intern Med* 1981; 95:257–282.
5. Roda E, Bazzoli F, Morselli M, et al: Ursodeoxycholic acid vs. chenodeoxycholic acid as cholesterol gallstone-dissolving agents: A comparative randomized study. *Hepatology* 1982; 2:804–810.
6. Ward A, Brogden RN, Heel RC, et al: Ursodeoxycholic acid: A review of its pharmacologic properties and therapeutic efficacy. *Drugs* 1984; 27:95–131.
7. Brink JA, Mueller PR, Simeone JF et. al: Morphologic characteristics of gallstones removed at cholecystectomy: Implications for shock wave lithotripsy. *AJR* (in press).

Extracorporeal Shock Waves: Properties and Principles of Generation

M. Delius, M. Müller,
A. Vogel, W. Brendel

Shock waves are single pressure pulses of high amplitude and short duration that can pass through living tissues with only minor side effects. It is now widely known that both kidney and gallbladder stones can be fragmented with shock waves generated outside the body. In all lithotripters, the shock waves are generated in water because water has the best acoustical matching to the body. Numerous methods based on different physical principles are employed to generate extracorporeal shock waves for medical purposes. They all have in common that the shock front is focused at a distance from the generator. The shock waves initially enter the body through the skin over a relatively large area. Focusing increases the wave amplitude up to 100 megapascals (1 MPa corresponds to about 10 atmospheres of pressure), and allows a rapid fall-off of energy and thus prevents damage to more distant tissues. Because shock waves destroy stones only in the focus, all lithotripters must have visualizing equipment, either ultrasound or x-ray, to accurately position the stone in the focal area.

SHOCK WAVE PROPERTIES

Shock waves are sound waves, that is, longitudinal pressure waves, with a large amplitude. In contrast to electromagnetic waves, shock waves need a medium in which to propagate. Shock waves usually occur as single pressure pulses. Very weak shock waves closely resemble sound waves and propagate without deformation at a constant velocity, just above the velocity of sound. This is not the case for stronger waves. Here, components in the wave with a higher pressure also have a higher velocity of propagation. As a consequence, these parts of the wave propagate faster than the parts with lower amplitude. This movement toward the head of the wave steepens the shape of the wave with increasing length of propagation to a steplike shockfront (Fig 1). The tail of the shock wave, including a compensating flat tensile phase, has an exponential pressure decay. Thus, a shock wave can be defined as a single, steplike increase in pressure, density, temperature, and particle velocity, which is always propagating faster than the sound velocity of the medium ahead of the shock front.

The behavior of sound waves is described by linear or geometrical acoustics. With increasing pressure of a shock wave, increasing deviations occur from this behavior and this is what gives the shock wave its unique properties. In addition to shock wave propagation, wave reflection and focusing differ from those of sound waves. The reflected pressure at a hard surface is always higher than is expected from linear acoustics, and the angle of a reflected oblique shock is not

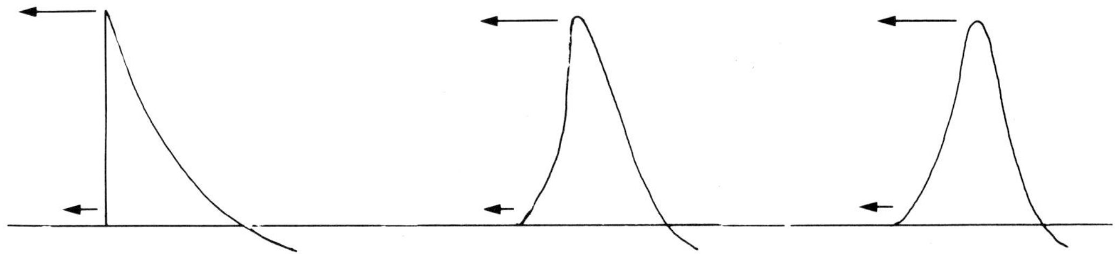

FIG 1.
Diagram of the steepening of a high pressure wave by higher velocity of sections of the wave with higher pressure. The direction of wave propagation is from the right to the left.

exactly the same as the angle of the incoming shock front. All these deviations increase with increasing shock wave pressure. The ratios between shock pressures, their propagation velocities, reflection angles, and other shock wave data in water have been previously set forth by Müller.[1]

The nonlinear behavior of shock waves can be investigated much easier in gases than in water. In air, the first nonlinear influence on the focusing process was found to occur when the shock wave velocity exceeded the sonic velocity by 3 percent.[2] Calculation revealed that in water the increase in shock wave velocity would be comparable and nonlinear shock wave effects would be relevant only beyond a shock wave pressure of about 30 MPa.[3] This was tested by Müller in experiments on focusing phenomena in water. He generated shock waves by underwater spark discharge and focused them by two different types of ellipsoidal reflectors:

The first type, a reflector similar to a spherical mirror with a short focal distance, reflects shock waves from a wide angle into the focus (Figs 2A and 3A).[3] The waves propagate only over a short distance as high-pressure waves with a pressure above the calculated threshold. No nonlinear effects are visible, as the concentration is reached on a very small area that leads to pressure levels over 100 MPa in the focus. The actual position of maximal pressure coincides with the geometric focus.

The second type, a reflector with a long focal distance, reflects shock waves from a narrow angle into the focus (Figs. 2B and 3B).[4] Nonlinear effects occur as focusing takes place at a high level of pressure over the long distance to the focus. The pressure gain from focusing is not as large and decreases considerably with increasing shock wave pressure; the focal pressure does not exceed 50 MPa. Thereby, the focal area is increased. The location of the pressure peak does not coincide with the geometric focus of the ellipsoid.

Some of the reflectors and shock wave energies of these experiments are comparable to settings used in lithotripters. Nonlinear effects can influence the focusing in lithotripters when pressures are high over long distances. The shortest distances that can be used in clinical lithotripters are predetermined by the distance of the stone from the body surface. This distance is relatively long if the shock wave focusing device has a small aperture. The pressure gain from focusing is lowered under this condition and the focal area increases.

The effects of nonlinearity on shock wave focusing can be calculated except in the highest pressure point in the focal region. The results of these calculations are in good agreement with the experimentally acquired data.[1,5] For a given design, it is possible to adjust for the nonlinear effects of shock waves during the construction of the shock wave reflector.

Wave transmission and reflection at an interface are determined by the acoustic impedances of the media. The impedance is the product of sound velocity and density. A sound wave in water is nearly completely reflected at a metal surface as the impedance of metals is higher than the impedance of water. Complete reflection

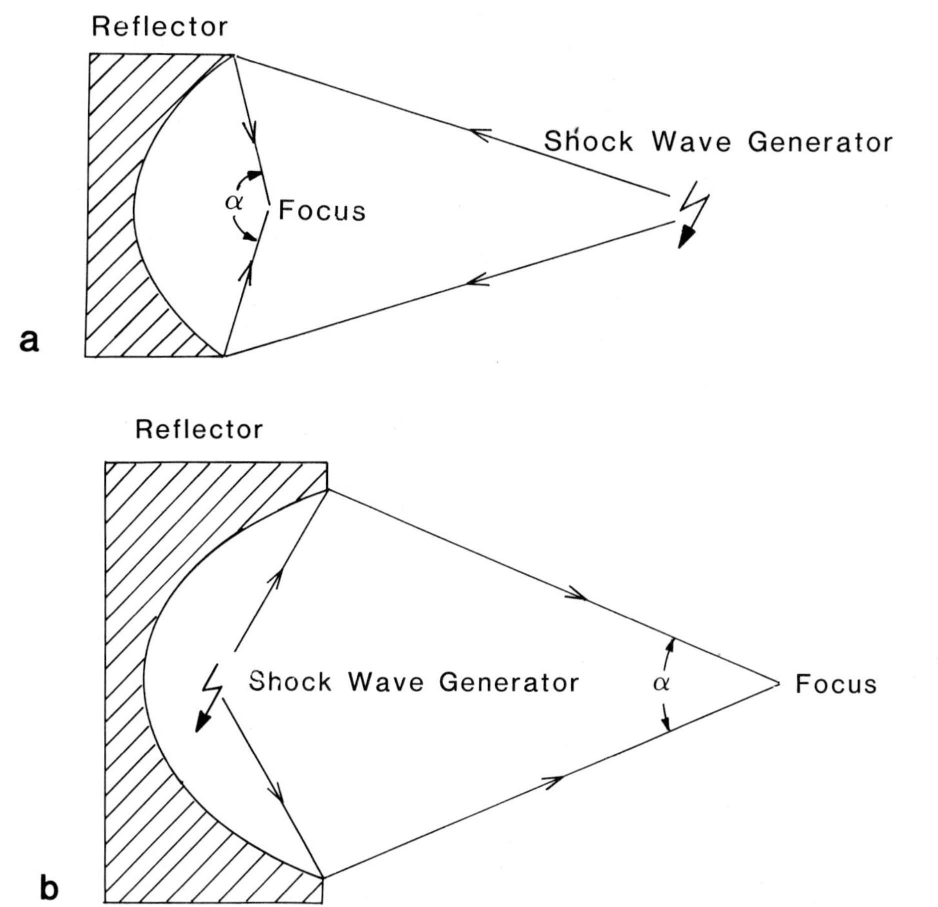

FIG 2.
Shock wave focusing with different arrangements of shock wave source and reflector. **A,** wide angle reflector with a distant shock wave source. **B,** narrow angle reflector with a shock wave source in close vicinity of the reflector.

also occurs at a gaseous interface but as the impedance of gases is lower the pressure changes its sign, that is, a positive pressure wave becomes a negative expansion wave. Wave propagation in biological tissues is not exactly the same as in water. Shock wave attenuation is higher in tissue than in water because tissue is inhomogenous and composed of structures of different density. Therefore, shock wave focusing should be worse in biological tissues, and the shock wave pressures are lower in tissue than in water.

In animal experiments with a Dornier HM 2 lithotripter, which has a relatively large focal area, a lower peak pressure was observed in tissue than in water at a comparable site. In the gallbladder, the shock wave pressure was reduced in the focus to 85 percent of the value obtained in water. When shock waves had passed the body wall and the liver, the pressure was reduced to 80 percent of the values obtained at the corresponding points in the shock wave field in water.[6]

TYPES OF SHOCK WAVE GENERATORS

Three different principles have been used to generate shock waves: point sources, electro-

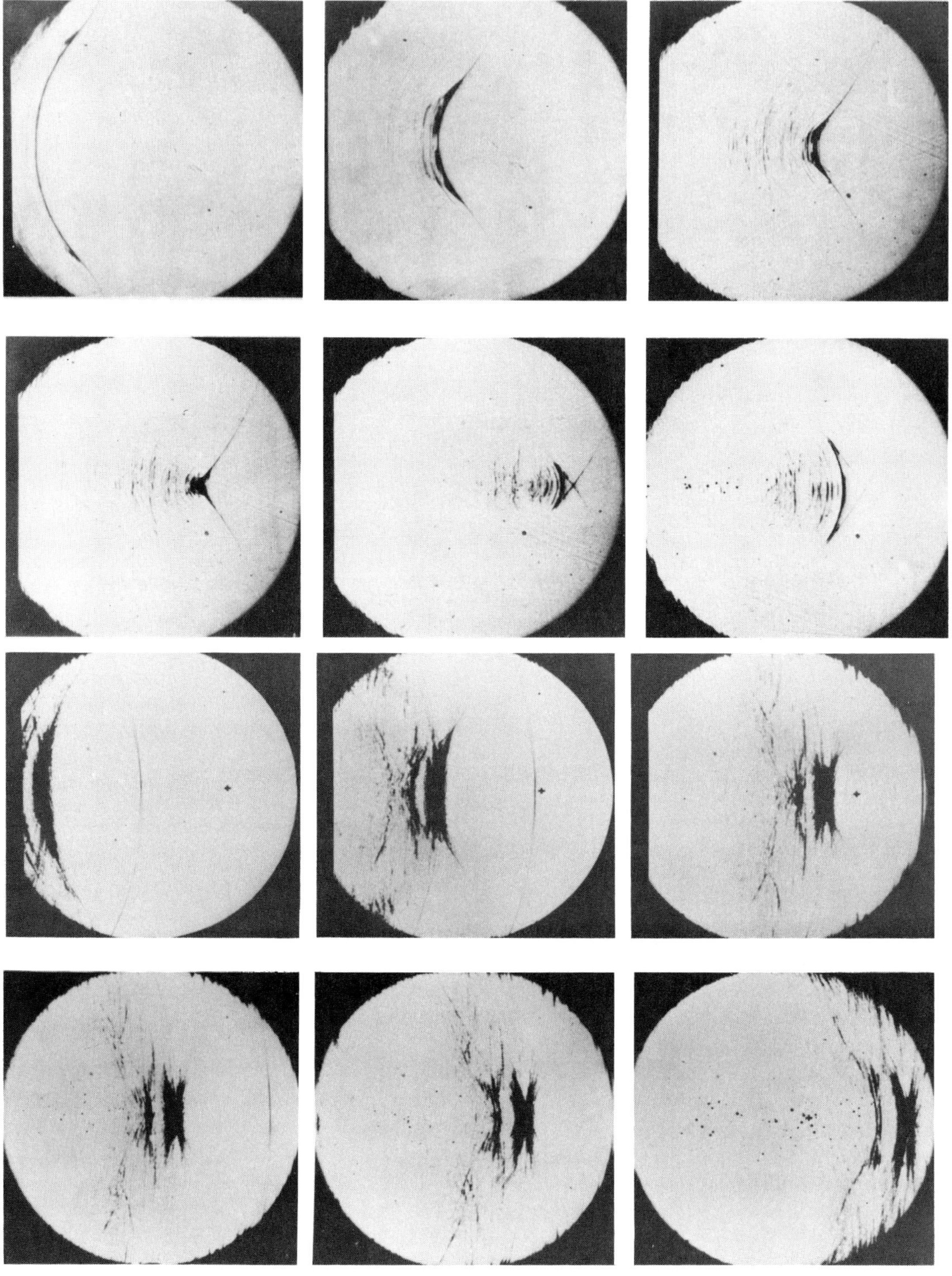

magnetic sources, and piezoelectric sources. Shock wave forms and peak pressures observed in clinical lithotripter systems are discussed in Chapter 3. Point sources generate spherical shock waves. The waves are generated by spark discharges or explosives. Their site of generation is located in one focus of a metal ellipsoid (Fig 4A). It reflects them to its second focus, where the stone must be positioned for fragmentation.

Dornier of West Germany introduced extracorporeal shock wave lithotripsy into medicine with an underwater electrode-ellipsoid system in which a capacitor is discharged via an underwater spark gap.[7] The expanding plasma between the electrode tips generates the shock wave. It has a steep shock front from the point of wave generation up to the second focus. The pressure gain from focusing and the focal area are dependent on the geometry of the ellipsoid. Technomed of France and Medstone of the United States use the same principle; Japanese workers employed microexplosive pellets instead of electrical discharges.[8]

An electromagnetic source for the generation of plane shock waves was developed in the 1960s by Eisenmenger to examine physical parameters of shock waves.[9] Siemens has since utilized the electromagnetic shock generator in its lithotripter system. A pulse of a strong electric current flows through a flat coil, where it induces a magnetic field (Fig 4B). In a metal membrane overlying the coil, the changing magnetic field induces a current associated with a magnetic field as in a transformer. The two magnetic fields influence each other, and the membrane is repelled from the coil just as similar poles of two magnets repel one another. The membrane movement generates a plane pressure wave in a water-filled tube attached to the device. When the plane wave is focused by transmission through an acoustic lens, it can be used for lithotripsy. The front of the wave generated at the metal membrane has a relatively long rise time. As its pressure is high, steepening occurs during wave propagation and the rise time shortens on the way to the focus.[9] The efficiency of transforming electrical into shock wave energy is lower with an electromagnetic system than with a spark-gap generator.

Piezoelectric sources use ceramic crystals, numbering between several hundred and several thousand, depending on the type of lithotripter. Edap of France, Richard Wolf of West Germany, and Diasonics of the United States employ piezoelectric sources in their systems. The crystals are mounted in a bowl-shaped dish array so they all have the same distance from the focus (Fig 4C). They generate converging, spherical shock waves needing no additional focusing devices. Discharge of a capacitor leads to crystal deformation, which induces a pressure wave in the adjacent water. The wave energy released per generator area is limited by the tolerance of the piezoelectric material and, in general, is lower with this method than with spark-gap or electromagnetic techniques. As a consequence, the total area of the shock wave generator must be larger for use in clinical lithotripsy. The angle in the focus between the outer waves of the generator is large when the focus has the same distance from the shock wave generator as in the other devices. The large angle and the completely homogenous pulse generation over the whole area of the shock wave generator (the reflected pulses from a point source at an ellipsoid

FIG 3.
Shadowgraphs of a focusing shock wave (visible diameter 178 mm). The wave is visualized as a dark line. **A,** Focusing at a shallow ellipsoidal reflector (diameter 195 mm, focal length 130 mm). The wave front shortly after reflection *(upper left)* increasingly converges during its propagation *(upper middle and right).* At the focal point *(lower left),* it is visible as a spot. Behind the focal point *(lower middle and right),* it diverges again. Note the cavitation bubbles generated along the center of the shock wave path *(lower right).* **B,** Focusing at a deep half ellipsoidal reflector (small diameter 180 mm, ratio of axes 0.6). The crossing marks the geometric focus. The wave front shortly after reflection *(upper left)* initially converges during its propagation *(upper middle and right),* but then in flattens *(upper right, lower left and middle),* owing to higher velocity of the central wave parts and does not converge any more in the focal area *(lower left).* Again, cavitation bubbles are visible in the center of the shock wave path *(lower middle and right).*

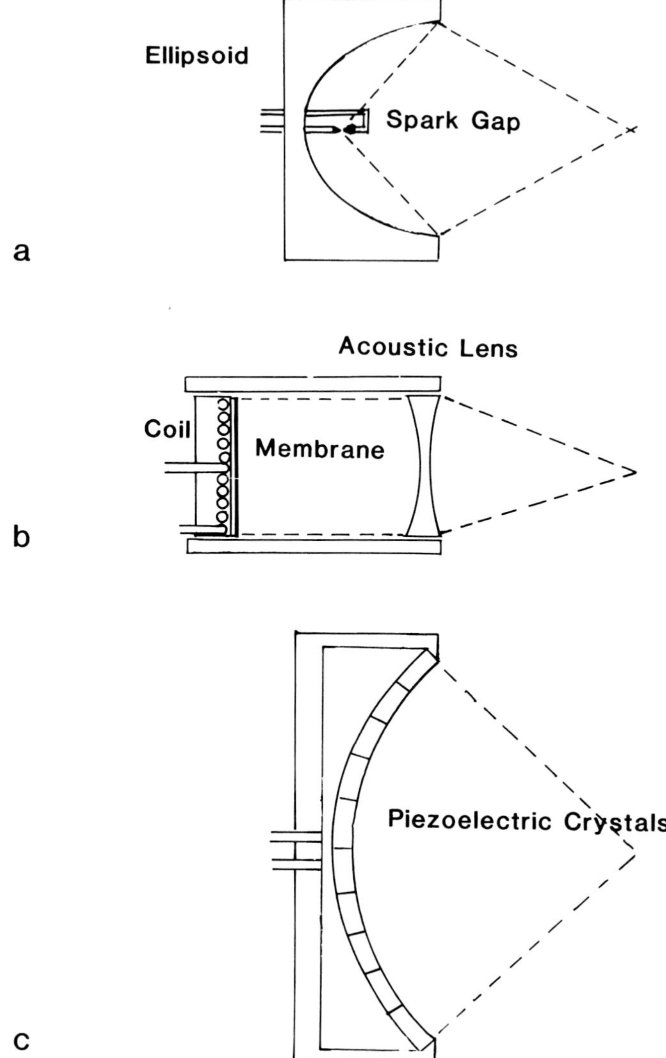

FIG 4.
A, shock wave generation with a point source (a spark gap is shown on the diagram). **B,** electromagnetic shock wave generation. **C,** piezoelectric shock wave generation.

wall do not have the same strength at each point of the wall) lead to good focusing, quite close to geometrical acoustics as in Figure 3A.[10] Owing to the limited tolerance of the crystals, the front of the wave at their surface has a relatively long rise time, shortening as parts of the wave with higher pressure propagate with a higher velocity than sound.

SUMMARY

Shock waves are single pressure pulses of high amplitude and short duration. In water, shock amplitudes over 100 MPa are easily reached by focusing devices, but deviations from linear acoustics occur during shock wave propagation, reflection and focusing if the shock wave pressure in water exceeds 30 MPa. These effects may be relevant in clinical lithotripters, leading to a decreased focal pressure and a larger focal area.

Shock waves are generated in lithotripters with point sources by spark-gap discharge or microexplosion, in lithotripters with electromagnetic devices by membrane movement and in lithotripters with piezoelectric devices by crystal motion. They are focused by an ellipsoid or an acoustic lens or are self-focusing.

REFERENCES

1. Müller M: Stoßwellenfokussierung in Wasser. Inaugural dissertation, Aachen 1987.
2. Sturtevant B, Kulkarny VA: The focusing of weak shock waves. *J Fluid Mech* 73, 651–71, 1976.
3. Müller M: Experimental investigations on focusing of weak spherical shock waves in water by shallow ellipsoidal reflectors. *Acustica* 1987; 64:85–93.
4. Müller M: Experimentelle Untersuchungen zur Fokussierung sphärischer Stoßwellen in Wasser durch tiefe ellipsoide Reflektoren. *Acustica* 1988; 67:
5. Sommerfeld M, Müller HM: Experimental and numerical studies of shock wave focusing in water. *Experiments in Fluids* 1988 6: 209-16.
6. Delius M, Enders G, Heine et al: Biological effects of shock waves: Lung hemorrhage by shock waves in dogs—pressure dependence. *Ultrasound Med. Biol.* 1987; 13: 61–7.
7. Forssmann B, Hepp W, Chaussy C, et al:Eine Methode zur berührungsfreien Zertrümmerung von Nierensteinen durch Stoßwellen. *Biomed. Tech.* 1977; 22: 164–8.
8. Kuwahara M, Kambe K, Kurosu S, et al: Extracorporeal stone disintegration using chemical explosive pellets as an energy source of underwater shock waves. *J. Urol.* 1986; 135: 814–7.
9. Eisenmenger W: Experimentelle Bestimmung der Stoßfrontdicke aus dem akustischen Frequenzspektrum elektromagnetisch erzeugter Stoßwellen in Fluessigkeiten bei einem Stoßdruckbereich von 10 atm bis 100 atm. *Acustica* 1964: 14, 188–204.
10. Coleman A, Saunders J: Comparison of extracorporeal shock wave lithotripters (based on measurements in the acoustic field), in Coptcoat MJ, Miller RA, Wickham EA (eds): *Lithotripsy II*. London, BDI Publishing, 1987, pp. 121-31.

Shock Wave Generators in Extracorporeal Shock Wave Lithotripsy

A. J. Coleman and J. E. Saunders

This paper describes the main differences between the shock wave generators of commercial extracorporeal shock wave lithotripters, using data extracted from the manufacturers' literature and our own measurements on commercial lithotripters.[1]

The differences between shock wave generators operated at (or near) their maximum output setting are described in terms of the relative values of four parameters:

1. The peak pressure
2. The beam area
3. The pressure gain
4. The energy per pulse

all measured in water at the shock wave focus. These terms will be defined below. Other parameters, including those that describe the shape of the pressure waveform, are ignored because it is difficult, at present, to relate them directly to clinical performance.

To compare the clinical performance (in the treatment of either renal or biliary stones) of different generators, we make the following assumptions:

1. Stone fragmentation occurs above a certain threshold value of peak pressure (dependent on the type of stone), and this fragmentation takes place only within the beam area measured at the focus.
2. The degree of stone fragmentation is greater when more acoustic energy is supplied to the stone in each pulse.
3. For low pulse repetition rates (less than about 20 Hz), pain is directly related to the value of the peak pressure at the skin where the beam enters the patient.
4. If tissue damage occurs, it is most significant in the focal region of the shock waves (defined by the beam area and also the depth of focus).

These assumptions will serve to link the measured parameters with some important aspects of clinical performance and enable us to draw some conclusions about the clinical performance of different shock wave generators.

The justification for their use is that, in most cases, they are supported by clinical experience and are not incompatible with the mechanisms that have been suggested to describe the interaction of shock waves with stones and tissue. As far as we know, however, they have not been directly verified by experiment and are, without doubt, oversimplified.

Our comments on the clinical performance of generators based on these assumptions are, therefore, open to question but may serve to encourage more critical examination of lithotripter performance.

CLASSIFICATION OF SHOCK WAVE GENERATORS

The commercial shock wave generators compared in this paper are listed in Table 1. Also

TABLE 1.

Classification of Commercial Shock Wave Generators: Relative Values of Peak Pressure, Beam Area, Gain, and Energy per Pulse

MANUFACTURER/LITHOTRIPTER	TYPE	PEAK PRESSURE	BEAM AREA	GAIN	ENERGY
A. Technomed Sonolith 2000	EH	Low	Large	Low	High
B. Dornier HM3	EH	Low	Large	Low	Medium
C. Siemens Lithostar	EM	Low	Small	Medium	Medium
D. Technomed Sonolith 3000	EH	Medium	Small	Medium	Low
E. Wolf Piezolith 2200 & 2300	PE	High	Small	High	Low
F. EDAP LT-01	PE	High	Small	High	Low

given in Table 1 is an indication of the generator type—electrohydraulic (EH), electromagnetic (EM), or piezoelectric (PE)—along with the relative magnitudes of the four parameters we have chosen to classify the generators.

This classification is described in more detail in the following sections. Further technical and clinical details of these lithotripters are given by Coptcoat and colleagues.[2]

PEAK PRESSURE AND BEAM AREA

The relative spatial-peak, temporal-peak positive pressure (referred to here as simply the peak pressure) and the relative half-amplitude beam cross-sectional area at the focus (the beam area) are plotted in Figure 1 for each lithotripter. The maximum peak pressure is produced by machine E (100 MPa), and the maximum beam area by machine A ($3.8 \times 10^{-4} m^2$).

Lithotripters that produce less than 50 percent of the peak pressure of machine E are classified (in Table 1) as low peak pressure and those above 80 percent (the PE type) as high peak pressure lithotripters. Between 50 percent and 80 percent is taken as medium pressure (litho-

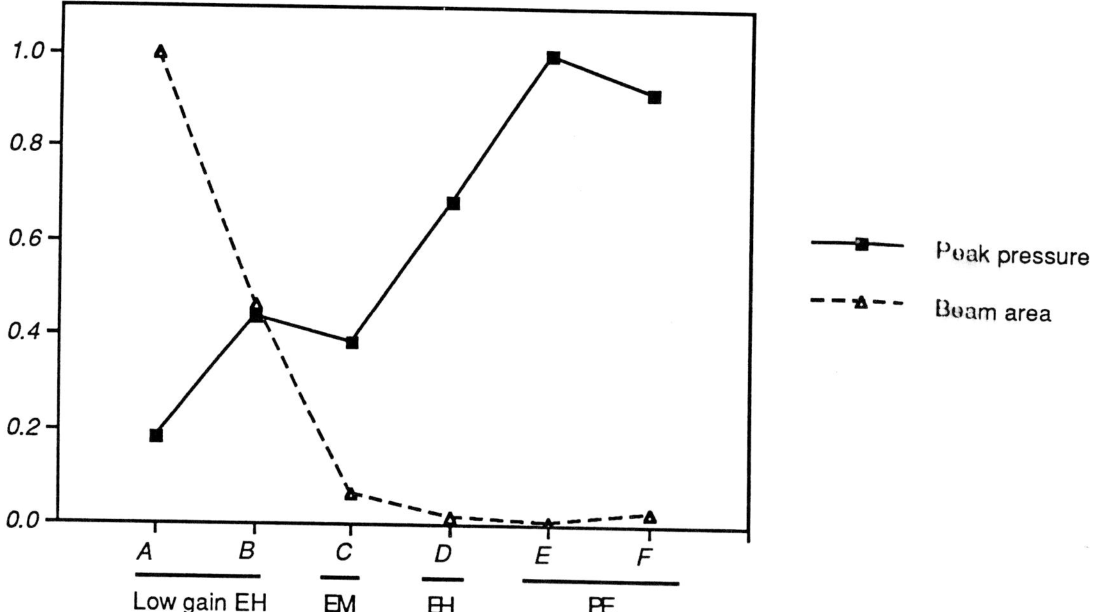

FIG 1.
The relative peak (+ve) pressure and focal beam area at the maximum output settings of different shock wave generators. (EH = electrohydraulic, EM = electromagnetic, PE = piezoelectric).

tripter D). The threshold for stone fragmentation is around 20 MPa.

The cross-sectional area of a typical 1-cm diameter stone represents about 20 percent of the beam area of machine A. This divides the group of lithotripters into those (A and B) where a 1-cm diameter stone would be situated well within the beam area and those lithotripters (C, D, E and F) for which the beam area would cover only a small fraction of the stone surface.

The peak pressure and beam area depend largely on the focusing geometry of and the total acoustic energy generated by the shock wave generator as described by the pressure gain and the energy per pulse.

GAIN AND ENERGY

The gain is defined here as the ratio of the temporal-peak pressure at the focus to that at the aperture of the shock wave source. The energy per pulse is defined as the energy passing through the focal plane of the acoustic source in water during one generator pulse. It can be estimated from the product of the integral over the pulse duration of the instantaneous intensity (obtained from the pressure waveform measured at the focus) and the half-amplitude beam area measured at the focus. Relative values of gain and energy per pulse are plotted in Figure 2.

Machine E produces the maximum gain (of about 200), and machine B the maximum energy per pulse (about 0.1 J).

The peak pressure at the skin, which we have assumed affects the degree of pain associated with ESL treatment, can be estimated from the peak focal pressure and the gain of the system. In practice, peak pressure at the skin (7 cm closer to the source than the focus) is approximately inversely related to the gain.

The degree of analgesia required on different lithotripters closely follows the skin pressure. On the low-gain lithotripters (A and B), a general or epidural anaesthetic is normally required. On the medium-gain lithotripters (C and D), a local anesthetic may be given; and on the high-gain lithotripters, it is possible to treat without anesthetic.

To correspond with the degree of analgesia required, low gain (in Table 1) is taken as less than 10, medium more than 20, and high gain more than 50.

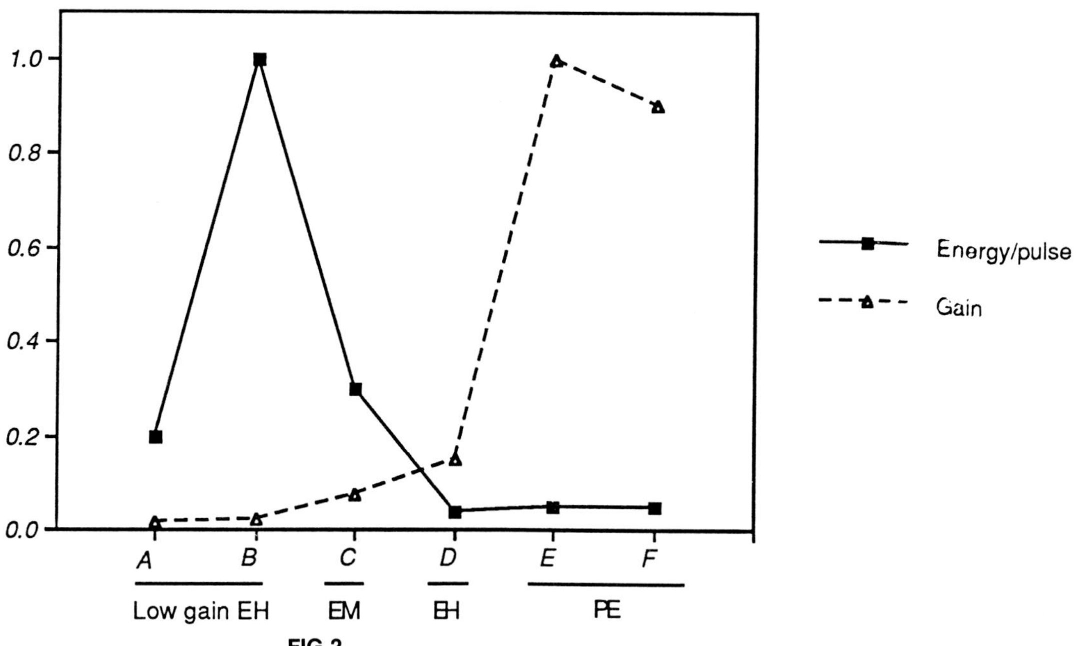

FIG 2.
The relative energy per pulse and peak pressure gain at the maximum output settings of different shock wave generators.

The shock wave generator on the Dornier HM3 (lithotripter B) produces the most energy and is termed a high-energy lithotripter; the EM type produces about 50 percent (medium energy) and the PE type about 10 percent of the energy from B. Those generators producing less than 15 percent are classified (see Table 1) as producing low energy.

THE IDEAL SHOCK WAVE GENERATOR

Before comparing the commercial shock wave generators, we will discuss the requirements for the ideal generator.

The ideal shock wave generator can, for the sake of argument, be taken to be one that rapidly fragments stones into grains with small linear dimensions, without pain and tissue damage.

The requirement for painless treatment indicates that the generator must give a small skin pressure; and, as we have shown, this is satisfied by machines with high gain. Tissue damage may be limited by making the beam area equal to or smaller than the cross-sectional area of the stone. Rapid fragmentation is achieved when the beam area is equal to or larger than the cross-sectional area of the stone and the energy per pulse is high. The peak pressure should be above a threshold value (which may vary from stone to stone) so that stone fragmentation takes place. The requirement for small fragment dimensions is taken to be related simply to the success in delivering the required energy to all parts of the stone. A large fragment, for example, that is outside the beam area for most of the treatment may remain large because it receives only a fraction of the total energy supplied during the entire treatment.

Subject to the validity of the basic assumptions, the ideal shock wave generator, therefore, has:

1. A high gain
2. A high energy per pulse
3. A peak pressure above a given threshold value
4. A beam area that is matched to the size of the stone or the distribution of stone fragments throughout the treatment

THE COMMERCIAL SHOCK WAVE GENERATORS

Shock wave generators A and B (the low-gain EH type) produce low peak pressures in a large area focus. Provided the peak pressure is above the threshold for stone fragmentation, these generators, therefore, may fragment the entire stone without the need to move the focal position. The high energy per pulse indicates that acoustic energy necessary to completely fragment the stone can be provided in a relatively small number of pulses. Because the beam area will generally be larger than the stone cross-sectional area, there is a potential for damage to tissues surrounding the stone. These types of generators produce significant pain because of the high skin pressure.

Shock wave generators E and F produce high peak pressures in a small area focus. Thus, only a small region of the stone is fragmented by each pulse. To fragment the whole of the typical stone, the small beam area at the focus has to be scanned over the stone. The energy per pulse is low, so that, for the same pulse repetition rate, the necessary acoustic energy to fragment the stone completely may be expected take longer to deliver than on machine A and B. For the same reason it is not possible by simply altering the beam geometry to increase the beam area, because this will reduce the peak pressure below the threshold for stone fragmentation. The potential for tissue damage will be greatly reduced because the beam area is almost always less than the cross-sectional area of the stone and, provided it is positioned correctly, will not include tissue. Generators E and F cause very little pain because they produce low peak skin pressures.

Machines C and D (the EM and medium-gain EH type) appear to be roughly intermediate in performance. They have a medium pressure gain and peak pressures that are low to medium.

CONCLUSIONS

Different types of commercial shock wave generators produce widely different peak pressures and beam areas. These differences result from the variations in beam geometries employed (described by the pressure gain) and the amount of energy generated by the acoustic source.

It is likely that these differences affect clinical performance; and, in order to speculate about the performance, some assumptions have been made which are justified by their plausibility.

The commercial lithotripters (listed in Table 1) each have certain clinical advantages and disadvantages, but none of them match the requirements chosen for the ideal generator. By combining the advantages of each type, however, it seems likely that some improvements could be achieved.

A lithotripter with the capability of providing a clinical performance that could be varied between the two extremes represented by the present low-gain EH and PE type generators and that had a beam area that could be altered to match the stone size may be suitable for clinics that treat a wide variety of stones. Such a lithotripter would be sufficiently flexible to limit pain and potential for tissue damage in each case to that compatible with efficient stone breaking.

REFERENCES

1. Coleman AJ, Saunders JE: A survey of the acoustic output of commercial extracorporeal shock wave lithotripters. *Ultrasound Med Biol* 1989;
2. Coptcoat MJ, Miller RA, Wickham JEA (eds): *Lithotripsy II: Textbook of Second Generation Lithotripsy*. London, BDI Publishing, 1987.

Shock Waves and Cavitation

M. Delius, M. Müller, A. Vogel, and W. Brendel

Cavitation, the formation or movement of bubbles in a liquid, is of importance for physicists and engineers since it is known to erode and destroy materials in a streaming fluid. Lithotripters generate cavitation in their focusing field. Evidence has accumulated during the last several years that cavitation is the major mechanism of tissue damage by extracorporeal shock waves and an important mechanism of gallstone destruction. Therefore, this chapter deals with the generation of cavitation bubbles, their movement in free fluid and near a surface, and the effects of their collapse on the surface. In addition, the effect of a shock wave on a gas bubble in free fluid and near a surface is described, and the effect of this bubble–shock wave interaction on the surface.

CAVITATION IN FREE FLUID

Cavitation involves the generation, expansion, and movement of new or preformed gas bubbles in a fluid.[1–3] The composition of cavitation bubbles is dependent on the ambient pressure, the pressures of the gases dissolved in the fluid, the vapor pressure of the fluid, and the diffusion velocities of the dissolved gases.[3]

GENERATION OF CAVITATION BUBBLES

Cavitation bubbles are generated in two different ways:

1. Expansion of a plasma leads to formation of a cavitation bubble. Underwater spark discharge, as in lithotripters, generates a plasma between the electrodes; optical energy from a laser also generates a plasma at the site of the laser focus.[1] The size of the cavitation bubbles ranged from millimeters to centimeters. In its initial stage, plasma expansion also leads to the emission of a shock wave, which in lithotripsy may be focused by an ellipsoid and used to treat patients.
2. Acoustic waves of negative pressure, so-called expansion waves, also generate cavitation. Expansion waves may occur when a shock wave is reflected in water at a water-air interface or in the tensile phase behind a shock wave. Expansion waves are also part of the shock waves in lithotripters. Here, they generate many cavitation bubbles during the focusing process. The bubbles are large enough to be visualized directly on shadowgraphs with a high-speed camera.

The peak pressures of the expansion waves generated in physical experiments in water and in clinical lithotripters do not exceed 10 MPa because abundant cavitation bubbles prevent a further pressure rise.[4,5] However, this tensile pressure amplitude would not have produced cavitation in pure homogeneous water, which has been shown to withstand even higher tensile stresses. The difference is due to the presence of cavitation nuclei, that is, small, undetectable, stabilized gas bubbles from which cavitation bubbles grow before the fluid itself fails to withstand the stress.[6] In one cubic centimeter of tap water thousands of nuclei are found. Some grow to a detectable size by an expansion wave. The generation of cavitation in fact usually means the expansion of preexisting nuclei and occurs at lower tensile stresses than 10 MPa.

MOVEMENT OF CAVITATION BUBBLES

Cavitation bubbles, independent of their mechanism of generation, are not stationary, but oscillating. One bubble oscillation takes place within a few hundred microseconds, depending on the bubble size and its surroundings; bubble movement can be studied only with high-speed cameras. After reaching the maximal size, the bubble collapses, driven by the ambient pressure in the liquid. At its minimum radius, the bubble rebounds and emits a shock wave. The bubble energy decreases greatly during this process; the major part of the energy is radiated from the bubble in the shock wave.[7] High temperatures and pressures are reached in the bubble in the compressed state. They are able to cleave chemical bonds and to generate free radicals. This can be shown, for example, by the oxidation of iodide to iodine, a reaction that also takes place during shock wave application in lithotripters.[8] Thus, shock waves are radiated during both cavitation phenomena:

1. The expanding plasma from optical or electrical energy input generates a shock wave.
2. The rebound of an oscillating bubble generates a shock wave.

As the optical or electrical energy input generates a shock wave and a cavitation bubble, a second shock wave from the bubble collapse will follow the first shock wave. When the bubbles are generated with a laser, the second shock wave has a peak pressure similar to that of the first wave.[7] However, the shock waves emitted at bubble collapse in lithotripters operated by electrical discharge are weaker. Their collapse is disturbed by the electrode tips in the bubble, and their bubbles are so large that they do not collapse spherically, which is a requirement for shock wave generation.[7]

GROWTH OF CAVITATION BUBBLES

The duration of cavitation bubble oscillations lasts up to several hundred microseconds. However, small gas bubbles can be detected up to a few seconds after shock wave generation with a lithotripter.[9] This means that previously undetectable gas bubbles have been expanded to a detectable size by lithotripter shock waves. The underlying process has been calculated for a typical lithotripter shock wave with a high positive pressure peak of short duration followed by a weaker expansion wave of longer duration.[10] During expansion of the bubble, its surface increases and the pressure in the bubble decreases below the ambient pressure. Therefore, gas dissolved in the liquid can easily diffuse into the bubble. During collapse, surface of the bubble decreases, and the time when the pressure in the bubble exceeds the ambient pressure is only a short part of the oscillation period. Therefore, less gas diffuses outward, and a considerably larger bubble is generated. This gas diffusion process explains why shock waves of a lithotripter generate gas bubbles of a detectable size.

CAVITATION NEAR A SURFACE AND EFFECT ON THE SURFACE

Cavitation is a powerful mechanism of considerable economic importance, as it can erode and destroy ship propellers and turbine blades. Erosion occurs due to bubble collapse at the surface of a solid. Here, bubble movement differs from the movement in free fluid.

CAVITATION BUBBLE COLLAPSE NEAR A SURFACE

If a cavity collapses near a hard surface, bubble collapse is not symmetrical because the movement of fluid around the bubble is disturbed by the surface. The bubble changes its shape during collapse, which primarily takes

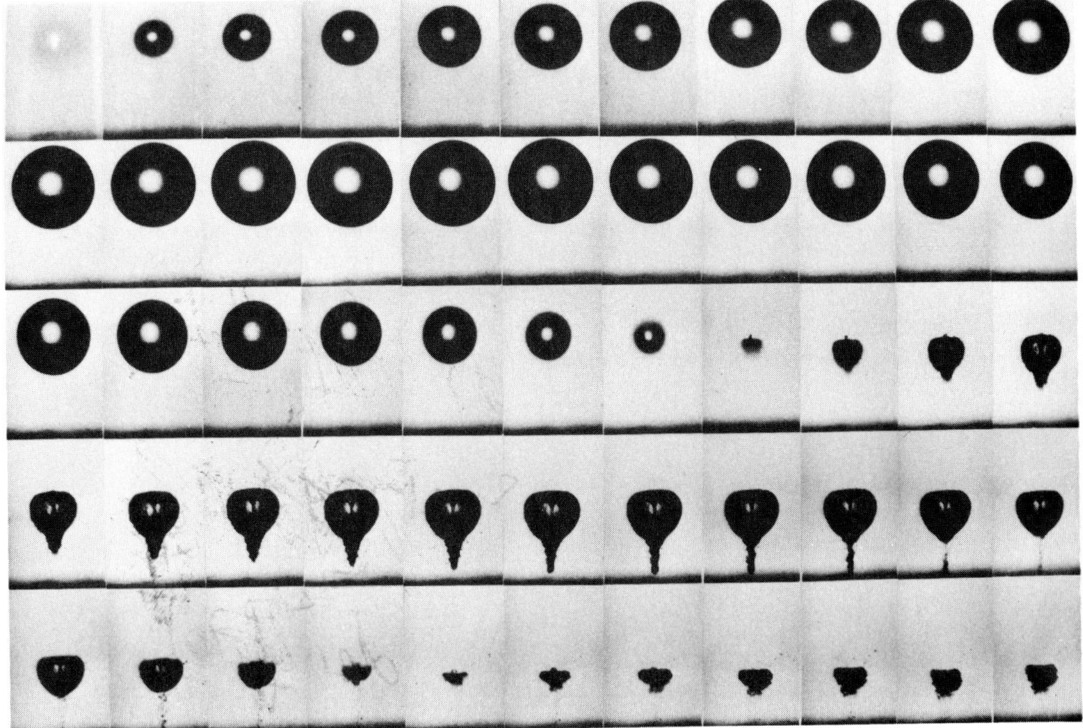

FIG 1.
Dynamics of a laser-produced single spherical bubble near a solid boundary. The size of each frame is 7.2 × 4.6 mm^2; the boundary is located at the bottom of the frame; and the framing rate is 75,000 per second. The sequence runs from the upper left to the lower right. A bubble is generated *(upper left),* expands and collapses *(up to the third row).* Jet formation in direction of the surface is observed in the end of the third and in the fourth row. Courtesy of Professor Lauterborn. (From Lauterborn W, Hentschel W: Cavitation bubble dynamics studied by high speed photography and holography: Part one. *Ultrasonics* 1985; 23:260.)

place from the side opposite the surface. A water jet is formed on the free side, which moves through the middle of the bubble in the direction of the surface (Fig 1). Again, a shock wave is emitted at rebound after the collapse, but it is weaker than that emitted by spherical bubble collapse. The ratio between the size of the bubble and its distance from the surface determines how much of the bubble energy is radiated as a shock wave. Asymmetrical bubble collapse at a surface is a very complex movement.[7] The duration of the whole process is in the microsecond range and can be followed only with high-speed cameras.

Asymmetrical bubble collapse is dependent on the properties of the surface where it occurs.[11] If the collapse occurs at a hard surface, the jet is directed onto the surface, as described above. If the bubble collapses near a very soft material such as soft rubber, or if it is located at a free surface like the interface between fluid and air, the movement of fluid during collapse is facilitated from the side of the surface. So, the direction of the jet points away from the surface into the fluid.

EFFECT OF CAVITATION BUBBLE COLLAPSE ON A SOLID

Easily deformable metals such as indium or aluminum have been used to study the impact of the bubble collapse on materials. In its first

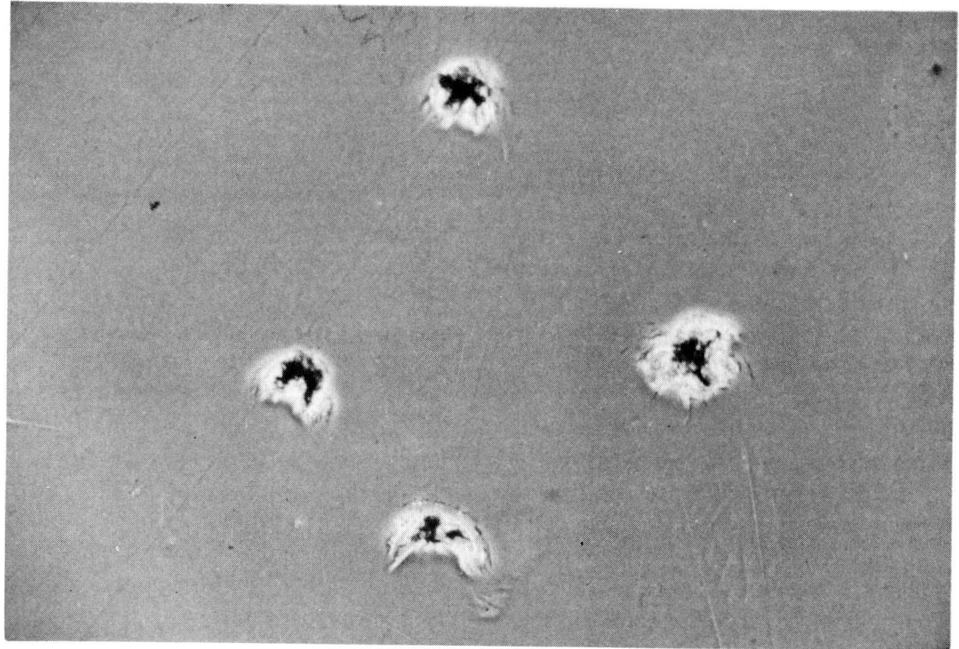

FIG 2.
Craters from cavitation bubble collapse on a polymethylmethacrylate surface.

stage, cavitation damage consists of small craters or circular indentations. Their size is in the micrometer range. It has been shown in a flow chamber that a pit was visible on a metal at the site of bubble collapse and jet formation when bubbles were flushed away from their site of generation.[12] This and other experiments established that bubble collapse was the mechanism of surface pit generation but could not determine with certainty how the destructive effect of the bubble collapse was mediated. Possible mechanisms were the jet impinging on the surface or the shock wave generated during cavitation bubble collapse.[13]

Lithotripters cause cavitation damage at surfaces. Aluminum foils exposed to shock waves in the pressure field of a lithotripter were sprinkled with small pits which again had the shape of craters and circular indentations.[14] Polymethylmethacrylate plates show similar signs of cavitation damage at their surface in the focus of the shock wave (Fig 2).

EFFECT OF SHOCK WAVES ON GAS BUBBLES

In the previous sections on the generation and movement of cavitation bubbles, their emission of shock waves and the growth of cavitation nuclei to detectable gas bubbles have been mentioned. In these cases bubble collapse was driven by the ambient pressure in the liquid. This section deals with the cavitation that occurs when a shock wave encounters a stationary gas bubble. Bubble collapse in this case is driven by the shock wave pressure.

EFFECT OF SHOCK WAVES ON GAS BUBBLES IN FREE FLUID

The interaction of an air bubble and a shock wave was studied years ago with a high-speed camera.[15] A shock wave hitting a gas bubble collapses it asymmetrically from the side where the wave approaches and generates a jet that penetrates the other side of the bubble. This asymmetric bubble collapse generates another shock wave that is so strong that it can repeat the same process in another gas bubble situated behind the first bubble.[16]

EFFECT OF SHOCK WAVES ON GAS BUBBLES AT A SURFACE

A shock wave hitting an air bubble attached to a surface collapses the bubble asymmetrically and induces jet formation onto the surface.[15] This collapse is more violent than the collapse of a spherical cavitation bubble of similar size as the movement of the bubble wall hit by the shock wave is faster and the collapse time is shorter. The jet velocities in air bubbles collapsed by shock waves are higher than the respective velocities during cavitation bubble collapse.[17]

EFFECT OF SHOCK WAVE-BUBBLE INTERACTION ON THE SOLID

The impact of an air bubble collapsed by a shock wave at a soft metal surface has been studied recently in detail.[17] The shock wave that was used to collapse the bubble did not damage the metal. However, when the shock wave hit the bubble, a crater was generated. The crater was larger if the bubble had a size that had been calculated to be collapsed intensely by the shock wave of the experiment. If the shock wave hit a bubble not in a straight angle as before but from an oblique direction, the jet also hit the surface in an oblique direction and the crater from this collapse had an elongated shape. The width of the crater corresponded to the jet diameter, supporting a causal relationship between the two phenomena. This experiment proved that the interaction between a shock wave and a bubble is a more potent mechanism of damage to metals than the sole action of the shock wave.

The jet velocities necessary for crater formation were much higher than the velocities expected from the static yield point of the metal.[17] The physical parameters that best describe the behavior of metals or other materials under cavitation are not known yet, and the forces acting during bubble collapse and jet impingement are difficult to determine directly. The proposal that the dynamic hardness is a more appropriate parameter than the static hardness[18] would be consistent with the experimental results.

Thus, there seem to be two different ways to generate cavitation damage at the surface of a solid:

1. Collapse of a cavitation bubble by the ambient pressure in the fluid.
2. Collapse of a gas bubble by a shock wave.

The latter can be very powerful, as a result of a high driving force. The impact of this new observation is not clear yet, and an examination of how much of the cavitation damage is actually due to bubble–shock wave interaction is needed.

The effects of bubble–shock wave interaction apply for lithotripter shock waves as well. Lithotripters generate detectable cavities and also provide the shock waves to interact with the cavities. So they are ideally suited to generate situations of bubble–shock wave interaction. The long lifetime of cavities generated with a lithotripter allows the interaction of a bubble with the subsequent shock wave at the operation frequency of the lithotripter. However, in contrast to evidence from tissue damage in in vivo experiments, there is only preliminary and indirect evidence that shock wave–bubble interaction is actually damaging solids in lithotripters. Polymethylmethacrylate surfaces showed fields of small straight lines, probably tears, exactly half way between craters from bubble collapse (Fig 3). They were most likely generated by waves radiated from the sites of crater formation. Their localization is evidence that crater formation must have occurred simultaneously. The simultaneous collapse of cavitation bubbles so close to each other is unlikely to be an independent event and is better explained by a shock wave collapsing preformed bubbles.

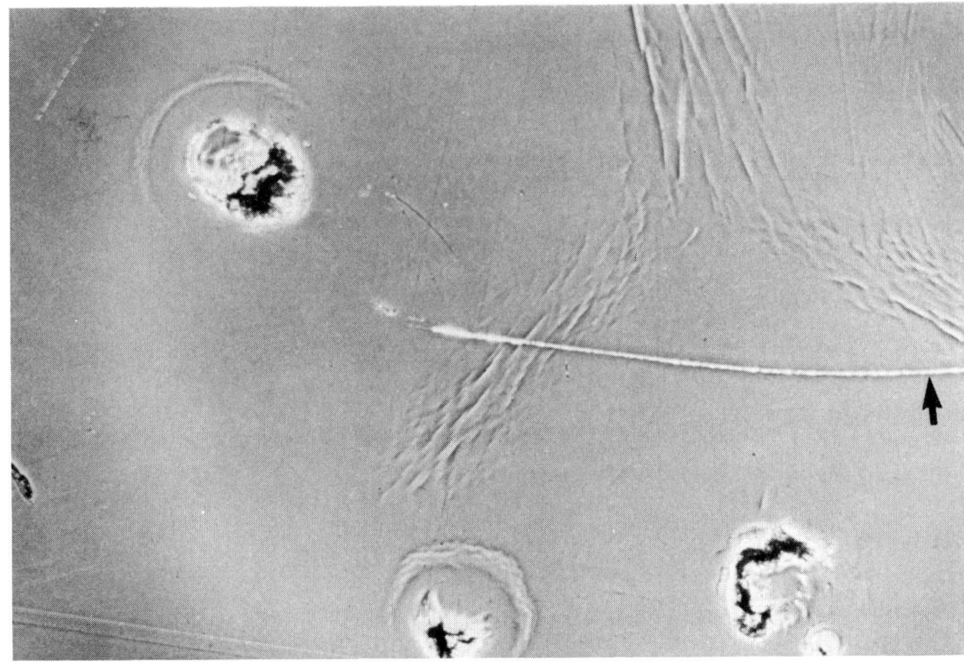

FIG 3.
Cavitation damage on a polymethylmethacrylate surface. Three craters are visible and three fields of small straight lines, one of them exactly halfway between two craters. The line *(arrow)* is a scratch not caused by shock wave exposure.

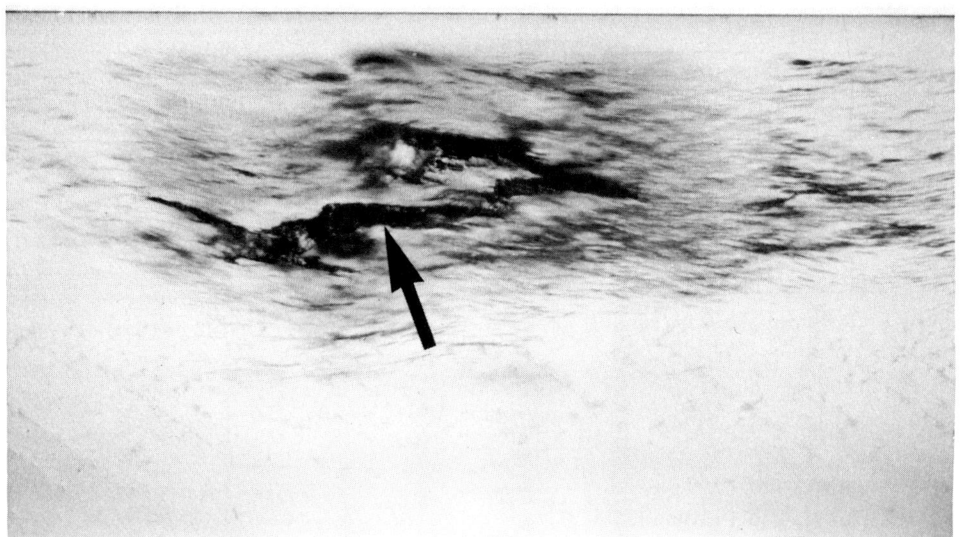

FIG 4.
Section through a Plexiglas plate exposed to extracorporeal shock waves. Tears in the material *(arrow)* run in parallel to the surface.

SHOCK WAVE EFFECTS IN SOLIDS INDEPENDENT OF CAVITATION

A shock wave generated in a solid by a high-speed water drop can induce material destruction.[19] If it is reflected at the interface to a medium of lower impedance, an expansion wave is generated in the solid. Strong expansion waves produce tears below the reflecting surface; the tears run in parallel to the surface and material is spalled off, that is, breaks off. The impact of high-speed water drops on ceramic plates demonstrates that in brittle solids, fracturing owing to expansion wave effects is a major mechanism of damage.[19]

Tears running in parallel to the surface can also be induced by lithotripter shock waves on polymethylmethacrylate plates if they are reflected at a free surface behind the plate (Fig 4). Considering the effect of a shock wave propagated in a brittle solid, there are two possible mechanisms of solid destruction by lithotripter shock waves:

1. A direct shock wave effect caused by lithotripter shock waves spalling off material.
2. A cavitation-dependent indirect shock wave effect.

The relative contribution of these mechanisms to lithotripsy is an important question for the optimization of the shock waves generated by lithotripters.

SUMMARY

Cavitation bubbles are generated by optical or electrical energy or by expansion waves expanding preexisting cavitation nuclei in the fluid. Shock waves are generated by optical or electrical energy or by cavitation bubbles collapse during rebound.

At a surface cavitation bubbles collapse asymmetrically under jet formation. A shock wave hitting a gas bubble collapses the bubble asymmetrically under jet formation. This bubble–shock wave interaction has been shown to induce material damage.

The expansion wave from a shock wave propagating in a brittle solid can damage the material at the side opposite to the wave entry. In lithotripters direct shock wave effects and cavitation-mediated effects can occur.

REFERENCES

1. Lauterborn W, Hentschel W: Cavitation bubble dynamics studied by high speed photography and holography: Part one. *Ultrasonics* 1985; 23:260.
2. Crum L: Acoustic cavitation, in Proceedings of the 1982 IEEE Ultrasonic Symposium. IEEE, New York, 1982, p 1–11.
3. Apfel RE: Acoustic cavitation, in *Methods of Experimental Physics,* vol 19, New York, Academic Press, 1981, pp 355–411.
4. Müller M: *Stoßwellenfokussierung in Wasser*. Inaugural dissertation, Aachen 1987.
5. Coleman A, Saunders J: Comparison of extracorporeal shock wave lithotripters (based on measurements in the acoustic field), in Coptcoat MJ, Miller RA, Wickham EA (eds): *Lithotripsy II,* London, BDI Publishing, 1987, pp 121–131.
6. Crum LA: Nucleation and stabilization of microbubbles in liquids. *Applied Scientific Research* 1982; 38:101–115.
7. Vogel A, Lauterborn W: Acoustic transient generation by laser produced cavitation bubbles near solid boundaries. *J Acoust Soc Am* 1988; 83:000.
8. Delius M: Unpublished observation.
9. Williams AR, Delius M, Miller DL, et al: Investigation of cavitation in flowing media by lithotripter shock waves both in vitro and in vivo. *Ultrasound Med Biol,* in press.
10. Church C: A theoretical study of cavitation generated by an extracorporeal shock wave lithotripter. *J Acoust Soc Am* 1988; 83(suppl 1):S72.
11. Gibson DC, Blake JR: Growth and collapse of bubbles near deformable surfaces. *Applied Scientific Research* 1982; 38:215–224.
12. Kling CL, Hammitt FG: A photographic study of spark-induced cavitation bubble collapse. Transactions ASME Series D, *J Basic Eng* 1972; 94:825–833.
13. Naudé CF, Ellis AT: On the mechanism of cavitation damage by nonhemispherical cavities collapsing in contact with a solid boundary. Transactions ASME Series D, *J Basic Eng* 1961; 83:648–656.
14. Coleman AJ, Saunders JE, Crum LA, et al: Acoustic cavitation generated by an extracorporeal shockwave lithotripter. *Ultrasound Med Biol* 1987; 13:69–76.
15. Lauterborn W: Kavitation durch Laserlicht. *Acustica* 1974; 31:51–78.

16. Dear JP, Field JE, Walton AJ: Gas compression and jet formation in cavities collapsed by a shock wave. *Nature* 1988; 332:505–508.
17. Tomita Y, Shima A: Mechanisms of impulsive pressure generation and damage pit formation by bubble collapse. *J Fluid Mech* 1986; 169:535–564.
18. Lush PA: Impact of a liquid mass on a perfectly plastic solid. *J Fluid Mech* 1983; 135:373–387.
19. Brunton JH: The physics of impact and deformation: I. High speed liquid impact. *Philos Trans R Soc Lond,* Series A 1966; 260:79–85.

Mechanisms of Action in Extracorporeal Shock Wave Lithotripsy: Experimental Studies

M. Delius
W. Brendel

This chapter details experimental, clinical, and theoretical observations on the effects of shock waves on living tissues.

BACKGROUND

The effect of shock waves on tissues was described 200 years ago in reports of blast injury sustained by miners.[1] Most information on the effect of shock waves from blasts was gained during World War I and II.[2] It was especially prominent in divers injured from underwater blasts, because shock wave propagation is less attenuated in water than in air and the waves enter the body with full intensity owing to the similar impedances of tissue and water. The major signs of blast injury were lung hemorrhage and multiple ruptures of the gut wall. Hemorrhages in the upper respiratory tract and effects on the central nervous system were also observed. Extracorporeal shock waves used for stone disintegrations differ from the shock waves causing blast injuries in at least two important respects:

They are usually weaker than the shock waves caused by blasts. For patient treatment, several hundred up to a few thousand extracorporeal shock waves are applied instead of the single strong blast wave causing the injury.

The waves are focused to the presumed point of their action in the body instead of passing through the whole body with similar strength. Only a very small part of the body is exposed to extracorporeal shock waves.

Yet, when the first biological experiments with extracorporeal shock waves were performed, lung hemorrhage was again the most prominent finding.[3] The experiments were done with rats, which were too small to keep the lungs out of the high-pressure field. No lung hemorrhage was noted in dogs when extracorporeal shock waves were targeted at canine kidneys for experimental kidney stone destruction, presumably because the larger animal model kept the lung out of the shock wave path.

LUNG DAMAGE

The lung is the most sensitive organ to shock waves. At the energy level employed for kidney stone destruction in patients, lung hemorrhage was detected in rats after application of only very few shock waves. No change in any other organ was observed under these conditions.

Lung hemorrhage was evaluated systematically in our laboratory in two experiments. In the first experimental series, the pressure threshold for hemorrhage was examined in rat lungs.

In the second, the critical distance between the lung and the shock wave focus at which lung hemorrhage occurred was determined in dogs. The shock wave parameters and conditions were relevant for gallstone destruction. This experiment, which had to be performed before gallstone destruction would be feasible in man, is reported in Chapter 60 of this book.

When shock waves generated with a Dornier HM 2 shock wave generator were focused directly to rat lungs, hemorrhage was detected after very few shock waves, even at the lowest energy setting of the machine.[4] Macroscopically, hemorrhage was homogenous, extending from the site of shock wave entry into the parenchyma. Its shape was not influenced by the lobar organization of the lung. Histologically, intra-alveolar blood was seen in most, if not all alveoli. At sites extensively affected, the alveolar septa were destroyed or necrotic; eventually, no septal architecture remained. Similar changes in the lung had been noted earlier with another type of shock wave generator that had been employed for experimental kidney stone destruction.[5] As the threshold for lung hemorrhage was located at far lower energy, the shock wave energy had to be further reduced. In a modified experimental setup, shock waves were again generated by spark gap discharge, but the spark gap was located free in the water bath and the waves were not focused. The shock wave pressure decreased with the distance from the spark gap. The lungs were normal after 10 shock waves, positioned at the largest possible distance from the spark gap with the lowest shock wave energy. The peak pressure registered at this site in water was below 5 MPa. However, the threshold for lung hemorrhage was even lower and could not be determined with this device as an increase in the number of shock waves to over 100 again generated lung hemorrhage in some rats.[4]

With the same experimental setup, lung hemorrhage was compared in rats under two conditions in which the total electrical energy of the shock waves applied was the same but their energy and number differed.[4] After few shock waves of higher energy, significantly more rats had hemorrhagic lungs than after many shock waves of lower energy. This showed that even above the threshold for lung hemorrhage, the energy or the peak pressure of the individual shock wave was a more important determinant of shock wave action that the total wave energy applied. However, in another experiment, the same was noted to be true for the shock wave effect on gallstones, and shock waves of too low energy or peak pressure could not be used for gallstone destruction.

The lung differs from other organs by its large air-tissue interface. Shock waves do not penetrate lung tissue but are reflected at the surface. This obviously plays an important role in the generation of shock wave damage as lung hemorrhage is detected at far lower shock wave energies than is damage to other tissues. Yet damage to other tissues differs only in quantity, not in quality. The general side effect of extracorporeal shock waves observed in all tissues examined to date is vascular damage and hemorrhage.

KIDNEY DAMAGE

Many investigators have studied the effect of shock waves in association with work on kidney stone destruction. All available types of shock wave generators have been used, and shock wave effects have been examined in at least four different animal species.[5-7]

We studied the effects of shock waves generated with a Dornier HM 2 lithotripter in dog kidneys using similar numbers of shock wave as in patient treatments.[8] Macroscopically, diffuse hemorrhages occurred in the perirenal fat and the inner renal capsule. Parenchymal changes were not detected at the kidney poles but were restricted to the part of the kidney that had been located in the high-pressure field of the shock waves. Within this area, they occurred focally and two types could be differentiated: hematomas and diffuse hemorrhages. Hematomas had a diameter of several millimeters. Diffuse hemorrhages covered larger areas and, in severely affected kidneys, extended from the cortex to the medulla. Histologically, they were shown to be due to hemorrhage into the interstitium and to red blood cell casts in dilated tubules. Venous walls were focally destroyed with hemorrhage into the adventitia, often with associated destruction of adjacent parenchyma. Thrombi were detected in interlobular and arcuate veins. Rarely, damage to arterial walls was documented with hemorrhage into the muscular layer or, on occasion, mural disruption with surrounding hematoma was noted (Fig 1). Electron microscopy disclosed tears in capillaries and small veins, which had led to diffuse extravasation of blood cells (Fig 2).

Vessel wall tears and hemorrhages were present in kidneys directly after shock wave application, suggesting that they were the primary changes caused by shock waves. The day following shock wave application, the kidneys looked swollen; interstitial widening and vacuolization of endothelial and tubular epithelial cells were additionally detected by electron microscopy. Follow-up of dogs up to 5 months after shock wave application revealed that hemorrhages healed by scar formation. Most of the scars were too small to be detected macroscopically. Histologically, they extended from the cortex into the medulla, or were smaller. A reduction in the renal parenchymal mass was not observed.

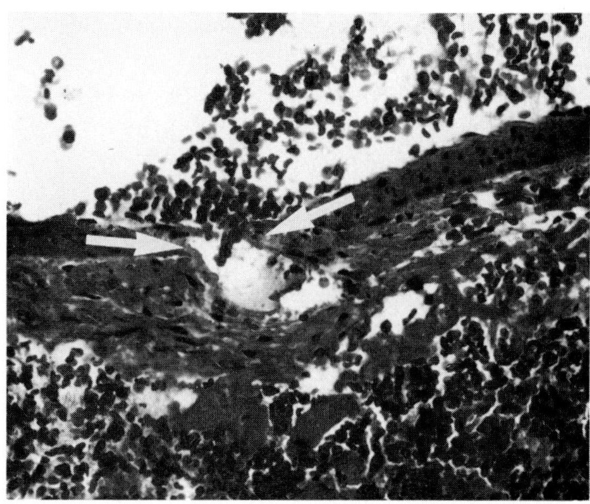

FIG 1.
Focal tear of the wall of an arcuate artery *(arrows)* after shock wave application to the kidney. The site was surrounded by a hematoma *(bottom)*.

OTHER ORGANS

Many different tissues have been exposed to shock waves, and hemorrhage was the most prominent finding in all of them. The effect of shock waves on the liver and gallbladder is described in Chapter 7; hemorrhage and venous

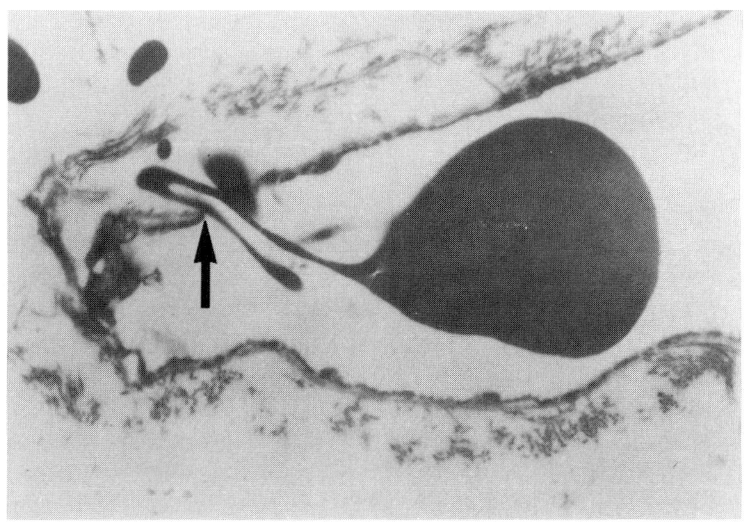

FIG 2.
Capillary wall tear with part of the red blood cell entrenched in the tear *(arrow)* while the major part is still in the vascular lumen (Courtesy of Professor Liebich, Institute for Veterinary Anatomy, University of Munich.)

damage occurred as well. Shock waves have also been focused to the heart and the bones. In the heart, focal hemorrhage was seen in the myocardium with destruction of cardiac muscle cells. Similar changes were seen in other muscles. When shock waves were applied to bones, the marrow became bright red owing to hemorrhage; there were associated changes in the trabecular organization. Hemorrhage also occurred around bones in the high-pressure field.

During shock wave application to the gallbladder wall or the kidney, the gut was in the high-pressure field of the wave. Petechial or confluent hemorrhages were seen in the mesentery and the gut wall. In the mesentery, they were typically located along the arcade vessels. Focal adhesions between bowel loops pointed to serosal changes. Hemorrhage into the peripancreatic fat with edema was seen, but the acini could not be shown to be affected. All these changes were minor; they had never led to extravasation of blood into the peritoneal cavity. Submucosal hemorrhage into the gut wall was uncommon, and mucosal ulceration was observed once. The influence of gas in bowel loops on the shock wave effect is not proven, but it can be expected to increase tissue damage as the tissue is exposed to the original as well as the reflected wave because the shock wave is totally reflected by bowel gas.

POSSIBLE MECHANISMS OF SHOCK WAVE DAMAGE

Shock waves caused vascular damage and hemorrhage in all organs examined to date. Shock wave damage occurred in the high-pressure field, where it had a focal distribution. Capillaries and veins were most heavily affected. This damage pattern was thought to point to the mechanism involved in the action of extracorporeal shock waves on tissues. Three possible mechanisms had to be considered as mediators of tissue damage: a thermal shock wave effect, a direct shock wave effect, and an indirect effect mediated by cavitation.

In the case of a thermal shock wave effect, significant tissue heating would have to occur. This would require enough energy to increase the tissue temperature. The energy of the shock waves, although high for periods of microseconds, is low in relation to the application time, which extends over several minutes. Its temporal average is only in the range of diagnostic ultrasound and too low to cause significant tissue heating, even if totally absorbed by the body.

In the case of a direct shock wave action, the pressure or tension generated by shock waves in certain tissue structures exceeded the forces they could withstand. The tissue failed and ruptured. The lack of information on the physical properties of tissues means not much is known about this process. Its evaluation is even more complicated, because shock wave pressures act only during very short periods in the microsecond range. Information on the forces needed to disrupt tissue is difficult to obtain as the magnitude of a short-acting force ultimately has to be larger than the magnitude of a longer-acting force.

In the case of an indirect shock wave action, tissue damage is mediated by cavitation, which is described in the preceding chapter. The formation of bubbles in vivo is a prerequisite for this mechanism. The movement of these bubbles, not the shock wave propagation through tissue, generates tissue damage. Basically, cavitation and a direct shock wave action do not exclude each other and, indeed, may act in common. Several factors point to cavitation as an important mechanism of tissue damage:

Cavitation is a focal event and easily explains the focal nature of tissue damage which is more difficult to explain by a direct shock wave action.

Cavitation could act nonspecifically on nearby structures without requiring a specific structure to fail. Around veins, damage to all nearby structures had been observed, which was difficult to explain by the flow of venous blood after rupture of the venous wall.

Shock wave damage was similar to damage after the application of high-intensity pulsed ultrasound. Focal vascular lesions generated by application of pulsed ultrasound to the brain have already been known to be secondary to cavitation.[9] Similarly, focal hepatic lesions from high-intensity ultrasound, which were probably induced by cavitation, had an appearance similar to focal hepatic lesions after shock wave application.[10]

CAVITATION IN VIVO

The pattern of tissue damage after shock wave application suggests that cavitation might play an important role. Previously, cavitation had been generated in vitro by shock waves. However, despite many experimental conditions that could generate cavitation in vitro, it was not possible to demonstrate cavitation in vivo. When we applied shock waves in vivo to the liver under ultrasound observation, it became obvious that cavitation occurred in vivo as well.

Administration of shock waves to pig liver under observation by real-time ultrasound revealed two clearly distinguishable changes in the liver: transient and longer lasting echogenic foci. Transient echogenic areas appeared in liver veins and were flushed away with the blood flow. They were assumed to be due to cavitation generated by shock waves and persisted up to several hundred milliseconds. This indicated that shock waves had generated quite stable, visible bubbles in the blood stream. After several hundred shock waves, the high-pressure field in the liver gradually brightened. The increased echogenicity lasted for minutes and generated shadowing behind it, suggesting that it was due to stable gas in this area. At dissection, hemorrhages were observed in the area where shock waves had been applied.

During gallstone destruction in patients, real-time ultrasound was used to localize the stones in the gallbladder or, rarely, in intrahepatic bile ducts. With increasing numbers of shock waves, some patients displayed similar sonographic changes in the high-pressure field. If part of a liver lobe was in front of the gallbladder in the high-pressure field, it became brighter after several hundred shock waves; this persisted for minutes. A focal bright transient flash could be seen with the administration of each shock wave. Intravascular reflections were rarely seen, but large hepatic and portal veins were not typically present in the high-pressure field. Changes of tissue reflectivity were especially prominent during the destruction of stones in intrahepatic bile ducts. In addition to the hepatic changes, the anterior abdominal wall became brighter with increasing shock wave number. In some patients, the increased echogenicity diminished gallbladder visibility during gallstone destruction, persisting for several minutes.

These findings indicate that cavitation by shock waves in vivo is easily detected by ultrasound. Bubbles appeared in liver vessels and were flushed away before longer lasting increases in reflectivity appeared. In addition, the same reflections indicating cavitation were also detected in bile when shock waves were administered to the gallbladder. The occurrence of cavitation in regions of tissue damage was further evidence that tissue damage by extracorporeal shock waves was mediated by cavitation.

RELATION OF SHOCK WAVE REPETITION RATE AND TISSUE DAMAGE

Shock waves are usually administered at a rate of one to three waves per second in our laboratory experiments on tissue damage and in clinical use as well. However, we have also studied tissue effects using a shock wave generator constructed by Dornier which could administer 100 shock waves per second without change of the peak pressures of the shock waves and their profile.[11]

Kidney damage and hemolysis were compared in groups of dogs after the administration of the same total number of shock waves. In one treatment group, the waves were administered at a rate of 100 waves per second; in the control group, they were administered slowly at a rate of one wave per second. The results differed widely between the two groups. Kidney hemorrhage was minor or absent when shock waves were administered slowly but was extensive when 100 shock waves were applied per second. In contrast to the control dogs, hemolysis was increased directly after the administration of fast shock waves.

The difference between the groups must have been due to interaction between shock waves in the group of fast shock wave administration. The duration of a shock wave was approximately 10 μs, while the interval between the shock waves was 10 μs when they were administered fast. A residual effect must have been left from the preceding shock waves over an interval that was 1000 times as long as the duration of the wave itself and influenced the effect of the following waves.

The question was further pursued in an experiment in which the rate of shock wave administration to dog kidneys was 15 waves per second (i.e., the time interval between the shock waves was 66 μs). The same number of shock waves was applied as in the previous experiment. Kidney damage was increased again as judged grossly by estimation of the hemorrhagic areas on kidney slices and comparison with the control group where the same number of shock waves had been administered at a rate of one wave per second. Hemolysis was significantly increased after shock wave application compared with the control group (Fig 3). No significant increase in hemolysis was seen in the control group relative to pretreatment values.

In another group of dogs, the same total number of shock waves was again administered, yet according to a different protocol. Two shock waves were administered per second with a time interval of 66 μs. This interval was the same as in the previous group, but only one shock wave followed the preceding shock wave. The interval between the shock wave pairs was long. In this group, there also was a tendency toward increased kidney hemorrhage compared with the control group. Most important, hemolysis was significantly increased compared with the control group and not much different from hemolysis after 15 shock waves per second.

The last experiment definitely excluded any thermal effect as the cause of these changes. The dependence on the administration rate could not be explained by a direct shock wave action. The last experiment showed that tissue damage was increased when two shock waves interacted with each other. The interaction occurred in

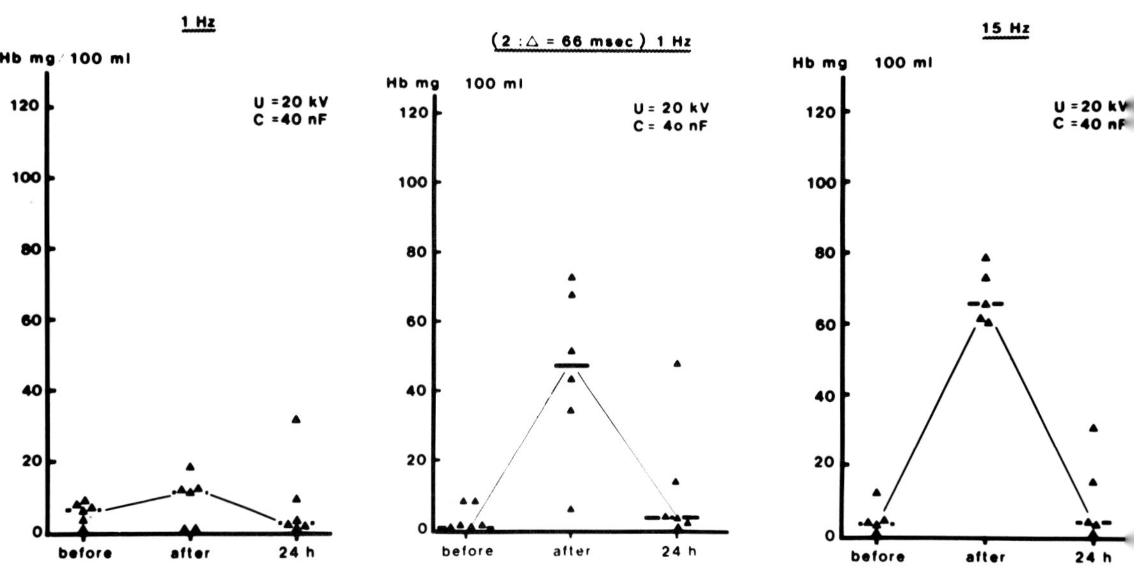

FIG 3.
Hemolysis in vivo after different rates of shock wave application. Blood was drawn before, directly after, and 24 hours after shock wave application.

spite of a time interval of 6600 times the wave duration between consecutive waves. The administration rate dependence also could not be explained by the generation of cavitation bubbles that caused damage by spontaneous collapse, as this did not take into consideration the interaction between shock waves.

MODEL OF SHOCK WAVE ACTION TO INDUCE TISSUE DAMAGE

Direct sonographic observation of the liver during shock wave administration had shown that bubbles persisted for up to several hundred milliseconds in the high-pressure field. In the group where shock waves were administered fast, with 10 or 67 μs intervals, bubbles would be encountered by the succeeding shock wave. This must have been the crucial event for the increase in tissue damage. At a wave administration rate of one shock wave per second, these bubbles could not be detected in the high-pressure field and were not encountered by the following shock wave. The administration of shock wave pairs indicated that the shock wave action on tissue was a two-stage process: the first shock wave generated bubbles. In accord with calculations, this was mainly done by the tensile (negative) wave of the shock wave which followed the positive pressure wave (see Chapter 4). The bubbles from the preceding shock wave were struck by the following shock wave and induced tissue damage. No information was gained from these experiments as to the fate of a bubble when it was hit by a shock wave.

Physical experiments have shown that a bubble hit by a shock wave collapsed asymmetrically under jet formation. This is independent of the presence of a hard surface, which is not present in blood and which is probably not even provided by the thin venous and capillary walls. Bubble collapse by shock waves had been demonstrated for bubbles in the range of several hundred micrometers or a few millimeters. With this information, a model of shock wave action in tissues could be derived as follows:

The bubbles persisting from the first shock wave collapsed under jet formation when they were hit by the positive pressure part of the following shock wave (Fig 4). This must have been the interaction leading to the increased tissue damage. It means that the first part of the second shock wave, the pressure wave, interacted with the second part of the first shock wave, the tensile wave. So shock waves had a tandem action in tissue.

As the interaction between shock waves and bubbles was a powerful mechanism of shock wave action at fast shock wave administration rates, it was considered that the shock wave damage in tissues after slow shock wave administration was caused in a similar way. This required bubbles in the high-pressure field at the slow shock wave application rate. In blood, this was not important as hemolysis was not significantly increased after slow shock wave application. Yet, such bubbles existed as stationary gas that had been observed by ultrasound in the liver after several hundred shock waves. They probably were located in the interstitium but an intravascular location with stasis in these vessels could not be excluded. It is not known whether

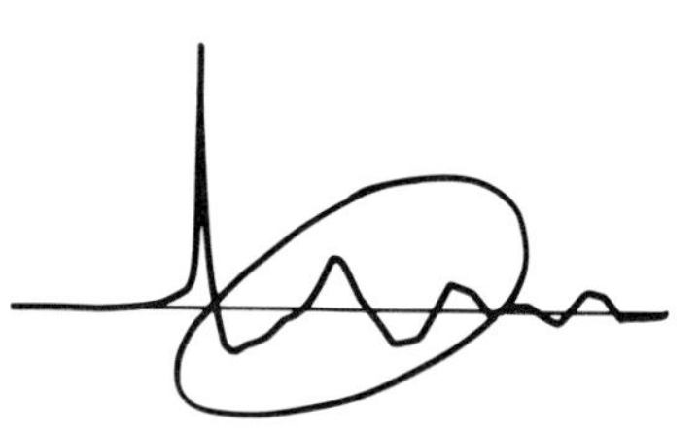

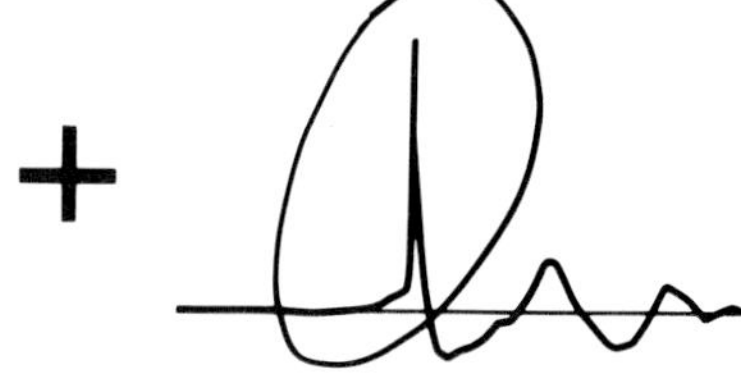

FIG 4.
Model of shock wave action in tissues: tandem action of shock waves. The waveform is from a pressure registration of G. Heine and H. Eizenhoefer from Dornier. Circles mark the parts of the wave acting synergistically.

in the latter case they were directly generated in the interstitium or whether they were transported into the interstitium, eventually by jets, through holes in blood vessel walls. So it is possible that the interaction of bubbles and shock waves also generated tissue damage at a slow shock wave administration rate.

The lung is different from other organs owing to its large air-tissue interface and is the organ most affected by shock waves. There are two different ways to consider the physical effect of shock waves on lung tissue. One is to view the lung as a planar air-tissue interface with reflection of the shock wave at the surface and the generation of considerable tensile force. The other is to consider the lung on the alveolar level as a densely packed field of stabilized interconnected bubbles. Shock wave interaction with bubbles could have occurred as described. As in this instance, bubbles did not have to be generated by the preceding wave, no tandem action of shock waves was required for lung hemorrhage. The consequence was that lung hemorrhage should be similar after slow and fast shock wave administration. We could not observe different degrees of lung hemorrhage after slow and fast shock wave administration when the lung was located in the periphery of the high-pressure field.

MECHANISM OF STONE DESTRUCTION

As mentioned earlier, extracorporeal shock waves caused several effects on solid materials such as plexiglass, aluminum foils, and model stones. The craters on aluminum foil and plexiglass were due to cavitation. Erosion of model stones at the anterior surface was observed by workers at Dornier and was believed to be also caused by this mechanism. In addition, spallation, that is, the removal of material from the rear side of a solid, was observed under certain conditions on plexiglass and other materials. The physical properties of gallstones have not been examined in detail, and it is not yet possible to compare them with the properties of better defined materials. Therefore, it is difficult to examine the mechanism of gallstone destruction by test materials.

Observations of gallstones during stone destruction in vitro have shown that the stones did not crumble diffusely or explosively. Indeed, stone fragmentation often followed typical patterns. It usually started at the anterior stone surface, the surface which was struck by the incoming shock wave. Small fragments were eroded from the anterior surface before the stone broke into major parts. Other stones, many of them larger, broke into a few large pieces in the beginning of stone destruction. Only a minimal amount of small fragments was generated up to that point. Generally, either the cracks in these stones were in parallel to the shock wave axis (i.e., they were directed from the anterior to the posterior stone surface) or they passed in another direction through the center of the stone. Selective destruction of the posterior side of the stone, which resembled the spallation effects observed in materials, could not be detected during gallstone destruction in vitro.

It has been claimed that the shock wave pressures generated by partial reflection of the shock wave at the anterior and posterior stone surfaces led to stone destruction.[12] According to this model, spallation at the posterior stone surface was an important mechanism of stone destruction. In general, reflection of a wave at an interface is dependent on the densities of and the velocities of sound in the media on both sides of the interface. The product of these two parameters, the impedance, would be a major determinant of stone destruction if it was caused by direct shock wave reflection at the stone surfaces. We therefore tested whether the impedance of the surrounding medium was really important for stone destruction.[13]

Gallstones of the same family were put into two different media of the same impedance, a cesium chloride solution and a glycerol solution. Gallstone destruction was completely different in these media (Fig 5). There was nearly no stone destruction if the stones were surrounded by glycerol, but they could be well destroyed in the cesium chloride solution. This showed that the impedance was not important for stone destruction. The type of fluid surrounding the

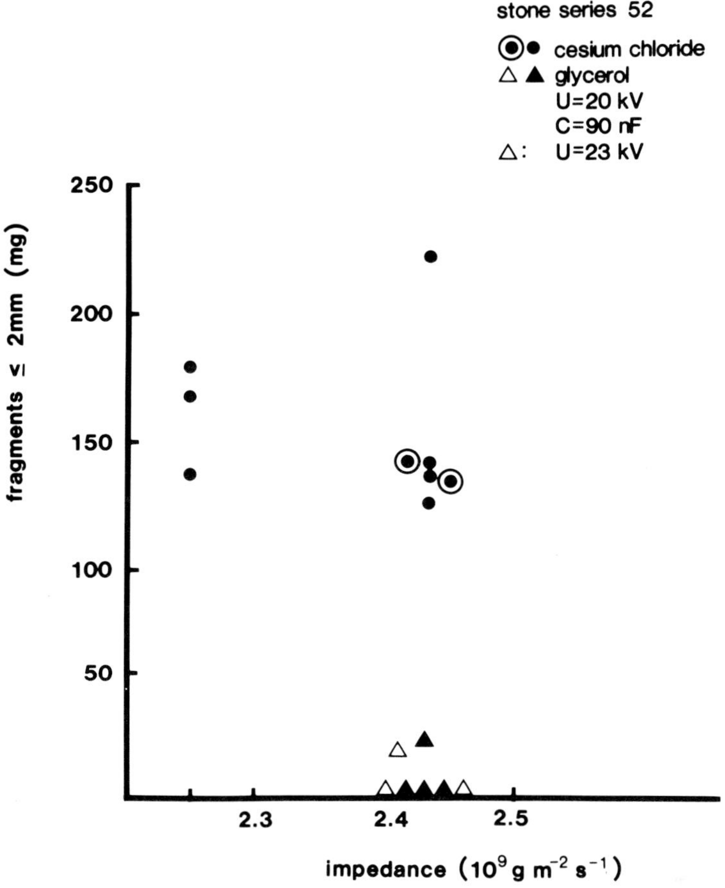

FIG 5.
Gallstone fragmentation in cesium chloride and glycerol. Stones of the same gallstone family were exposed to the same number of shock waves, and fragments of up to 2 mm were weighed to record the destructive effect quantitatively. Double rings denote stones in cesium chloride which were destroyed by shock waves that had to run through a layer of glycerol before they reached the stone.

stone was more important as stones could be destroyed in cesium chloride solutions of different impedance. In conclusion, the mechanism of stone destruction must have been located in the surrounding fluid. Cavitation was considered the most probable mechanism of gallstone destruction. Cavitation has been shown to occur in vitro and in vivo with shock wave administration. Using aluminum foils as an indicator for cavitation, cavitation pits were detected on foils in cesium chloride solution but not on foils in glycerol.

Cavitation is dependent on the surrounding pressure of the medium and is suppressed by hyperbaric pressure. Aluminum foil deformation by shock waves was completely suppressed in a pressure chamber pressurized to 100 atmospheres. Gallstone destruction in the chamber under this pressure was greatly reduced compared with stone destruction at atmospheric pressure (Fig 6). This supports cavitation as the major mechanism of gallstone destruction. However, the experiment itself was not unequivocal evidence that cavitation was the mechansim, be-

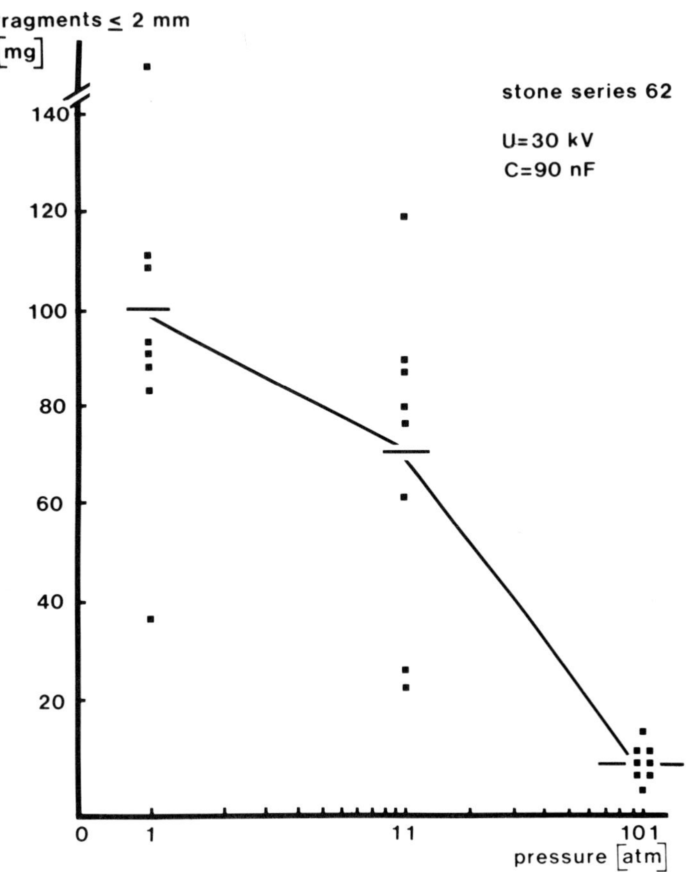

FIG 6.
Gallstone destruction of stones of a gallstone family in a pressure chamber. The amount of fragments up to 2 mm size was determined again.

cause stone destruction as a result of spallation might have been suppressed as well by hyperbaric pressure. This was, however, improbable due to the previous experiment as the mechanism of stone destruction is mediated by the surrounding fluid.

Not much is presently known about the involvement of other mechanisms in gallstone destruction by extracorporeal shock waves. Gallstones are heterogenous and, in some stones, a mechanism other than cavitation may play a greater role. Some stones contain enough air to reflect the shock wave in the stone and to generate a stronger tensile wave. The role of the water content in these pre-formed stone cracks is not known either. The examination of these effects is complicated, as some gallstones are naturally under tension and self-destruction of gallstones without shock wave application occurs relatively often.[14] Interestingly, the preformed cracks run always through the stone center just at the fragment lines when stones initially break into large fragments.

These results were obtained with the relatively weak extracorporeal shock waves applied in medicine today. They certainly do not exclude that shock waves of higher peak pressure will be able to destroy gallstones by a direct wave effect. The mechanism of stone destruction may be important for the definition of the wave characteristics that determine stone destruction and may play a role in optimizing the parameters of shock waves used to destroy stones.

MODEL OF SHOCK WAVE ACTION FOR STONE DESTRUCTION

According to the above experiments, cavitation was a major mechanism of stone destruction. Therefore, the same mechanism can be said to have contributed to stone destruction as well as tissue damage. In tissue, shock waves exerted their effect by interaction with bubbles.

As mentioned already, Tomita and Shima showed that a soft metal surface could be damaged by a shock wave if the wave encountered a gas bubble in front of the surface. A water jet was formed by the wave, which impinged on the surface. The surface was not damaged if it was hit by a similar shock wave without an adherent bubble. This showed that shock wave damage to metals was also mediated by interaction of a shock wave with a bubble. Preliminary evidence from the administration of extracorporeal shock waves to plexiglass suggested that the craters on the plexiglass surface were also caused by interaction of shock waves with bubbles. There was a hint that multiple bubbles were involved and interacted to generate damage when they were struck by a shock wave. It is highly probable, although it has not been shown, that a similar interaction occurs during the destruction of gallstones. This would mean that shock waves act according to the same mechanism when they destroy stones and cause tissue damage. The combined action during stone destruction could explain two observations which were difficult to explain by simple collapse of a bubble:

It has been shown that a focused tensile wave generated more cavitation in the focal area than positive pressure shock waves.[15] However, it was not able to destroy stones.[16] The explanation according to the model would be that there was no shock wave to collapse the bubbles forcefully.

In some shock wave generators, the tensile wave that generated cavitation was less sharply focused than the positive pressure wave. The area of stone destruction by focused shock waves, however, was restricted to the area of the peak positive pressure. Again, the explanation would be that there was no shock wave to collapse the bubbles forcefully.

The interaction between shock waves and bubbles, which may explain some experimental results on tissue damage, may also explain some observations made during stone breakup. It remains to be seen whether there will be significant implications for lithotripter design.[17]

SUMMARY

Shock waves caused hemorrhages and vascular changes in all tissues examined. Tissue damage occurred focally; capillaries and veins were most affected by wall damage and thrombus formation. Tissue damage by shock waves was especially prominent in the lung, where the threshold for damage was lowest. Shock wave energy or peak pressure was a better determinant of lung hemorrhage than the temporally averaged shock wave energy applied to the organ.

Shock waves exert a direct and an indirect effect on the tissue, the latter being mediated by cavitation. Cavitation was considered a probable mechanism of tissue damage owing to the focal nature of the tissue damage and the similarity to cavitation-mediated ultrasonic lesions.

Sonographically, cavitation was shown to occur in vivo during shock wave application to the liver. First, it was detected intravascularly and the bubbles were flushed away with the blood flow; later, stationary gas was seen in the high-pressure field.

Renal tissue damage and hemolysis were increased when shock waves were applied with fast administration rates, either 15 or 100 waves per second. Hemolysis was increased after administration of pairs of shock waves. This led to a model of shock wave tandem action in tissues: the tensil wave of the first shock wave generates bubbles that are hit by the positive pressure part of the following shock wave. Gallstone destruction by shock waves was dependent on the medium surrounding the stone and not on the impedance of the surrounding fluid. Hyperbaric pressure suppressed gallstone destruction, supporting cavitation as a major mechanism of gallstone destruction. It is suggested that bubble-shock wave interaction causes tissue effects and side effects of shock waves.

REFERENCES

1. Clemedson, CJ: Blast injury. *Physiol Rev* 1956; 36:336–54.
2. Desaga, H: Blast injuries, in: *German Aviation Medicine: World War II,* vol. II, Washington DC, U.S. Government Printing Office, 1950, pp 1274-1293.
3. Chaussy C: *Extracorporeal Shock Wave Lithotripsy*. Karger, Basel, 1982
4. Brendel W: *Grundversuche zur Sroßwellentherapie*. Forschungsbericht T 86-093, Bundesministerium für Forschung und Technologie, Bonn, 1986.
5. Konrad G, Ziegler M, Häusler E, et al: Fokussierte Stoßwellen zur berührungsfreien Nierensteinzertrümmerung an der freigelegten Niere. *Urologe [A]* 1979; 18:289–293.
6. Thibault T, Bory J, Cotard JP, et al: Lithtripsie à impulsions ultra-courtes. Étude expérimentale sur une lithiase rénale du chien. *Ann Urol (Paris)* 1986; 20:20–25.
7. Newman R, Hackett R, Senior D, et al: Pathological effects of ESWL on canine renal tissue. *Urology* 1987; 29:194–200.
8. Delius M, Enders G, Xuan Z, et al: Biological effects of shock waves: Kidney damage by shock waves in dogs—dose dependence. *Ultrasound Med Biol* 1988; 14:117–22.
9. Fry F, Kossoff G, Eggleton R, et al: Threshold ultrasonic dosages for structural changes in the mammalian brain. *J Acoust Soc Am* 1970; 48:1413–1417.
10. Chan SK, Frizell FA: Ultrasonic thresholds for structural changes in the mammalian liver. 1977 Ultrasonic Symposium Proceedings, IEEE, New York, 1977, pp 153–156.
11. Delius M, Jordan M, Eizenhoefer H, et al: Biological effects of shock waves: Kidney haemorrhage by shock waves in dogs—administration rate dependence. *Ultrasound Med Biol,* in press.
12. Forssmann B, Hepp W, Chaussy C, et al: Eine Methode zur beruehrungsfreien Zertruemmerung von Nierensteinen durch Stosswellen. *Biomed Tech* 1977; 22:164–168.
13. Delius M, Heine G, Brendel W: A mechanism of gallstone destruction by extracorporeal shock waves. *Naturwissenschaften* 1988; 75:200–201.
14. Bauer KH: Über die Selbstzertrümmerung von Gallensteinen und Neubildung von Steinen auf der Grundlage von Steintrümmern. *Archiv f Klin Chir* 1931; 165:53–80.
15. Müller M: Stoßwellenfokussierung in Wasser. Inaugural dissertation, Aachen 1987.
16. Müller M: personal communication.
17. Delius M, Brendel W: A model of extracorporeal shock wave action: Tandem action of shock waves. Letter to the editor. *Ultrasound Med Biol*, in press.

Second-Generation Extracorporeal Shock Waves for Gallstone Lithotripsy: In Vitro Experiments and Clinical Relevance

M. Staritz, A. Rambow, P. Mildenberger, M. Goebel, P. Schäfe, Th. Junginger, R. Hohenfellner, M. Thelen, and K.-H. Meyer zum Büschenfelde

ABSTRACT

First-generation shock wave sources are approved to disintegrate gallstones effectively, but require immersion of the patient's body in a tank of water. A recently developed second-generation shock wave source (Lithostar®, Siemens, Erlangen) generates shock waves electromagnetically. It presents several novel features. In particular the waterbath can be omitted, and because of lower shock wave pressure general anesthesia is not required. In vitro studies showed that 36 out of 38 gallstones (11 to 30 mm in diameter) could be disintegrated. Two concrements resisting lithotripsy were pure cholesterol stones.

Independent of shape, size, and composition (cholesterol or pigment) the maximum diameter of remaining fragments after lithotripsy was between 1 and 8 mm. For sufficient disintegration precise focusing (± 1 cm) of the stone and maximum power of the shock wave generator were required. Second-generation shock wave technique is a major advance in clinical practice. Efficiency, however, is not superior to the conventional device. Further improvement must be stimulated.

INTRODUCTION

Recently shock wave lithotripsy of gallstones has been reported[1] to be suitable for therapy for selected patients. So far, the shock wave technique meets several disadvantages. Particularly, the immersion of the patient's body in a tank of degassed water makes the procedure inconvenient, time-consuming, and relatively expensive. The high pressure of the shock waves (up to 1000 bar) causes pain and requires general or epidural analgesia in 60 percent of patients.[1]

Recently developed second-generation shock wave sources have several novel features. Administration of shock waves is possible without water bath, and, therefore, more convenient for the patient. Owing to lower shock wave pressure and a larger area serving for penetration of the pressure waves through the skin shock wave application causes only slight discomfort and general anesthesia is not necessary. However, "painless" lithotripsy has lower efficiency as a typical disadvantage. Particularly piezo-generated shock waves demonstrated such problems.[2] Although renal calculi are easier to disintegrate than gallstones only 40 percent of patients with renal calculi were treated successfully after one single

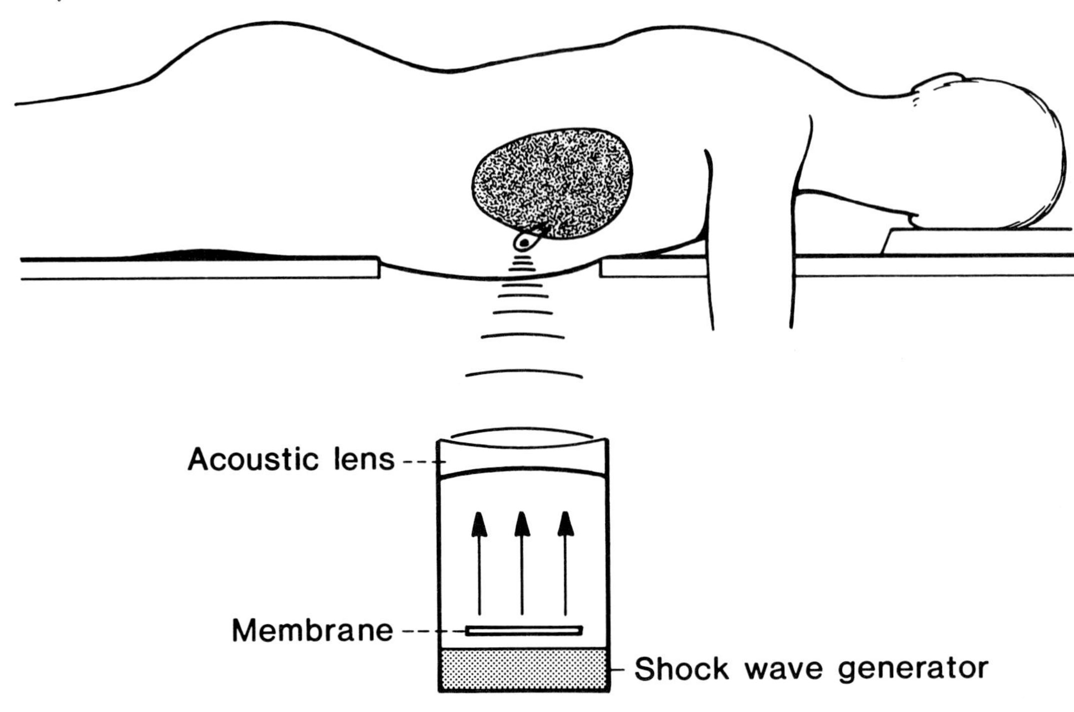

FIG 1.
Second-generation shock waves source generating shock wave energy by discharging an electromagnetical coil.

session by the Piezolith (Wolf, Knittlingen, FRG). The remaining patients received between two and eight treatments.[2] The third technique available so far is acoustically generated shock waves (Lithostar®, Siemens, Erlangen). In kidney stones the machine was as effective as the water bath device, however, required more shocks to disintegrate kidney stones.[3]

The experience gathered with renal calculi in our department encouraged administration of second-generation shock waves on gallstones. Therefore, the aim of this study was to investigate the effect of second-generation electromagnetically generated shock waves on gallstones of different sizes, shapes, and compositions in order to use this experience for subsequent clinical application.

METHODS

SHOCK WAVE SOURCE AND STONE DISINTEGRATION

The second-generation shock wave source used for our studies is commercially available (Lithostar®, Siemens, Erlangen, FRG) and generates shock waves electromagnetically. An electromagnetic coil discharging between 15 and 20 kV moves a special membrane. This membrane causes a pressure wave in an internal water pathway transmitting the pressure wave on to an acoustical lens that provides focusing of the pressure wave (Fig 1). In the focus a maximum pressure of about 300 bar is available. The focus zone has the shape of a cigar that is 8 cm long and 1.5 cm broad. The surface of the cigar represents the 50 percent isobar of the maximum pressure, which is present only in an inner zone measuring approximately 2 mm in diameter.

For our in vitro experiments, shock waves were transmitted into a water bath that acted as an acoustical model of a patient's body. The gallstones to be disintegrated were placed in a latex container and slightly fixed by a stone basket. The wire of the basket was visible by two-dimensional fluoroscopy and served to align the stones with the focus of the shock sources. Stone disintegration was defined to be complete when all stone fragments were removed from the basket.

EXPERIMENTS AND RESULTS

SHOCK WAVE ENERGY AND STONE DISINTEGRATION

Treatment of kidney stones has demonstrated that the discomfort caused by shock wave administration correlates with shock wave pressure. The aim of this study was to investigate which minimal energy expressed as voltage is required for disintegration of gallstones. For that purpose, 12 stones out of a stone family from the gallbladder of one patient were studied. These stones were very similar in shape and size (diameter 10 to 11 mm) and were typical cholesterol-pigment-gallbladder stones. The voltage used to generate shock waves was varied between 15 and 22.3 kV.

The experiment showed that the number of discharges required for complete lithotripsy increased exponentionally with decreasing voltage (Fig 2). It also showed that disintegration of gallstones required very high energy, close to the upper range of the capacity of the machine.

ACCURACY OF STONE FOCUSING AND SUCCESS OF DISINTEGRATION

According to the technical discription of the Siemens Lithostar, a maximum pressure of 300 to 500 bar is present in the focus of the shock waves. This focal region has the form of a cylinder 80 mm long and 8 mm broad. Respiration of the patient, however, causes a deviation of the stone by 1 to 2 cm.

The aim of this study was to show whether spontaneous respiration of the patient is allowable or whether it is preferable to apply shock waves only during apnea. Twelve stones out of a stone family (diameter 10 to 11 mm) were included. Shock waves were always applied to three of these stones at a time which were either focused exactly, or deviated from the focus by 1 cm, 2 cm and 3 cm, respectively.

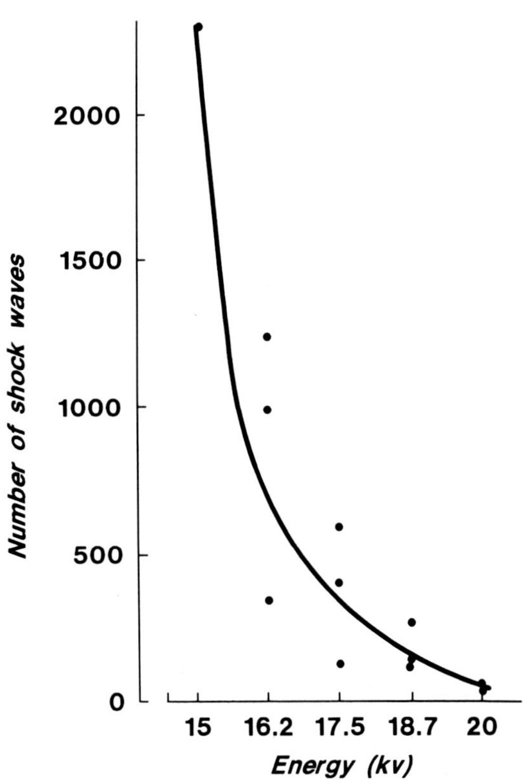

FIG 2.
Correlation between number of shock waves required for complete stone disintegration and energy. Voltage (kV) is a linear measure for extracorporeal shock wave energy. Each point (●) represents one individual stone out of a stone family removed from the gallbladder of one patient.

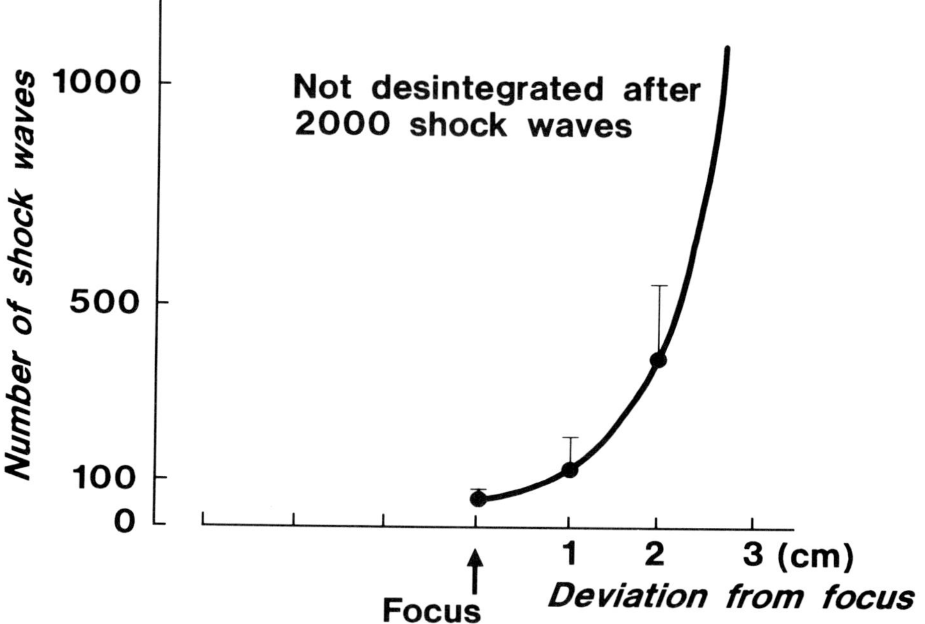

FIG 3.
Correlation between number of shock waves required for complete stone disintegration and deviation of the calculi from the focus. Each mean value (± SEM) represents the number of shocks required for three stones.

The results showed that the number of shocks required for disintegration of the stones increased exponentially with the deviation from the focus. Deviation by 1 cm, however, caused only mild increase in the number of discharges required for complete lithotripsy. Stones 3 cm from the focus could not be disintegrated (Fig 3).

CORRELATION BETWEEN SHAPE, SIZE, AND COMPOSITION OF THE STONES AND NUMBER AND SIZE OF THE FRAGMENTS

The fragments of all 36 gallstones which had been disintegrated in-vitro were examined. Stone composition (cholesterol, pigment, or mixed stones) was estimated by visual inspection of the stones. Two stones had a calcium rim and an inner core formed from cholesterol. We found that none of the stone characteristics, such as composition (cholesterol, pigments, or mixed stones), except for stone size (11 to 30 mm) could be correlated to either the number or size of the fragments produced. In particular, in each of these typical and representative gallstones, the size of the fragments varied between 1-mm particles and large fragments up to 8 mm in diameter (Fig 4). Only the concrements with calcium rim showed another disintegration pattern. From these stones the rim was first dissolved as big calcium particles, and then the core of the concrement was disintegrated.

FAILURE OF LITHOTRIPSY AND COMPUTED TOMOGRAPHY

All 38 concrements were investigated by computed tomography.[5] The radiological density of the stones varied between −40 and +170 Hounsfield units (HU). Only two of the calculi could not be disintegrated even after administration of 3000 shocks. These were pure white cholesterol stones that had been removed from young female obese patients. All other stones disintegrated successfully demonstrated density values above 0 Hounsfield units. Amazingly the two stones could be fractured in our Dornier lithotriptor at 20 kV after 500 and 700 shocks, respectively.

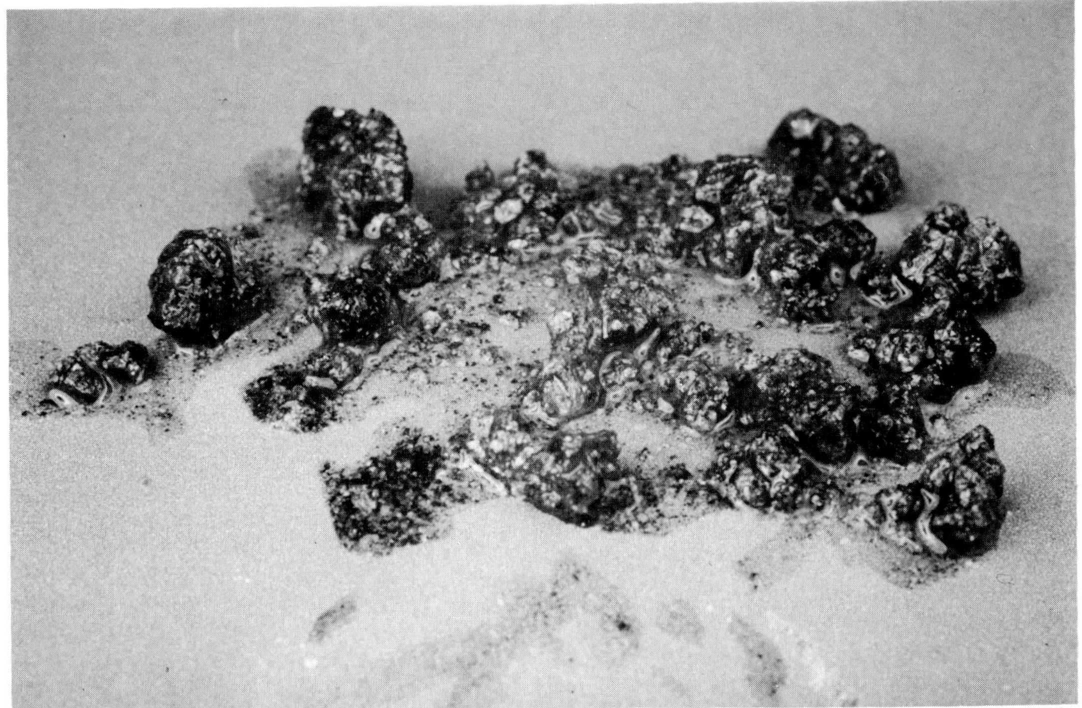

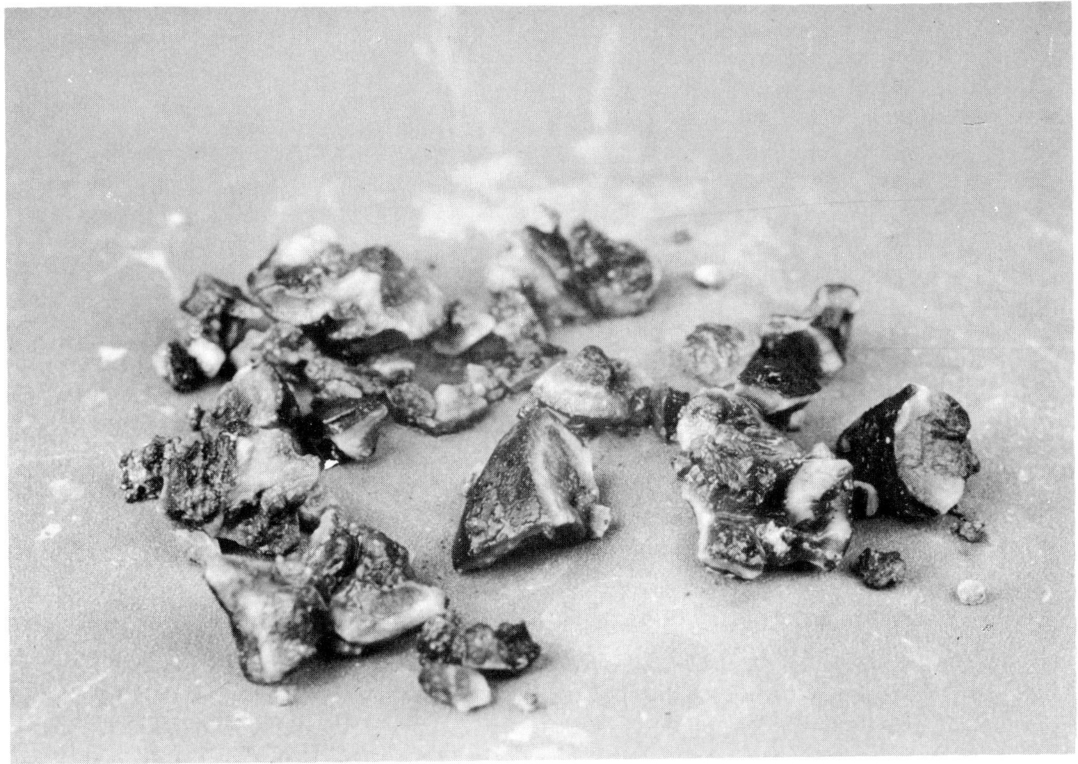

FIG 4.
Two samples for in-vitro fragmentation of A, pigment and B, cholesterol gallstones.

DISCUSSION

Second-generation extracorporal shock wave generators are proved to effectively disintegrate renal calculi.[2, 3] In vitro studies presented in this paper and recently reported in vivo experience[4] demonstrate that gallstones can also be disintegrated.

However, gallstone fragmentation is much more difficult than disintegration of kidney stones. Whereas soft pure cholesterol stones are likely to resist second-generation shock waves, disintegration of typical gallbladder stones required much more energy (voltage) than renal calculi. According to our clinical practice,[3] they were easily broken at 15 kV; gallstones were not, not even in vitro. Energy (voltage) that is close to the upper range of the available capacity of the second-generation device is required. Therefore, transmission of shock wave energy onto the stone must be ideal and particularly precise focusing is necessary.

Shock wave administration onto gallstones is obviously less effective than that onto kidney stones, which can be disintegrated into tiny fragments comparable to sand. The fragmentation pattern of gallstones is quite different. In the individual stone, it comprises tiny particles as well as large fragments having a diameter up to 8 mm and more. The size of the stone is not dependent on stone composition.

According to our experience we consider second-generation acoustically generated shock waves to be a major advance in the management of therapy. Application is easier, faster, and presumably less expensive, and general anaesthesia is not necessary.[3, 4] The efficiency, however, is not superior to the conventional device.[1] Fragments remaining after lithotripsy are too big for spontaneous passage through the biliary systems, and subsequent medical dissolution therapy is still required.

ACKNOWLEDGMENT

The authors wish to thank Ms. Barbara Paus for careful secretarial assistance.

REFERENCES

1. Sackman, M, Delius, M, Sauerbruch, T, et al: Shock-wave lithotripsy of gallbladder stones: The first 175 patients. *New Engl J Med* 1988; 318:7.
2. Philip, T, Kellett, MJ, Whitfield, HN, et al: Painless lithotripsy: Experience with 100 patients. *Lancet* 1988; 41–43.
3. Wilbert, DM, Riedmiller, H, Alken, P, et al: Zweite Generation der extrakorporalen Stoβwellenlithotripsie (Lithostar). *Dtsch Med Wschr* 1987; 112:1637–1640.
4. Staritz, M, Floth, A, Rambow, A, et al: Extracorporeal shock waves (device of the second generation) for therapy of large common bile duct stones: Success and problems. *Gastroenterology* 1987; 92:1652(A).
5. Hickman, MS, Schwesinger, WH, Bova, JD, et al: Computed tomographic analysis of gallstones. *Arch Surg* 1986; 121:289–291.

In Vivo Parameters of Gallstone Fragmentation: Experimental Basis

M. Delius and W. Brendel

This chapter details the series of experiments carried out to elucidate the clinical phenomena associated with fragmentation of human gallstones by extracorporeal shock waves.

BACKGROUND

When the idea to use contact-free shock waves for stone destruction was born in the late 1960s, the destruction of kidney stones was considered the primary clinical application. However, at least from the technical point of view, it seemed there was no reason why destruction of other types of stones should not be possible as well. Gallstones have a high prevalence in the general population, and the number of operations to remove stones from the gallbladder and the bile ducts is also high. Therefore, the potential for wide clinical application prompted testing of gallstone destruction by shock waves as an alternative to operative treatment. However, the clinical implications for the surgical treatment of kidney stones differ in several respects from the situation in patients with gallstones:

1. The perioperative mortality of open surgery for kidney stone removal is high compared with the mortality of surgery for an elective cholecystectomy. The risk of losing the kidney at reoperation for a recurrent stone is even higher. The gallbladder, of course, can be removed at operation since obviously there is no necessity to preserve it as a functioning organ.

2. The stone mass and the number of stones are usually higher in the gallbladder than in the pelvocalyceal complex.

3. The upper urinary tract is flushed with large urine volumes and has an outflow tract in a gravity-dependent position, which favors the passage of stone fragments. The gallbladder is a blind sac with an outflow tract of a size and position not well suited for the passage of stone fragments.

4. Passage of small kidney stones or gravel via the urinary tract is a common clinical observation. Passage of stones or stone fragments from the gallbladder is less easily observed, and it is not known how often small gallstones pass spontaneously. Yet some gallbladders are filled with a high number of very small stones that obviously did not pass via a narrow cystic duct. A similar situation in the kidney is not known.

5. Obstruction of the ureter or the biliary tract could lead to ureteral or biliary pain, but only in the biliary tract is there a risk of pancreatitis. The risk could increase when many fragments acquire a size that enables them to pass the bile ducts.

6. The risk of stone recurrence in the kidney exists after surgery as well as after stone destruction by shock waves. Cholecystectomy eliminates the risk of stone recurrence in the gallbladder. The incidence of recurring stones in the gallbladder was high if the gallbladder was preserved, as had been shown with oral bile acid dissolution, certainly higher than the incidence of recurrent stones in the kidney.

So in contrast to the therapeutic gain from the

application of extracorporeal shock waves for kidney stone destruction, the gain from the application of shock waves for gallstone destruction was expected to be lower and the risk of complications from obstruction of the common bile duct by fragments higher. The application of shock waves for kidney stone destruction in humans had been predicted to fail owing to obstruction of the ureter by the large mass of fragments. The same was again predicted to happen in the common bile duct, even with small stone fragments. Yet in both cases it was unknown, and it could not be estimated from known clinical situations what happened to stone fragments after stone destruction and how dangerous they were.

The first experiments on extracorporeal shock wave destruction of gallstones in animals were carried out at the Institute for Surgical Research in Munich in cooperation with Dornier Medizintechnik at a time when extracorporeal shock waves had just been shown to be effective for kidney stone destruction in humans.

GALLSTONE DESTRUCTION IN VIVO

In the first series of experiments human gallstones were implanted surgically into the gallbladders of dogs or monkeys to test gallstone destruction in vivo. The size of the stones ranged from 1 to 2 cm; the number of stones implanted was between one and four. Extracorporeal shock waves were administered after varying intervals from directly after stone implantation up to several days.

Shock waves were applied with a Dornier HM 1 lithotripter.[1] This was the first kidney stone lithotripter used for patient treatment. It was equipped with a 90-nF capacitor and operated with a voltage of 20 kV. Shock waves were generated under water by electric discharge between the two tips of an electrode and focused by a metal ellipsoid. Shock waves generated with this electrical energy and focused with this ellipsoid had already been successfully used for kidney stone destruction. The dogs were fixed on a moveable stretcher and were partially immersed into the water of the tank. Their gallstones were positioned into the shock wave focus by two intersecting x-ray beams, which were marked on monitors (Fig 1). The same system had been used to visualize the position of the kidney stones. As most gallstones were radiolucent, they could be seen only with a contrast agent. Success of stone fragmentation after shock wave application was judged from the size of the fragments in the gallbladder at dissection. Dissection was performed directly after shock wave application or during the following days.

In the first group of 9 dogs 300 to 750 shock waves were applied. Stone destruction was achieved in over two thirds of them. In the second group of 18 dogs and 3 monkeys the number of shock waves was increased to 800 to 1200. Stone destruction was achieved in 90 percent of these animals. Although the high rate of stone destruction especially in the latter group was satisfactory, the size of the fragments was not. In some animals the result was very good, with fragments of a few millimeters maximal size only in their gallbladder. In most of them, however, at least one particle larger than half a centimeter maximal diameter was left in the gallbladder, and even stone fragments larger than 1 cm were recovered. In four dogs no fragments were found in the gallbladder. It could not be decided whether the fragments had passed via the bile duct or had been dissolved, as dog bile has a very high litholytic activity and dogs have the ability to pass even several grams of fragments of 6 mm maximal size from their gallbladders.

In the third group of five dogs small gallstones of several millimeters size only were implanted into the common bile duct. A clip had to be placed at the lower end of the duct to prevent stone passage. Contrast agent was injected via T-drain. Directly after stone implantation 1000 shock waves were administered to the stones. As had been expected stone destruction into very small fragments was achieved in this experimental setup.

This first series of experiments showed that gallstones could be destroyed by shock waves in vivo in most cases, but the resulting fragments in the gallbladder were quite large. This was in

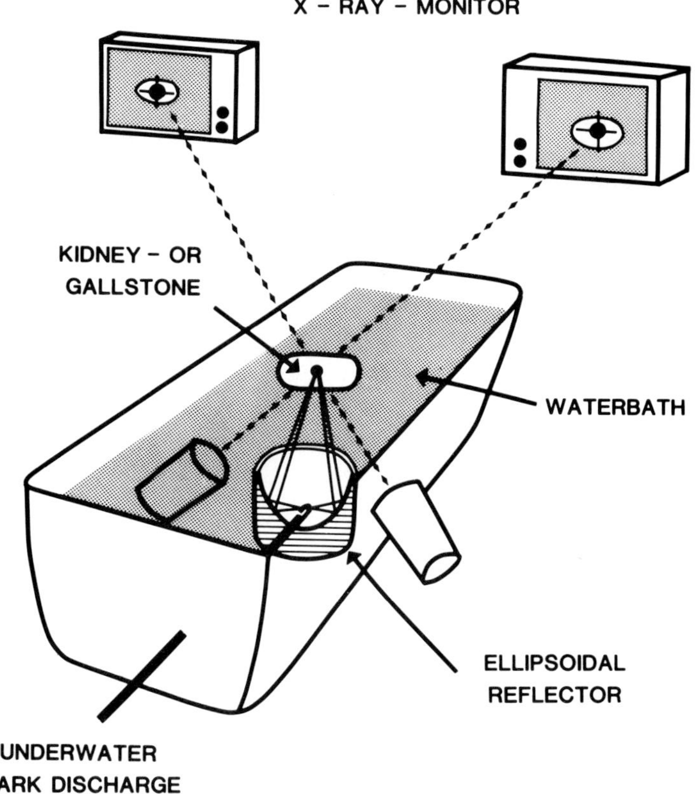

FIG 1.
Design of the Dornier HM 2 lithotripter. The central beams of two x-ray systems which are marked on monitors intersect in the waterbath at the point where the shock waves are focused by the ellipsoidal reflector. Any object positioned on both central beams is in the focus.

contrast to what had been expected from in vitro data. The reason was the difficulty in localizing stone fragments in the gallbladder. After the initial stone breakup no fragments could be detected with the x-ray system employed, and shock waves had to be administered randomly without clear radiographic guidance in a large gallbladder volume. Localization of gallstone fragments by x-ray control was inadequate in contrast to kidney stone fragment localization. An alternative explanation of the poor results might have been that the shock wave pressure in the gallbladder was too low to destroy gallstones, as the shock wave might have been absorbed and diffracted by tissue. However, direct pressure registration by implantation of a pressure probe into the gallbladder showed that tissue absorption was not high enough to explain the discrepancy between the in vitro and in vivo data.

No stone destruction could be achieved in at least one instance where the stone was well visualized in the gallbladder, and all shock waves were focused on the stone according to the x-ray positioning system. Additional in vitro experiments showed that there was a group of gallstones that could not be pulverized into smaller fragments with the number of shock waves and the wave energies employed. This group was not homogenous with respect to the chemical composition of the stones as it included typical cholesterol stones and stones with a calcified rim.

Two modifications of the lithotripter design were made as a result of this first series of experiments. As localization of stone fragments by x-ray in the gallbladder was inadequate, ultra-

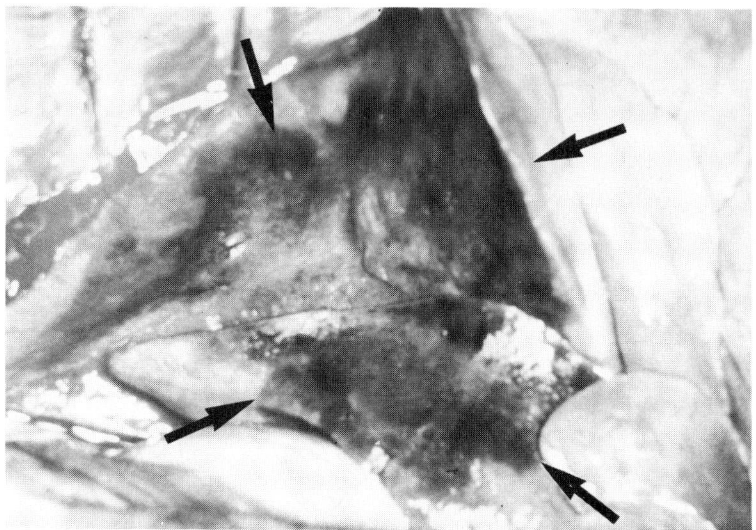

FIG 2.
Lung hemorrhage in the right lower lobe of the lung *(arrows)*. View of the diaphragmatic surface of the lung in situ.

sound was considered a better way to localize gallbladder stones. The lithotripter therefore was equipped with an ultrasound positioning system. In addition, since some gallstones proved difficult to fragment, Dornier modified the ellipsoid to better concentrate the shock wave energy and fragment stones more readily. The similarity between gallstone destruction in vivo and in vitro made it possible to examine the destructive capability of the shock wave device separate from its biological effects.

TISSUE EFFECTS

The side effects of shock wave application in this experiment were lung hemorrhage and comparably minor changes in other organs in the focal region. They were investigated in more detail in the following experiments. No stones were implanted which could impede the detection of tissue damage by shock waves and complicate a defined experimental setup.

LUNG HEMORRHAGE DURING GALLSTONE DESTRUCTION

Lung hemorrhage was the most serious side effect observed after gallstone destruction in vivo. It was detected in over 80 percent of the animals at autopsy. Hemorrhage was located at the diaphragmatic surface of the lung (Fig 2). The diaphragmatic surface of the right lower lobe and the accessory lobe were the most affected, while the right middle lobe and the left lower lobe were only slightly hemorrhagic or not at all. Hemorrhage always extended in continuity from the surface up to 1.5 cm into the parenchyma. This was not surprising because shock waves were reflected at the interface between tissue and gas in the lung and could not penetrate the lung parenchyma. Owing to the anatomical position of the gallbladder in relation to the lung it was probable that the lung had been in the high-pressure field of the shock wave, not very far from the focus, when shock waves were administered to the gallbladder of dogs or monkeys. The degree of lung hemorrhage was considered intolerable for shock wave application in humans although no animal had died and no hemoptysis was noted after shock wave application.

The risk of patients suffering lung hemorrhage had to be known before shock waves could be administered. Therefore, the conditions leading to lung hemorrhage had to be investigated in more detail in a separate experiment.[2]

In this experiment the distance of the lung tissue from the focus of the shock wave which prevented the occurrence of lung hemorrhage was determined. By pressure registrations at the lung surface the pressures associated with hemorrhage were directly registered. With these data the prediction of lung hemorrhage in humans was considered possible in spite of the different anatomical setting.

Pressure probes were implanted between the lung and the diaphragm in dogs. The position of the probe in relation to the pressure field of the shock wave was determined with the x-ray positioning system. Shock waves were administered with the Dornier HM 2 lithotripter equipped with the same ellipsoid as in the previous experiment. Its high-pressure field had an elongated shape along the long axis of the ellipsoid and was rotationally symmetrical around the long axis (Fig 3). Because of the asymmetry, pres-

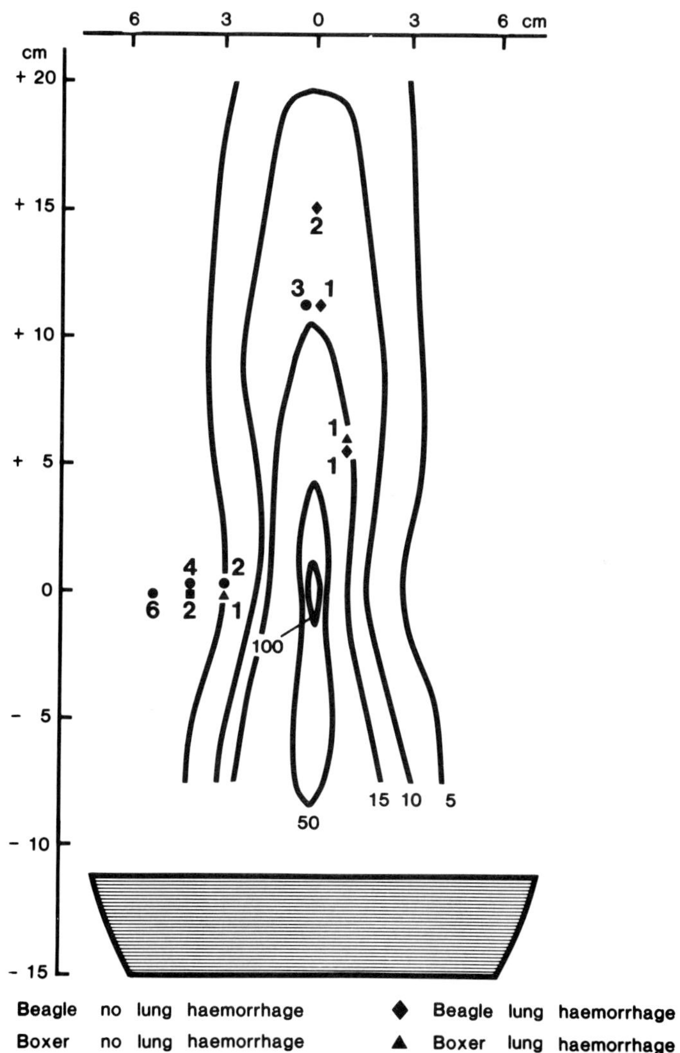

FIG 3.
Lung hemorrhage in dogs. The lines denote the rotationally symmetrical isobars (relative units) as determined in water; the focus is on 0 position on both axes of the pressure field. Symbols denote the position of the pressure probes. Lung hemorrhage was restricted to the high-pressure field of the shock wave, which extends along the long axis of the ellipsoid.

sure probes were positioned on two axes in the field at various distances from the focus: on the long axis and on an axis perpendicular to it through the focus. A thousand shock waves were administered under conditions similar to the previous experiment. The lung was examined for hemorrhage at the site where the probe was located.

On the long axis of the shock wave field lung hemorrhage was detected as far as 15 cm from the focus. The shock wave pressures registered on this axis were in the range of several MPa. On the axis perpendicular to the long axis through the focus, no hemorrhage was seen at 4 or 5 cm from the focus. Hemorrhage at 3 cm was only questionable and might have been due to spillover of blood from sites closer to the focus. The shock wave pressures registered on this axis were between 15 and 30 percent of the values registered at the other axis and did not exceed 2 to 3 MPa.

The experiment suggested that with this shock wave device the lung should not be on the long axis of the shock wave field during shock wave application in humans. Yet lung hemorrhage could be prevented by keeping a distance of more than 3 cm from this axis. The results could be transferred to pressure distributions of different geometry as the shock wave pressures at the lung surface were registered. The ellipsoid currently used for gallstone destruction in the clinical system now in use (MPL 9000) has a pressure distribution with a smaller focal region.

EFFECT OF SHOCK WAVES ON THE LIVER AND GALLBLADDER

Hemorrhages of the liver and gallbladder and of the other upper abdominal organs were of only minor significance in the experiment on gallstone destruction in vivo. The liver capsule showed subcapsular hemorrhagic blisters in the high-pressure field of the wave; capsular adhesions between liver lobes were observed in the high-pressure field in front of the gallbladder. Petechial hemorrhages occurred on the serosal surfaces of the pancreas and duodenum, but mucosal ulceration or hematomas were not observed. Petechial hemorrhages were also noted on the gallbladder wall; sometimes the submucosa of the gallbladder appeared hemorrhagic. In some dogs clotted blood was detected in the gallbladder. It could not be determined whether it was due to stone implantation or hemorrhage into the gallbladder caused by shock wave application. Elevations of liver enzymes, which had been observed after shock wave application, returned to normal during the following days.

Experiments on gallstone destruction had shown that the destructive capability of shock waves had to be increased for certain types of gallstones. Dornier achieved this by fashioning an ellipsoid with a much smaller focus. Using model stones Dornier achieved the same destructive capability with this ellipsoid at an operating voltage of 15 kV as with the ellipsoid from the previous experiments at an operating voltage of 20 kV. Stones which were difficult to destroy before could be fragmented more easily with the new ellipsoid at 20 kV. Stones that were easily fragmented could be either fragmented now at the lower energy level as before or with less shock waves at a higher energy level. As a result the question arose whether to treat all patients with the higher shock wave energy or whether it would be more appropriate to adjust the shock wave energy to the level necessary for an efficient stone destruction and to keep it as low as possible. Stone destruction was considered efficient if the stone could be fragmented within an acceptable time. The biological effects of shock waves of higher destructive capability were considered one criterion for the decision as to the optimal patient treatment regimen.

The biological effects of the two ellipsoids were compared in a preliminary experiment with groups of dogs consisting of three animals. Tissue damage in the upper abdomen after shock wave application to the gallbladder was examined according to an experimental protocol without stone implantation. The gallbladders were visualized by x-ray after contrast opacification. Shock waves were focused to a single point in the wall of the gallbladder neck. They passed through liver tissue overlying the gallbladder before they reached the bladder wall and then re-entered the liver in the hilar area behind the focus (Fig 4). In this position the duodenal wall

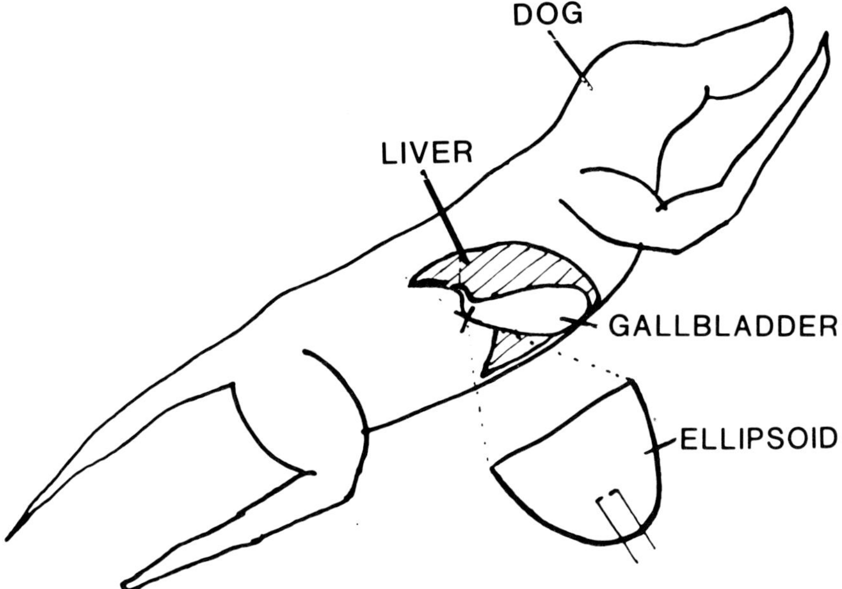

FIG 4.
Positioning of the dogs for shock wave application to the gallbladder wall in the region of the gallbladder neck.

and pancreatic head were close to the focus. Fifteen hundred shock waves were administered. In analogy to the examination of kidney damage by shock waves the dogs were dissected the day following shock wave application and tissue damage was examined.

Tissue damage was similar in dogs when shock waves were administered either with the old ellipsoid at 20 kV or with the better focusing ellipsoid at 15 kV, that is, at similar destructive capability.

Macroscopically, the liver surface disclosed small subcapsular hemorrhages or blood-filled blisters that were at times confluent. The area where they occurred had a diameter of 2 to 4 cm and corresponded to the high-pressure field of the shock wave. The largest subcapsular hemorrhage observed was a blood blister of over 3 cm diameter. In a few cases there was destruction of the liver capsule. If the capsule had been damaged between liver lobes, they were adherent.

Changes in the liver parenchyma were again restricted to the high-pressure field of the shock wave. Two types could be differentiated: the first was hemorrhage. Hemorrhages up to 4 mm diameter or less were seen in all dogs. In a minority of them hemorrhages were larger, up to 1 cm in diameter (Fig 5). Most of the small hemorrhages were very small and had a diameter of 1 to 2 mm only. The second change were thrombi in single liver veins in the high-pressure field. They were seen in half of the animals.

Histologically, small hemorrhages were seen in the liver parenchyma in the high-pressure field. They could not be shown to originate from a certain type of vessel or to be restricted to areas around portal or central veins. Many of the hemorrhages were very small foci only. Hemorrhage into the connective tissue of portal veins was common and could be associated with venous wall destruction and thrombus formation or extend beyond portal fields and affect the adjacent liver parenchyma. When thrombi were detected, they were nearly always located in portal fields and not in liver veins. Rupture of hepatic arteries was not detected; the bile ducts were usually intact as well.

Macroscopically areas of the outer gallbladder

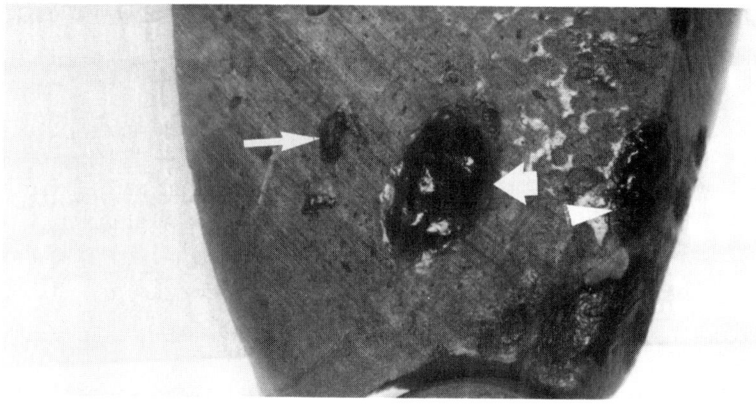

FIG 5.
Hemorrhage in the liver after shock wave application. A larger hemorrhage *(large arrow),* a small hemorrhage *(small arrow),* and flat subcapsular hemorrhages *(triangle)* at the site of shock wave entry into the liver. Scale in centimeters.

surface were covered with confluent subserosal petechiae. On the inside the gallbladder mucosa directly in the focus of the shock wave was ulcerated in nearly all dogs (Fig 6). Hemorrhage had occurred into the gallbladder lumen with blood clot formation. The gallbladder wall was hemorrhagic and swollen below this area. The amount of blood oozing from the injured mucosa must have been low as blood in the gut was never detected.

Histologically the gallbladder mucosa in the focus was ulcerated with destruction of the mucosal layer or destruction of the villous tips with hemorrhage into the mucosa. These sites were covered with fibrinoid material. The underlying gallbladder wall was edematous and hemorrhagic. No destruction of collagen fibers was noted. The biological effects of the better focusing ellipsoid were also examined with the higher destructive capability at 20 kV. There were hints that tissue damage might have been increased. Damage to the gallbladder wall had not been observed to such extent in the previous experimental series where the focus had not been kept at one point in the gallbladder wall.

The findings of this experiment suggested a need to be cautious and to restrict the destructive capability in patients to the effects actually needed for stone destruction. This approach was later shown to be of advantage when nearly all treatments were performed without general or epidural anesthesia. However the experiments also showed that it was possible to administer shock waves of higher destructive capability if needed for stone destruction.

Certain extrapolations to the clinical situation in humans can be made. Shock waves are administered to gallstones with humans lying in prone position. Waves are administered from below, and the gallbladder wall is located directly at the same position as the stones in the focus. The position of the wall in relation to the shock wave focus is probably similar to the animal experiment. In contrast to this similarity the setup of the experiment differed from the situation during gallstone destruction in humans in several respects:

The focus was positioned at a single site in the gallbladder wall. Gallstone fragments in humans were usually spread over a larger area in the gallbladder, and not all shock waves were administered to a single site in the wall. However in humans several hundred shock waves were also administered to single areas of the gallbladder wall. So it was likely that gallbladder wall changes occurred in some patients during gallstone destruction.

In the majority of patients shock waves entered the gallbladder directly and did not pass through the liver en route. No liver damage was expected to occur as the liver was not in the high-pressure field.

Gallstones were located in the fundus in the vast majority of treatments. So the liver hilus was not as close to the focus as in the experimental setup. It has been shown that blood vessels were less exposed to the high-pressure field in patients. This means that thrombi were also less likely to occur.

Gallstones absorbed part of the shock wave energy. This reduced the effect of shock waves on tissues behind the stone.

Altogether the results on tissue damage with this experimental setup showed what could happen but not what had to happen. They also suggested that with a patient positioned as performed today, tissue damage should be at a minimum.

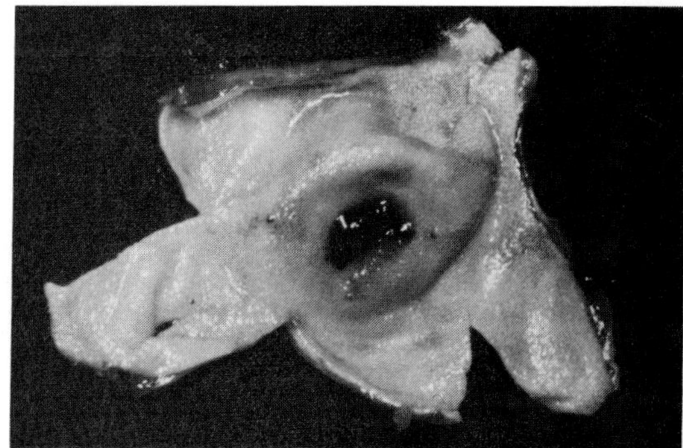

FIG 6.
Mucosal hemorrhage in the gallbladder neck at the point that had been in the shock wave focus. Scale in centimeters.

PASSAGE OF STONE FRAGMENTS FROM THE GALLBLADDER

Up to this point only the problems of gallstone destruction had been addressed. It was obvious from the therapeutical situation that this was only a minor question compared with the problem that arose after the generation of hundreds or thousands of stone fragments in the gallbladder. The potential of these fragments to cause obstruction was not known. It was not even known whether it was advantageous to fragment stones down to a minimum size as small as sand. Perhaps the potential of these fragments to obstruct the bile ducts was higher compared with the potential of larger fragments, since small fragments could reach the papilla more easily and form a solid block in front of it. If such fragments had a high potential for obstruction, intervention to remove them might be necessary and had to be tested before the application of shock waves for gallstone destruction in humans. An unknown risk would arise from this additional procedure and impede the proper evaluation of complications arising from the application of shock waves. Fragment passage had not been addressed in the experiment on gallstone destruction in vivo. The size of the fragments after shock wave application had been highly variable, and dogs have been shown to dissolve cholesterol stones in their gallbladders. Furthermore, there had not been enough time to observe fragment passage as autopsy could be delayed for only a few days after shock wave application to gain information about the fragment size. Otherwise, differentiation between passage and dissolution had not been possible.

Fragment passage was approached in an experiment in which a defined amount of stone fragments with a maximal size of 2 or 4 mm was implanted into the gallbladders of two groups of dogs.[3] Gallstone fragments had to be replaced by kidney stone fragments that had a similar shape and were insoluble in canine bile. The amount of fragments that had left the gallbladder after 5 weeks was determined. Hepatic and pancreatic enzymes were also monitored regularly to detect obstruction.

Five weeks after fragment implantation, about two thirds of the fragments of 2 or 4 mm maximal size had left the gallbladder (Table 1). No difference was detected between the groups, but each group was divided into dogs that had no or only very few fragments left in their gallbladders and dogs that had retained over half of the implanted amount. The reason for this difference could not be detected. Obstruction of the common bile duct was observed at autopsy in only one dog with 4-mm fragments, but all dogs of this group had transient enzyme elevations

TABLE 1.
Passage of Stone Fragments from Canine Gallbladders

MAXIMAL FRAGMENT SIZE MM	NUMBER OF ANIMALS	RESTING FRAGMENTS, %	PAPILLARY OR DUCTAL LESIONS	LIVER ENZYME ELEVATION
2	11	36 (0–68)	–	+
4	5	32 (0–59)	+	++

pointing to transient obstruction of the common bile duct. In the dogs with 2-mm fragments no obstruction was detected. Elevations of their pancreatic and hepatic enzymes occurred significantly less often and were borderline increases of very short duration only. Stone fragments passed from the gallbladder without any sign of obstruction in the majority of animals of this group. The results of this experiment suggested that in contrast to common opinion there seemed to be a chance that fragments could pass in patients without severe obstruction. Smaller fragments caused less obstruction than larger fragments, and this suggested that fragments after gallstone destruction should be as small as possible. In practice it was difficult even in vitro to obtain a maximal fragment size smaller than 2 mm with extracorporeal shock waves. Yet it was also evident that fragment clearance was slow in a large number of dogs. No experiment with a longer follow-up was performed, but the result suggested that additional litholytic therapy might be required in at least a subset of patients.

All the factors relevant for the clearance of fragments from gallbladders are not known. All kidney stone fragments used in the experiment did not float. Gallstones nearly always behaved in a similar way. When floating stones were destroyed by shock waves, the vast majority of fragments sank to the bottom, which pointed to the importance of air entrapped in the stones. In general, only fragments located in the outflow tract could be expected to have a chance to be expelled by a contracting bladder. As the cystic duct in the experiment was passed equally well by both stone sizes the position of the indundibulum could have been important for mechanical fragment clearance. With the clinical application of gallstone destruction these questions can be better examined in humans.

SUMMARY

It was shown by implantation of gallstones into gallbladders of dogs that gallstone destruction in vivo was possible. The major side effect was lung hemorrhage, which was in addition to minor changes in the liver and gallbladder. The pulmonary damage could be prevented by keeping the lung away from the high pressure field, that is, keeping the pressure below 2 to 3 MPa. Tissue damage to the liver was shown to consist of hemorrhage and damage to veins; in the gallbladder mucosal ulceration and oözing of blood into the lumen were observed. These changes indicated a need to restrict the energy for stone destruction to the actually needed level, which had to be high for some gallstones. The passage of stone fragments implanted into dog gallbladders was associated with more signs of obstruction when the fragments were larger. Small fragments caused little obstruction, but fragment passage was not complete in many dogs.

REFERENCES

1. Brendel W, Enders G: Shock waves for gallstones: Animal studies. *Lancet* 1983; 1:1054.
2. Delius M, Enders G, Heine G, et al: Biological effects of shock waves: Lung hemorrhage by shock waves in dogs—pressure dependence. *Ultrasound Med Biol* 1987; 13:61–67.
3. Delius M, Enders G, Brendel W: Passage of stone fragments from the gallbladders of dogs. *Surgery Gynecol Obstet* 1988; 166:241–244.

The Short-Term Effects of Extracorporeal Shock Wave Lithotripsy on the Human Gallbladder

Alan G. Johnson, Bryan Ross, and T.J. Stephenson

The tissue effects of extracorporeal shock wave lithotripsy (ESL) are poorly characterized. Although the short-term local tissue response in animals to spark-percutaneous lithotripsy for gallstones has been described,[1] and more distant effects including pulmonary hemorrhage have been reported,[2] the effects in human tissue of piezoelectric ESL are unknown. Following local ethical committee approval, a group of patients was, therefore, treated by ESL before planned cholecystectomy and detailed histological analysis of the gallbladder were performed. We considered it was important to check for damage before starting a controlled trial of lithotripsy for gallstones.

This work was supported by the Department of Health and Social Security and Trent Regional Health Authority.

MATERIALS AND METHODS

Fifteen patients (5 male and 10 female; ages 23 to 84 years) with gallstones demonstrable by ultrasound scan were subjected to a standardized treatment from the Wolf 2300 Lithotripter of 2000 to 2500 shocks at setting 3 to 4 at intervals between 4 hours and 5 days before cholecystectomy. One patient was treated on two consecu-

TABLE 1.
Histological Changes (Light Microscopy)

	TREATED (TOTAL 15)	CONTROL (TOTAL 6)	ASSOCIATION WITH ESL
Rokitansky-Aschoff sinuses	10	1	NS
Chronic inflammation	13	4	NS
Mucosal fibrosis	9	3	NS
Muscular hypertrophy	7	2	NS
Acute inflammation	2	0	NS
Vascular dilatation	13	0	p = 0.005*
Edema	12	0	p = 0.005*
Mucosal denudation	13	0	p = 0.005*

(NS = not significant.
*Fisher's exact probability test.

tive days. One observer (T.J.S.) examined these gallbladder patients together with six untreated control patients, unaware of which patients had been treated. Opened gallbladders were photographed in the fresh state before selection of tissue blocks from the tip, equatorial region, and the neck of each for histological examination. A separate sample of mucosa was fixed and processed by critical point drying and gold coating for scanning electron microscopy. The removed gallstones were assessed for degree of fragmentation.

RESULTS

Gallbladders removed within 6 hours of ESL confirmed the impression from real-time ultrasound scanning of mural edema (Fig 1) and, additionally, showed vascular dilatation and several petechial hemorrhages on microscopic examination. Edema and vascular dilatation were absent from two gallbladders excised at 48 hours and 5 days after ESL, but variable mucosal denudation remained. Scanning electron microscopy at a magnification of 512 confirmed the presence in all cases of mucosal denudation seen by light microscopy and revealed many foci of denudation of patches of about 50 epithelial cells in regions that had appeared intact by light microscopy (Fig 2). The approximate proportion of mucosal denudation in treated cases ranged from 10 to 90 percent. In all cases where the crypt mouths of Rokitansky-Aschoff sinuses were seen by scanning electron microscopy, they were lined by intact epithelium.

CONCLUSION

ESL produces transient mural edema and vascular dilatation in the stone-filled gallbladder,

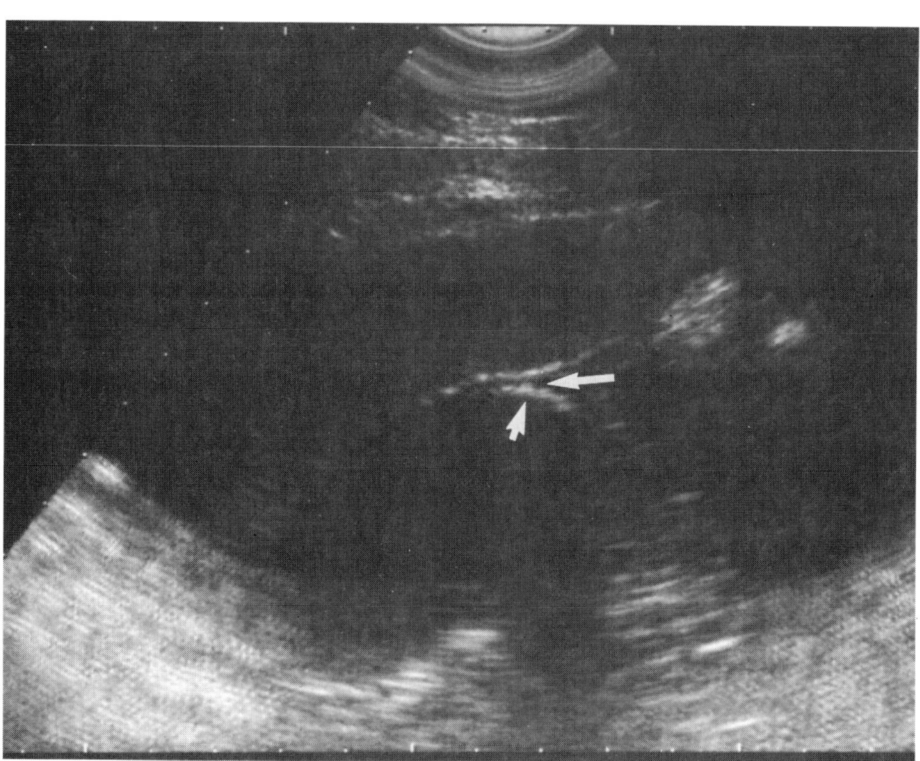

FIG 1.
Ultrasound scan of gallbladder during lithotripsy treatment of stones *(short arrow)*, showing development of wall edema *(long arrow)*.

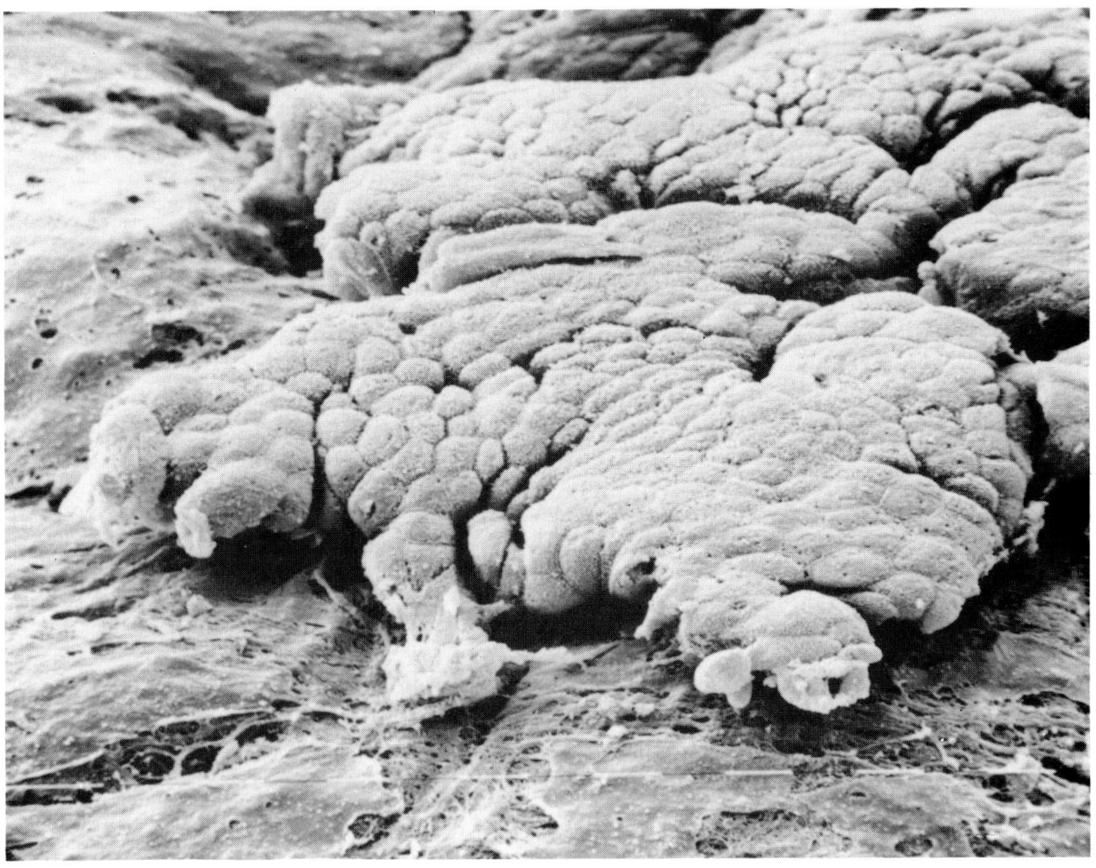

FIG 2.
Scanning electron micrograph of gallbladder mucosa after lithotripsy, showing islands of epithelial cells surrounded by denudation (x640).

but these changes do not suggest any risk of perforation. There is also epithelial denudation, which spares the crypts. The causes of this need further study. However, the presence of intact epithelium in the mouths of mucosal crypts may serve as a source of viable cells for re-epithelialization.

REFERENCES

1. Brendel W, Enders G: Shock waves for gallstones: Animal studies. *Lancet* 1983; 1:1054.
2. Delius M, Enders G, Heine G, et al; Biological effects of shock waves: Lung hemorrhage by shock waves in dogs—pressure dependence. *Ultrasound Med Biol* 1987; 13:61–67.

Extracorporeal Shock Wave Lithotripsy of Gallstones: The Munich Experience

Gustav Paumgartner

Since the first cholecystectomy in 1882 by Carl Langenbuch,[1] a number of nonsurgical treatments of gallbladder stones have been developed, lithotripsy by extracorporeally generated shock waves being one of the most recent innovations.[2] After animal studies had been performed by Brendel and his group,[3, 4] and in vitro experiments had been carried out by Neubrand and associates,[5] an interdisciplinary group in Munich[2] treated the first patients with gallbladder stones by extracorporeal shock wave lithotripsy in 1985.[2] Up to now, more than 400 patients with gallbladder stones and more than 60 patients with bile duct stones have been treated by our group.

GALLBLADDER STONES

METHODS AND SELECTION OF PATIENTS

The first 175 patients were treated with a Dornier prototype lithotripter;[2] all further patients were treated with a Dornier lithotripter MPL 9000. These lithotripters employ a high-voltage generator and underwater electrodes to discharge sparks that cause a sudden evaporation of water and the formation of a plasma between the electrodes. This creates a pressure wave of high velocity and energy. The electrodes are mounted in the first focus of an ellipsoidal metal cavity. The pressure wave is reflected from the walls of this cavity and condensed in the remote focus, where a pressure of about 1000 bar can be generated within nanoseconds.

Most of the tissues of the human body have an acoustic impedance very similar to that of water; therefore, the shock waves can be transmitted from the shock wave source into the body with negligible attenuation through a water bath or a water bag that is interfaced with the skin by an ultrasonic coupling gel. The shock waves travel practically unimpeded through the body's soft tissues, because they have an acoustic impedance similar to that of water. When they reach the stone, energy is liberated owing to a change in accoustic impedance and to cavitation phenomena on the surface of the stone causing stone destruction.[6] Tissue damage may occur if focused shock waves enter the lungs.

For fragmentation of gallbladder stones, the patient is treated in the prone position, so that the shock waves enter the abdomen from the ventral side. In the early phase of the development of the method, the patient was partially immersed in a tank of water.[2] Advanced technology in the Dornier lithotripter MPL 9000 now uses a compressible water bag to transmit the shock waves into the body (Fig 1).

Ultrasound is used to guide the positioning of the stones and to monitor the process of fragmentation. Up to 1600 shock wave discharges are delivered to the patient within about 40 min-

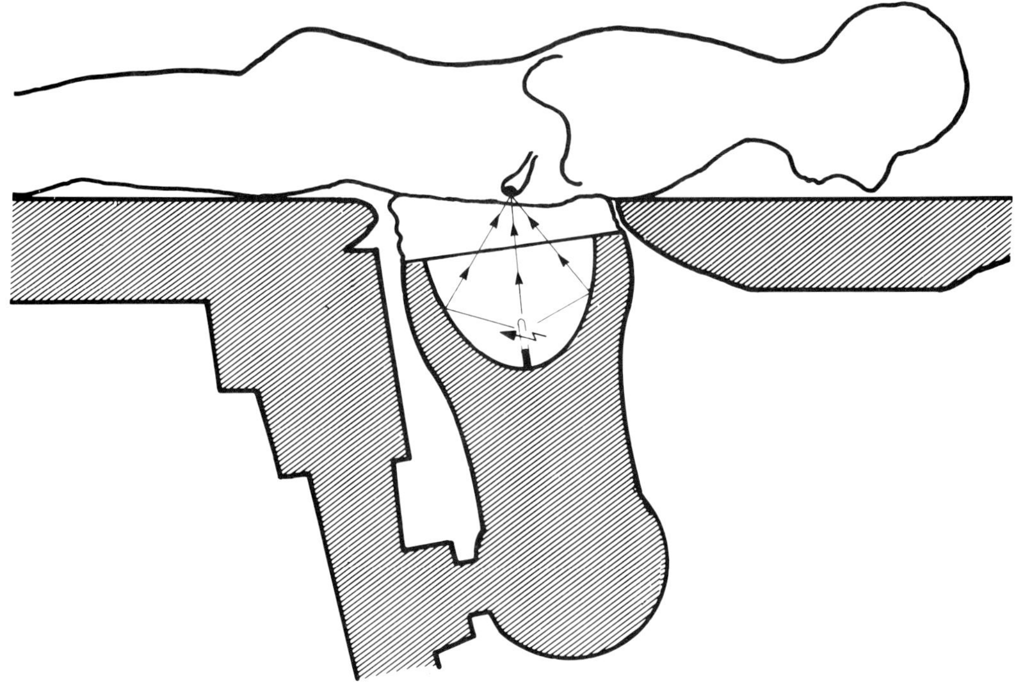

FIG 1.
Shock wave lithotripsy of gallbladder stones. The shock waves are reflected to a focal point where the stone is positioned.

utes. They are triggered by the continuously monitored R-wave of the patient's electrocardiogram.[7, 8] The path of shock waves must avoid lung and bone.

In the early phase of the development of the method,[2] the treatment was performed under general or peridural anesthesia. More recently, about two thirds of the patients received intravenously administered analgesics,[9] the rest are treated without any medication.

It cannot be expected that all stone fragments are expelled from the gallbladder; only patients with radiolucent stones that presumably were cholesterol stones were selected for shock wave treatment and all patients received adjuvant litholytic therapy with bile acids. A combination of ursodeoxycholic acid and chenodeoxycholic acid (7 to 8 mg/kg body weight each per day) was given with the evening meal. Bile acid therapy was started at least 1 week (median: 12 days) before shock wave treatment and continued for 3 months after complete disappearance of stone fragments.[8]

The criteria used by our group for selection of patients with gallbladder stones for extracorporeal shock wave lithotripsy are listed in Table 1. Of all patients with gallbladder stones referred to our institution for treatment, 28 percent met these selection criteria. The most frequent reasons for exclusion of patients from shock wave lithotripsy were too numerous and/or calcified stones. In a separate, still on-going study, we are also exploring shock wave lithotripsy in patients with gallbladder stones that exhibit a calcified rim.

RESULTS AND DISCUSSION

In the treatment of more than 400 patients, we were able to fragment the stones in nearly all pa-

TABLE 1.

Selection of Patients with Gallbladder Stones for Extracorporeal Shock Wave Lithotripsy

INCLUSION CRITERIA
1. History of biliary pain.
2. Solitary radiolucent stone with a diameter up to 30 mm or up to 3 radiolucent stones with similar total stone volume.
3. Gallbladder visualization on oral cholecystography.
4. Clear detection of stone(s) by ultrasound and positioning in the shock wave focus must be possible.

EXCLUSION CRITERIA
1. Acute cholecystitis or cholangitis.
2. Biliary obstruction or bile duct stone.
3. Acute pancreatitis.
4. Coagulopathy or current medication with anticoagulants, aspirin, or nonsteroidal antiinflammatory drugs.
5. Vascular aneurysms in the shock wave path.
6. Pregnancy.

tients selected according to the above criteria. The success rate, defined as complete disappearance of fragments on repeated ultrasound examinations, varied according to the number and the size of the stones.[8] Although complete disappearance of stones can occur within days after shock wave application in individual patients, it took 2 to 4 months until half of the patients were completely free of fragments (Fig 2). After shock wave treatment, about 80 percent of the patients were free of stones 8 to 12 months later. Both dissolution as well as passage of fragments contribute to this outcome.

Shock wave treatment was tolerated wtihout serious adverse effects. There were no signs of tissue damage except cutaneous petechiae in 12 percent and transient hematuria in 3 percent. No signs of hepatocellular damage or hepatobiliary dysfunction could be detected by laboratory tests such as measurements of aminotransferases, alkaline phosphatase, and bilirubin.

Approximately one third of the patients experienced transient biliary pain related to stone fragments. It must, however, be noted that all patients have had biliary pain prior to shock wave treatment. About 2 percent of the patients developed mild pancreatitis between 2 weeks and 6 months after shock wave treatment, and in one patient endoscopic sphincterotomy was necessary to remove stone fragments from the common bile duct. Elective cholecystectomy has been performed in about 1 percent of the patients because of insufficient stone fragmentation; no further operations were necessary.

Comparable results have been reported by another group[10] in 157 patients using the same device, but the follow-up of these patients was too short to permit a definite evaluation of the percentage of patients with complete disappearance of fragments. Preliminary results in 24 patients have recently been reported from a French group[11] employing a different lithotripter with a similar method of shock wave generation. Using

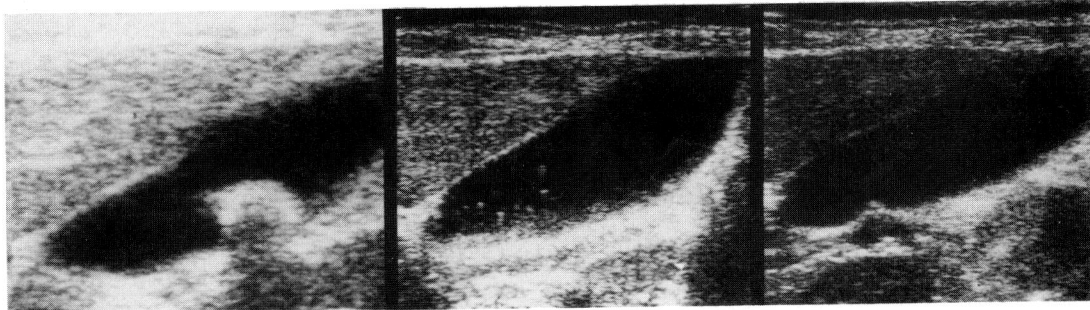

FIG 2.
Ultrasound of the gallbladder showing a solitary stone before extracorporeal shock wave lithotripsy *(left)*, multiple small fragments 1 day after lithotripsy *(center)*, and disappearance of fragments 6 weeks after lithotripsy and adjuvant bile acid therapy *(right)*. (From Paumgartner G, Sauerbruch T: Heutiger Stand von Litholyse und Lithotripsie von Gallensteinen. *Chirug* 1988; 59:190. Used by permission.)

a different principle for shock wave generation, namely a piezoceramic system, Hood and colleagues[12] have achieved fragmentation of gallbladder stones in 34 of 38 patients. The efficacy of this technique (which has also been combined with oral bile acid therapy) with respect to complete stone disappearance is still unknown. A combination of extracorporeal shock wave lithotripsy of calcified cholesterol gallstones with direct solvent dissolution by methyl-tert-butyl ether (MTBE) has been reported by Peine and associates.[13]

The results indicate that, in selected patients with gallbladder stones, extracorporeal shock wave lithotripsy is a safe and effective alternative to cholecystectomy. With the present criteria for patient selection, about 25 to 30 percent of the patients with symptomatic gallbladder stones referred to our department appear to be suitable candidates for this new nonsurgical treatment. Further improvements of the technique may permit us to extend the applicability of the procedure to patients with gallstones who have been excluded so far.

BILE DUCT STONES

The technique for fragmentation of bile duct stones is somewhat different from that used to fragment gallbladder stones.[7, 14] Most patients have been treated in a Dornier kidney lithotripter (HM3) in the supine position and the shock waves entered the body from the rear. This position is chosen because intestinal gas is often interposed between the shock wave source and the stones. A nasobiliary catheter is placed in these patients in order to inject contrast medium into the common bile duct for visualization of the stones. The positioning of the stones and the disintegration of the stones are monitored by fluoroscopy using a two-dimensional x-ray system.

Patients with bile duct stones were selected for extracorporeal shock wave treatment if their stones could not be removed by endoscopic procedures including mechanical lithotripsy. This was the case in about 20 percent of the patients with bile duct stones who had been referred to our department for nonsurgical treatment. The stones in these patients were either too large or impacted, or stenosis of the common bile duct or intrahepatic location made stone extraction impossible. In about 80 percent of these patients, shock wave lithotripsy resulted in stone fragments that passed spontaneously or could easily be extracted endoscopically[15] (Fig 3).

Present experience in patients with bile duct stones shows that the procedure is relatively safe. No signs of tissue damage could be detected by computed tomography, ultrasound, x-ray, and laboratory investigations. About 25 percent of the patients exhibited transient hematuria, probably caused by traversal of the shock waves through the right kidney.[15]

A multicenter study[16] has recently confirmed our early experience and several other groups have reported successful treatment of bile duct stones by extracorporeal shock wave lithotripsy[17–19]

REFERENCES

1. Langenbuch C: Ein Fall von Exstirpation der Gallenblase wegen chronischer Cholelithiasis. *Berliner Klin Wschr* 1882; 18:725–727.
2. Sauerbruch T, Delius M, Paumgartner G, et al: Fragmentation of gallstones by extracorporeal shock waves. *N Engl J Med* 1986; 314:818–822.
3. Brendel W, Enders G: Shock waves for gallstones: Animal studies. *Lancet* 1983; 1:1054.
4. Brendel W, Delius M, Enders G: Experimental destruction of gallstones by shock waves, in Paumgartner G, Stiehl A, Gerok W (eds): *Enterohepatic Circulation of Bile Acids and Sterol Metabolism*. Lancaster, England, MTP Press, 1985, pp 381–385.
5. Neubrand M, Sauerbruch T, Stellaard F, et al: In vitro cholesterol gallstone dissolution after fragmentation with shock waves. *Digestion* 1986; 34:51–59.
6. Delius M: Extracorporeal shock-wave lithotripsy of gallstones, in Baethmann A, Messmer K (eds): *Surgical Research: Recent Concepts and Results*. Berlin, Springer-Verlag, 1987, pp 77–81.
7. Paumgartner G: Fragmentation of gallstones by extracorporeal shock waves. *Semin Liver Dis* 1987; 7:317–321.
8. Sackmann M, Delius M, Sauerbruch T, et al: Shock-wave lithotripsy of gallbladder stones: The first 175 patients. *N Engl J Med* 1988; 318:393–397.

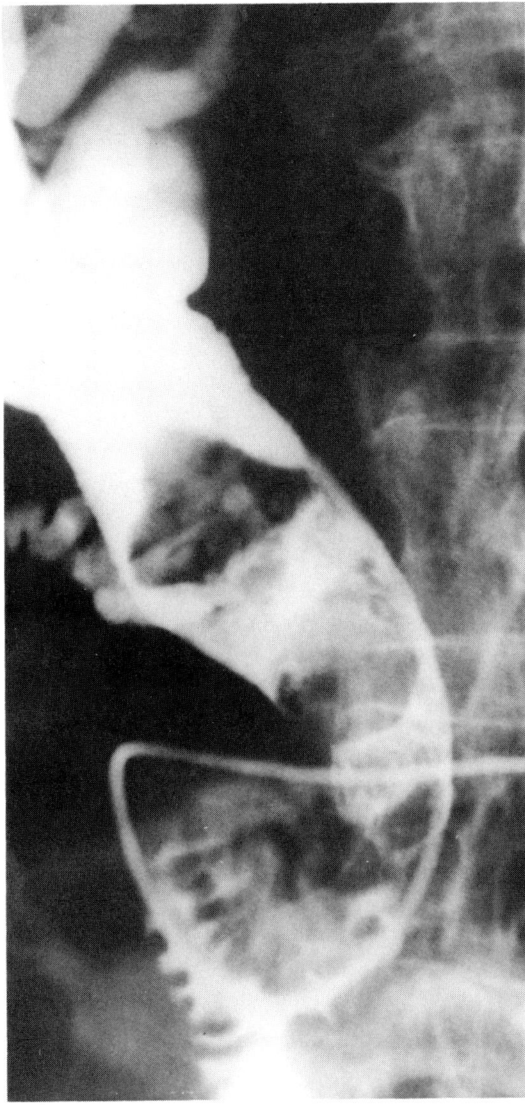

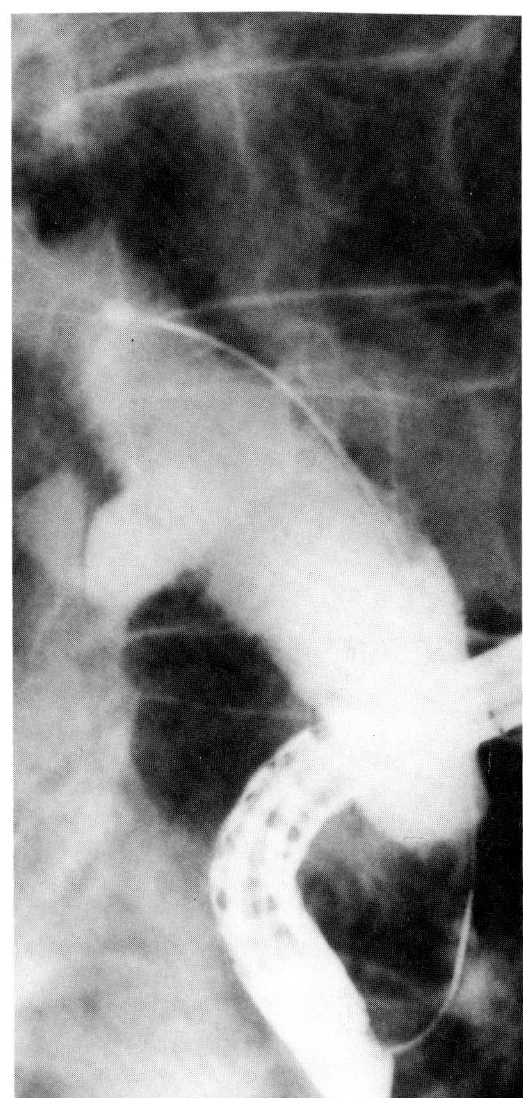

FIG 3.
Retrograde cholangiogram before *(left)* and after *(right)* extracorporeal shock wave lithotripsy of stones in the common bile duct and endoscopic extraction of the fragments. (From Paumgartner G, Sauerbruch T: Heutiger Stand von Litholyse und Lithotripsie von Gallensteinen. *Chirug* 1988; 59:190. Used by permission.)

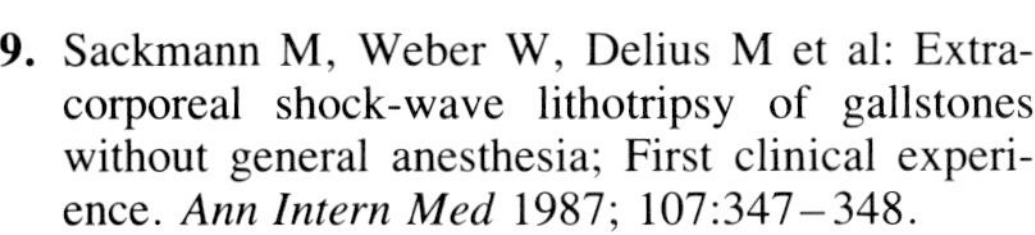

9. Sackmann M, Weber W, Delius M et al: Extracorporeal shock-wave lithotripsy of gallstones without general anesthesia; First clinical experience. *Ann Intern Med* 1987; 107:347–348.

10. Greiner L, Wenzel H, Jakobeit Ch: Biliaere Stoss-wellen-Lithotripsie. Fragmentation und Lyse—ein neues Verfahren. *Dtsch med Wschr* 1987; 112:1893–1896.

11. Ponchon T, Martin X, Mestas JL, et al: Extracorporeal lithotripsy of gallstones. *Lancet* 1987; 2:448.

12. Hood K, Keightley A, Dowling RH, et al: Piezoceramic lithotripsy of gallbladder stones: Initial experience in 38 pateints. *Lancet* 1988; 1:1322–1324.

13. Peine CJ, Petersen BT, Williams HJ, et al: Fragmentation and dissolution of calcified cholesterol gallstones (CGS) using extracorporeal shock wave lithotripsy (ESWL) and methyl tert-butyl ether (MTBE) in humans. *Hepatology* 1987; 7:1113.

14. Paumgartner G, Sauerbruch T: Heutiger Stand

von Litholyse und Lithotripsie von Gallensteinen. *Chirurg* 1988; 59:190–196.

15. Sauerbruch T, Holl J, Sackmann M, et al: Treatment of bile duct stones by extracorporeal shock waves. *Semin Ultrasound, CT, MR* 1987; 8:155–161.

16. Sauerbruch T, Stern M, and the Study Group for Shock Wave Lithotripsy of Bile Duct Stones: Fragmentation of bile duct stones by extracorporeal shock waves: A new approach to biliary calculi after failure of routine endoscopic measures. *Gastroenterology* 1988 (in press).

17. Gelfand DW, McCullough DL, Myers RT, et al: Choledocholithiasis: Successful treatment with extracorporeal lithotripsy. *AJR* 1987; 148:1114–1116.

18. Liguory CL, Lefebvre JF, Beaugerie L, et al: Lithotritie biliaire extra-corporelle: Resultats preliminaires a propos de 5 cas. *Gastroenterol Clin Biol* 1987; 11:209.

19. Meyer WW, Hottenrott Ch: Lithotripsie intrahepatischer Gallensteine. *Dtsch Med Wschr* 1987; 111:1280–1282.

Technical Considerations in Performance of Extracorporeal Shock Wave Lithotripsy (ESWL) of Gallstones

T. Sauerbruch, M. Sackmann, J. Holl, and G. Paumgartner

KEY CONCEPTS

1. Most gallstones can be disintegrated by extracorporeally induced shock waves.
2. The particle size achieved may vary considerably, dependent on the number of stones, stone size, stone matrix, total shock wave dosage, the characteristics of the shock wave generator, structures in the shock wave path, and the medium surrounding the stone.
3. Disintegration of stones is only of therapeutic interest if the fragments can be successfully cleared, either spontaneously, by dissolution, or in certain cases by extraction.
4. The aim of shock wave lithotripsy of gallstones is the effective, safe, and quick disappearance of gallstones from the biliary tract with low morbidity. In order to achieve this, the careful selection of patients with regard to symptoms, stone characteristics, and gallbladder function is of prime importance.

PRINCIPLE OF EXTRACORPOREAL SHOCK WAVE LITHOTRIPSY OF GALLSTONES

Shock waves are high-pressure waves. They are generated outside the body in a water bath or a water cushion, and owing to the approximately equal acoustic impedance of tissue and water, they are transmitted almost reflection-free into the body. Since the acoustic impedance of stones differs from that in the tissue, the energy is reflected when the waves meet the stone, creating a compressive wave that propagates into the calculus. Also a tensile wave is created after reflection from the back surface of the stone. In addition, cavitation around the stone may cause erosion and damage of the surface. These combined forces will result in disintegration of most human calculi.[1–4]

DIFFERENT SHOCK WAVE MACHINES

Extracorporeal shock wave lithotripsy machines may vary in the energy source (spark gap, peizoelectric array, or electromagnetic membrane movement), the focusing system (ellipsoidal reflector, shaped array, or lens) and location system (x-ray, ultrasound). At present, no clinical trials have been published that would allow a direct comparison of these different systems and machines.

SHOCK WAVE GENERATORS

Unfortunately, we have little knowledge of

the threshold of the peak positive pressure, the peak negative pressure, or the time pressure profile of the shock waves and the focal dimensions necessary to disintegrate gallstones. A small, in vitro study showed that, using the old kidney machines, spark-gap systems were more potent than electromagnetic generators.[5] At present, no in vivo data are available comparing the efficacy and the extent of tissue damage using the various systems, information that could be of considerable clinical significance.

All present machines employ focused shock waves and create a limited area of high pressure in which the stone must be positioned. In the surrounding tissue, the pressure is relatively low, and therefore tissue damage can be kept to a minimum. The focusing systems (ellipsoidal reflectors, lenses, or shaped arrays) mainly determine the focal dimensions. The older kidney machines (Dornier HM 3, Siemens Lithostar, Technomed Sonolith) have a relatively large focal region with a length of several centimeters and width of 1 to 3 cm. In comparison, the piezoelectric systems and the more recent spark-gap systems with an altered geometry of the ellipsoid (larger aperture) have smaller focal volumes. A large focal dimension needs less accurate stone location and probably allows treatment of a larger stone burden. However, it exposes a large volume of normal tissue to high pressures and therefore may cause more pain and tissue damage. Small focal dimensions, on the other hand, while allowing treatment with low discomfort and negligible tissue damage, require a more precise location of the stone, which may be inefficient or time consuming in the treatment of a large stone.

According to our own experience, common bile duct stones with a large stone volume require a large focal volume with high energies (e.g., Dornier HM 3 with a capacitance of 80 nF).

COUPLING OF SHOCK WAVES

In the currently available machines, shock waves are generated in water. Acoustic coupling to the patient's body is achieved either by immersion of the patient into a water basin or a water bath or by a compressible water bag that is coupled to the body using ultrasonic gel.

Although a mobile water cushion allows the most variable shock wave entry into the patient's body from different directions, possible interface problems with these membrane systems, especially in patients with atypical anatomy, should be taken into account. On the whole, however, the increased maneuverability gained by using a mobile water cushion may outweigh the advantages of the ideal coupling by direct water contact.

LOCATION SYSTEM

For the treatment of gallbladder stones, ultrasound is required for locating the stone, positioning of the stone into the focal area, and monitoring of the treatment. Ultrasound allows an accurate linking between stone images and the shock wave focus and minimizes positioning errors. For this, the ultrasound system should be mounted along the axis of the shock wave path. Treatment of common bile duct stones usually requires x-ray for adequate positioning and monitoring of fragmentation because bile duct stones often are overshadowed by the duodenum when using ultrasound.[6]

POSITIONING OF THE PATIENT DURING TREATMENT

For the treatment of gallbladder stones, shock wave entry from the ventral side (Fig 1) with the patient in the prone position is probably most convenient.[3, 7] In this position, the fundus of the gallbladder is very close to the body wall, and there is only a small layer of tissue attenuating the shock waves. The shock wave path can be easily monitored by an integrated ultrasound system. This, however, is not the case with common bile duct stones. Based on the anatomy shown by CT sections (Fig 2), a dorsal route of entry of shock waves with the patient in supine postion appears to be optimal for the treatment of bile duct stones. With the patient in this posi-

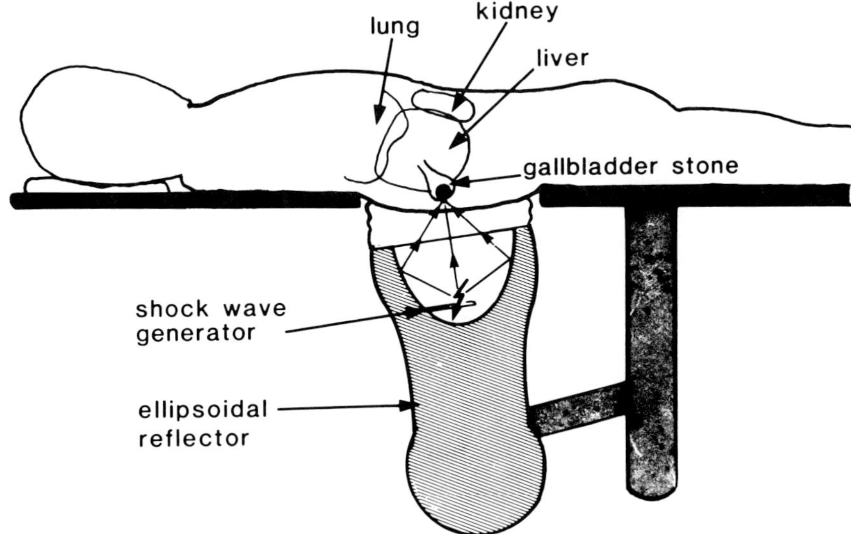

FIG 1.
Treatment of gallbladder stones by extracorporeally induced shock waves using the Dornier system (MPL 9000). Shock waves are generated by high-voltage spark-gap discharge in a water cushion and reflected by an ellipsoidal cavity to an area of high energy (focal point). The stone is located into this point by an ultrasound system mounted in the shock wave axis. The patient is in prone postion.

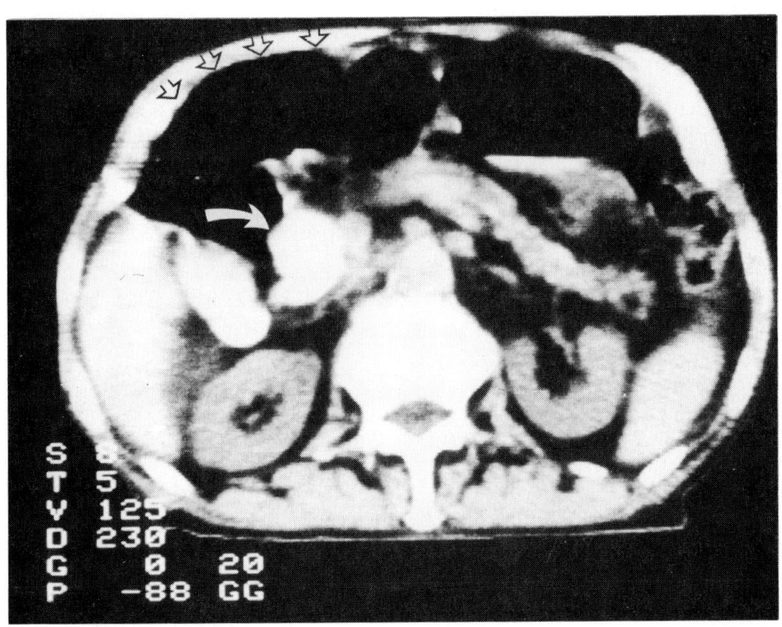

FIG 2.
Computed tomography of a patient with common bile duct stones. It is obvious that the dilated common bile duct *(arrow)* may be shadowed by gas-filled bowel loops *(arrow)* that reflect the shock waves when coming from the ventral side. Contrary to this, when coming from the rear with the patient in supine position (see Fig. 3), shock waves may travel relatively unimpeded through the body to a stone in the common bile duct.

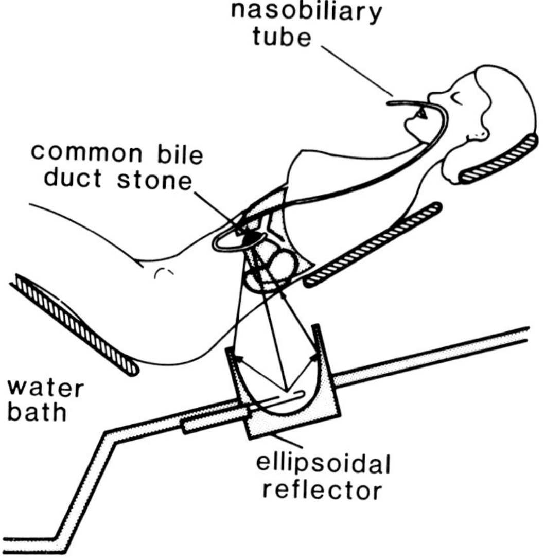

FIG 3.
Treatment of bile duct stones by extracorporeally induced shock waves: The patient is partly immersed in a water bath in supine position using a kidney lithotriptor (HM3, Dornier). Location of the stone into the shock wave focus is achieved by x-ray. The stones are visualized by giving contrast through an endoscopically placed nasobiliary tube. (From Sauerbruch T, Holl J, Sackmann M, et al: Treatment of bile duct stone by extracorporeal shock waves. *Semin Ultrasound, CT, MR* 1987; 8:155. Used by permission.)

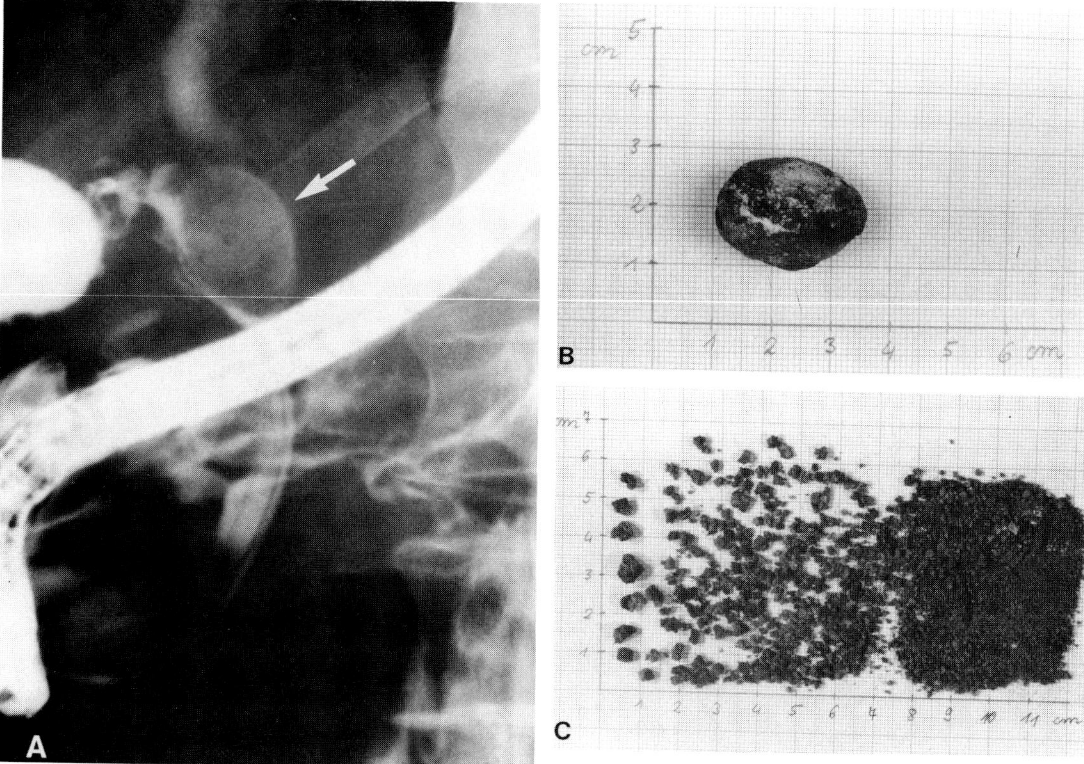

FIG 4.
Retrograde cholangiogram of a patient with an impacted bile duct stone (*arrow*) at the junction between the cystic duct and common bile duct, **A.** The stone was treated twice by ESWL (total of 2600 shocks: HM 3). After failure of repeated ESWL, the stone was removed surgically, **B,** and immediately placed into a bag filled with physiological saline. **C,** It was then easy to disintegrate the stone using the same lithotripter (1000 shocks) the patient had been treated with. This anecdotal report demonstrates the influence of the surrounding medium on the effect of disintegration. It may be speculated that total impaction of the stone, **A**, without surrounding fluid prevented successful disintegration in vivo.

tion, the shock waves travel relatively unimpeded through the body, whereas shock waves may be reflected by gas-filled bowel loops when coming from the ventral side toward the common bile duct (Figs 2 and 3).

There are situations, however, where changing the patient's position may be useful. For example, floating stones or stones with a very low sedimentation rate may move around in the gallbladder during ESWL. This can be prevented by placing the patient in supine position and applying the shock waves from the ventral side so that the stones move to the dependant gallbladder wall and do not float freely in the gallbladder lumen. On the other hand, bile duct stones may be located by ultrasound and treated with ventral shock wave entry when they are located intrahepatically. Thus, it is desirable to have a machine which allows one to move both the patient and the shock wave generator in different directions.

MEDIUM SURROUNDING THE STONES

It has been shown by Delius and coworkers[8] that the medium surrounding the stone could have an important influence for adequate disintegration. Cavitation may be an important factor for stone destruction. Therefore, the medium surrounding the stones should allow the development of cavitation bubbles. It has yet to be elucidated whether a change in the composition of the bile (e.g., postprandial versus fasting status) is important for improvement of stone disintegration by changing viscosity and generation of cavitation in bile. In addition, the large difference in the acoustic impedance between the stone and the surrounding bile is probably important for gallbladder stone disruption. The situation with gallbladder stones is nearly ideal: the stone rests in a relatively large volume of fluid that has acoustic characteristics close to those of water.

The medium surrounding bile duct stones, however, is less conducive to shock wave transmission. There is less fluid surrounding the stones or the stones may be even impacted, a possible explanation for the less successful fragmentation of many bile duct stones (Fig 4) compared with gallbladder stones. In patients with bile duct stones, therefore, instilling fluid into the biliary tree (e.g., physiological saline) may improve the effectivity of ESWL.

TYPE OF STONES

In vivo, most gallbladder stones are more easily shattered than bile duct stones. One explanation may be the difference in the surrounding medium (see above). A further reason may be a different stone structure. The pure cholesterol crystalline stones (Fig 5) are probably more easily disintegrated than pigment stones (Fig 6), which may be bound together by a glycoprotein matrix. This, however, up to now, is poorly documented by in vitro studies.[9]

Unfortunately, very little is known about the pressure threshold necessary for the disintegration of the different stone types, such as cholesterol stones, black pigment stones, brown pigment stones, or mixed stones. However, considering the numerous variables in stone composition, stone size, and stone volume, systematic examinations, even in vitro, are difficult. From our own in vitro study,[9] using a spark-gap system at 16.5 kV with a focal volume of about 2 ml and 1500 discharges or a fragment size $\leq$ 2 mm as endpoints, we know that stone volume is a more important factor for stone disintegration than cholesterol content or calcification of the stones. After the treatment of solitary stones with a diameter of about 25 to 30 mm (i.e., a volume of about 10 ml) at least one fragment larger than 5 mm always remained. Therefore, it is advisable to treat solitary stones no larger than 25 to 30 mm, if only one session of shock wave lithotripsy is planned.

Although most gallbladder stones, irrespective of their cholesterol content, can be shattered by shock waves,[9] only cholesterol stones are amenable to adjuvant oral litholytic therapy using chenodeoxycholic and ursodeoxycholic acid. These cholesterol stones are best identified by

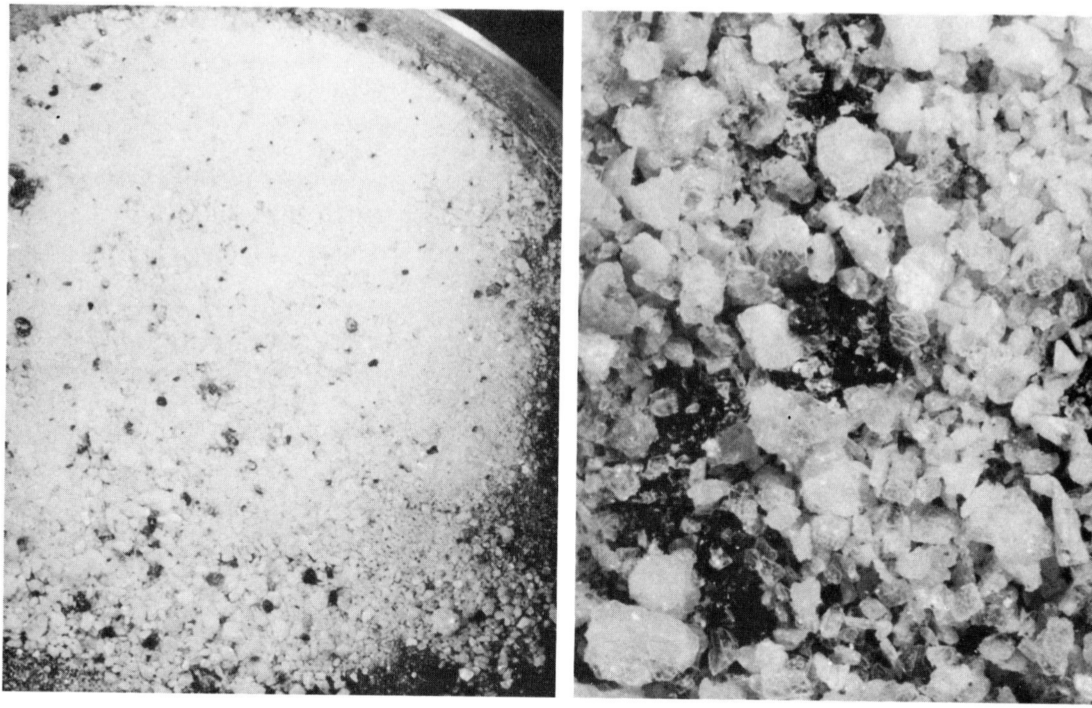

FIG 5.
Left: fragments after in vitro disintegration of a large solitary cholesterol stone (6.5 ml, >95% cholesterol content). Right: magnified view.

their radiolucency in the oral cholecystogram and by a low CT density.[9]

From our own clinical experience, it may be inferred that solitary radiolucent stones can be treated more effectively than multiple stones (Fig 7). This finding has not been corroborated by in vitro studies, possibly for the following reason: in the case of multiple stones, it is more difficult to detect and position all calculi in the shock wave focus one after another in the in vivo situation. There is a further reason to prefer solitary stones for ESL: stone recurrence probably occurs less frequently in patients with multiple stones than in those with solitary stones.[10]

Stones with a calcified rim, often cholesterol stones with a shell that prevents oral litholytic therapy, may be treated successfully with oral bile acids after shock wave lithotripsy.[11] The success rate, however, is considerably lower than in the pure radiolucent stones.

In common bile duct stones, stone composition, location, and size are not of prime importance. Treatment of all stones not amenable to routine endoscopic measures should be attempted, irrespective of their number, size, or location in the biliary tree. However, despite the encouraging overall results, a treatment failure rate of about 20 percent at the first session may occur.[12]

FRAGMENT SIZE

With common bile duct stones, even production of coarse fragmentation may be sufficient to allow extraction after endoscopic sphincterotomy.[3, 6, 12] With gallbladder stones, on the other hand, the best results are probably achieved when the particles are no larger than 2 mm. In this case, most fragments may pass spontane-

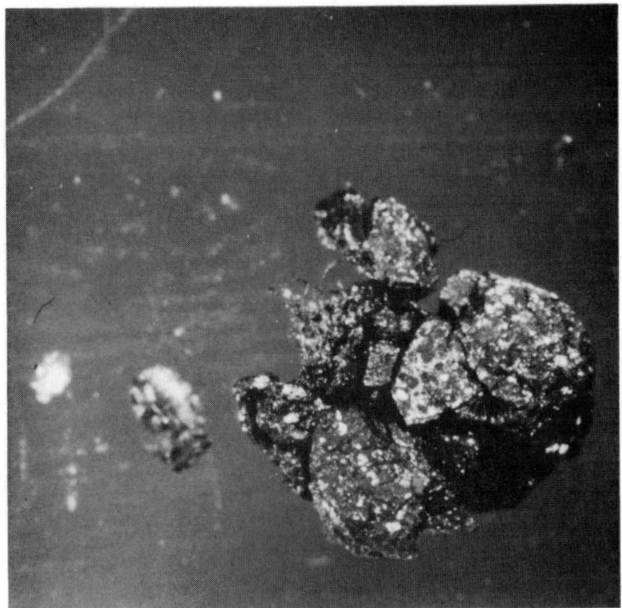

FIG 6.
Only partial in vitro fragmentation of a black pigment stone (0.07 ml, < 10 percent cholesterol, 31 percent calcium bilirubinate) after application of 1500 shocks (Dornier MPL 9000 ellipsoid at 16.5 kV without inline ultrasound).

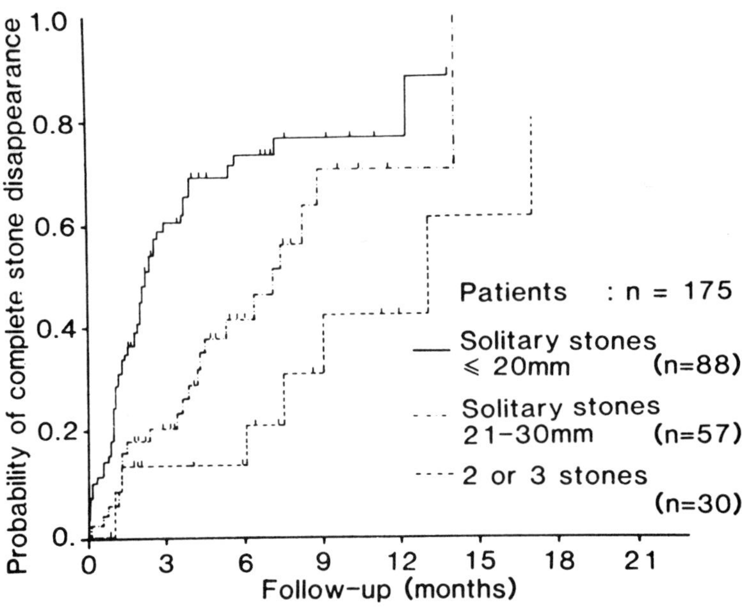

FIG 7.
Probability of complete stone disappearance of large and small solitary gallbladder stones and of multiple gallbladder stones after ESWL and adjuvant medical dissolution therapy. (From Sackmann M, Delius M, Sauerbruch T, et al: Shock wave lithotripsy of gallbladder stones: The first 175 patients. *N Engl J Med* 1988; 318:393. Used by permission.)

ously along the cystic duct and the common bile duct through the papilla of Vater into the duodenum without causing major adverse effects. In addition, adjuvant litholytic therapy may be most effective with this particle size. However, for stones larger than 2 cm, fragmentation to particles not larger than 2 mm is rarely achieved.[9]

It is difficult, if not impossible, to determine the size of very small fragments during ESL. We, therefore, stop treatment when acoustic shadows can no longer be detected in the gallbladder or when the upper limit of shock waves, which may be applied without major tissue damage (about 1600 discharges in the Dornier system), has been reached. Fragments larger than 5 mm that persist longer than 3 months probably warrant retreatment.

ANESTHESIA

Shock wave lithotripsy may induce a dull, heavy pain, the degree of which probably is dependent on the shock wave pressure and focal volume. In addition, some generators may induce arrhythmias when the myocardium during its hyperexcitable phase is in the electromagnetic or pressure field of the shock waves. Shock waves are triggered by the R-wave of the ECG in some machines. Therefore, at least in the older devices, it is the task of the anesthesiologist to handle the patient's pain and potential arrhythmias.

In the early stages of the treatment of gallstones, all patients received shock wave lithotripsy under general anesthesia.[3, 7] This has the advantage of minimal stone movement when high-frequency jet ventilation is used and results in a shorter treatment time. However, the development of new systems with a smaller focal volume and increasing experience of the physicians treating the patients have obviated the necessity for general anesthesia[13] in the treatment of gallstones, and ESL of gallbladder stones is becoming an out-patient procedure. Occasional pain may requre either sedation or analgesia.

Although general anesthesia is no longer applied for patients with gallbladder stones, one be more stone movement and because lower pressures in a smaller focal area are applied.

Bile duct stones may be treated without general anesthesia. However, our own experience showed that a large focal volume with high energy (e.g., Dornier HM 3) is generally necessary for adequate stone disintegration; therefore general anesthesia may be advisable.

ADJUVANT TREATMENT

Disintegration of gallbladder stones may warrant adjuvant treatment for two reasons. First, even after optimal disintegration of stones, fragments may persist in the gallbladder,[14] owing to sedimentation of the particles and owing to incomplete contraction of the gallbladder. It is not clear whether positioning of the patient after treatment, for example, left lateral decubital position during the night, improves clearance of fragments from the biliary system by simple gravitation. Second, in most patients some fragments too large to allow spontaneous passage through the biliary system will persist.[7]

Disintegration of stones results in an enormous increase in the surface-area-to-volume relationship and disruption of noncholesterol stone layers. Both factors should considerably enhance stone dissolution by drugs that decrease the cholesterol saturation of bile. This was shown by our initial in vitro experiments[15] and by our initial clinical experiences.[3] Since it has been shown[16] that stone dissolution occurs more rapidly with a combination of ursodeoxycholic and chenodeoxycholic acid (7 to 8 mg/kg per kilogram each of substance nightly), we start this treatment at least 1 week prior to ESL and continue for 3 months beyond disappearance of fragments as assessed by ultrasound. This prolonged treatment is performed to dissolve even those small fragments that are not detectable by ultrasound.

Direct instillation of solvents (e.g., MTBE) after ESL has also been performed. Fragmentation may, according to in vitro studies, halve the treatment time.[17] It must be realized, however, that with the use of adjuvant procedures involving gallbladder puncture, the advantage of the treatment as a whole may no longer be considered noninvasive.

GALLBLADDER FUNCTION

Since ESWL is combined with adjuvant bile salt therapy and since also some spontaneous passage of fragments is anticipated, a patent cystic duct should be documented in patients undergoing ESWL for gallbladder stones by a positive oral cholecystogram. The degree of gallbladder contraction after an oral stimulus neccessary for succesful ESWL of gallstones is ill-defined. In our own studies, we have seen patients with impaired function of the gallbladder in whom total clearance of fragments can nevertheless be achieved.[18] Further clinical trials must define whether these patients have a high risk of gallstone recurrence.

SHOCK WAVE DOSAGE AND RETREATMENT OF STONES

Little is known about the total dosage of shock waves that may be delivered to the patient at one session or about the schedule for retreatment. Using a spark-gap system, we confine the dosage to 1600 shocks in order to prevent tissue damage. Using these limitations, we experienced no severe tissue damage directly attributable to shock waves and no deterioration of gallbladder function. We advise re-treatment when fragments larger than 5 mm persist after 3 months. Piezoceramic systems probably require a higher initial shock wave dosage and more retreatment sessions.[19]

STONE RECURRENCE

Stone recurrence is likely as with other types of nonsurgical treatment. It is possible that the cumulative rate of stone recurrence could reach 50 percent within 5 years.[20] Clinical follow-up studies are necessary to define patients with a high risk of recurrent gallbladder stone disease. At present, patients receive ultrasound examination every 6 months. When stone recurrence is detected, oral bile acid therapy is started because these calculi are probably very young, newly formed cholesterol stones.

SELECTION OF PATIENTS

Only symptomatic patients with a history of biliary pain should be treated. Prophylactic therapy of gallstones would achieve only a very slight gain in life expectancy. Patients with asymptomatic stones also have little desire for treatment. Therefore, we believe that ESWL should not be performed in these patients despite the low morbidity rate. The ideal patient should have a radiolucent solitary stone no larger than 30 mm in a functioning gallbladder as assessed by a positive cholecystogram. In these patients, the probability of total clearance of the stone and fragments under an adjuvant oral litholytic therapy after 1 year is about 80 percent. The patients should have normal coagulation parameters to prevent larger, shock wave–induced hematoma, and they should have no signs of chronic gallbladder inflammation, bile duct stones, or bile duct occlusion. Contraceptive treatment should, if appropriate, be carried out during the treatment period.

All patients with bile duct stones in whom routine endoscopic measures have failed are eligible for shock wave lithotripsy, provided they have normal coagulation parameters and there are no structures in the shock wave path that are susceptible to shock wave–induced tissue damage.[21] With these restrictions, at present probably no more than 20 percent of all symptomatic gallbladder stone patients and less than 10 percent of patients with common bile duct stones are suitable candidates for shock wave lithotripsy.

SUMMARY

Radiolucent solitary gallbladder stones and bile duct stones not amenable to routine endoscopic measures may be treated succesfully by extracorporeal shock wave lithotripsy.[20] An ideal lithotripter for gallbladder stones should have a generator with a variable shock wave energy output, variable dimensions of the focus, and a variable position. It should have an ultrasound system mounted in the shock wave axis, together with x-ray for the treatment of common bile duct stones. This type of lithotripter may be succesfully used for the treatment of gallstones providing careful patient selection has been carried out.

ACKNOWLEDGEMENT

I am indebted to M. Stern for review of the manuscript and Ms. M. Bäurer for secretarial help.

REFERENCES

1. Chaussy C, Brendel W, Schmiedt E: Extracorporeally induced destruction of kidney stones by shock waves. *Lancet* 1982; 2:1265–1268.
2. Brendel W, Enders G: Shock waves for gallstones: Animal studies. *Lancet* 1983; 1:1054.
3. Sauerbruch T, Delius M, Paumgartner G, et al: Fragmentation of gallstones by extracorporeal shock waves. *N Engl J Med* 1986; 314:818–822.
4. Sauerbruch T, Holl J, Sackmann M, et al: Disintegration of a pancreatic duct stone with extracorporeal shock waves in a patient with chronic pancreatitis. *Endoscopy* 1987; 19:207–208.
5. Petersen BT, Segura JW, Thistle JL: Gallstone lithotripsy: In vitro comparison of four different shock wave generators. *Gastroenterology* 1988; 94:A581.
6. Sauerbruch T, Holl J, Sackmann M, et al: Treatment of bile duct stones by extracorporeal shock waves. *Semin Ultrasound CT, and MR* 1987; 8:155–161.
7. Sackmann M, Delius M, Sauerbruch T, et al: Shock wave lithotripsy of gallbladder stones: The first 175 patients. *N Engl J Med,* 1988; 318:393–397.
8. Delius M, Heine G, Brendel W: A mechanism of gallstone destruction by extracorporeal shock waves. *Gastroenterology* 1988; 94:A93.
9. Schachler R, Sauerbruch T, Wosiewitz U, et al: Fragmentation of human gallstones using extracorporeal shock waves: An in-vitro study. *Hepatoloy*, in press.
10. Hood KA, Gleeson D, Ruppin H, et al: Can gallstone recurrence be prevented? The British/Belgian post-dissolution trial. *Gastoenterology* 1988; 94:A548.
11. Sackmann M, Sauerbruch T, Holl J, et al: Results of ESWL in gallbladder stones with radiopaque rim compared to radiolucent calculi. *J Hepatol* 1988, in press.
12. Sauerbruch T, Stern M, and the Study Group for Shock-Wave Lithotripsy of Bile Duct Stones: Fragmentation of bile duct stones by extracorporeal shock waves: A new approach to biliary calculi after failure of routine endoscopic measures. *Gastroenterology* 1988, in press.
13. Sackmann M, Weber W, Delius M, et al: Extracorporeal shock-wave lithotripsy of gallstones without general anesthesia: First clinical experience. *Ann Intern Med* 1987; 107:347–348.
14. Delius M, Enders G, Brendel W: Passage of stone fragments from the gallbladders of dogs. *Surg Gynecol Obstet* 1988; 166:241–244.
15. Neubrand M, Sauerbruch T, Stellaard F, et al: In vitro cholesterol gallstone dissolution after fragmentation with shock waves. *Digestion* 1986; 34:51–59.
16. Podda M, Zuin M, Fazio C, et al: Comparison of the efficacy and safety of ursodeoxycholic acid in patients with radiolucent gallstones: A randomized controlled trial, in Paumgartner G, Stiehl A, Gerok W (eds): *Bile Acids and the Liver*. Lancaster, MTB Press, 1987, in press.
17. Smith BF, Murray S: Laser fragmentation of human gallstones: Effect on stone dissolution in methyl-tert-butyl ether (MTBE) in vitro. *Gastroenterology* 1988; 94:A592.
18. Spengler U, Sackmann M, Sauerbruch T, et al: Gallbladder motility before and after extracorporeal shock wave lithotripsy (ESWL). *Gastroenterology*, in press.
19. Hood KA, Keightley A, Dowling RH, et al: Piezo-ceramic lithotripsy of gallbladder stones: Initial experience in 38 patients. *Lancet* 1988; I:1322–1324.
20. Lanzini A, Jazrawi RP, Kupfer RM, et al: Gallstone recurrence after medical dissolution: An overestimated threat? *J Hepatol* 1986; 3:241–246.
21. Paumgartner G: Fragmentation of gallstones by extracorporeal shock waves. *Semin Liver Dis* 1987; 4:317–321.

Dissolution of Gallstones Following Extracorporeal Lithotripsy of the Gallbladder: Preliminary Clinical Data

T. Ponchon, X. Martin, J. L. Mestas, E. Krawitt, and R. Lambert

Although there are diverse methods available for the treatment of gallstones (*i.e.*, surgery, solubilizing agents, endoscopic sphincterotomy, transhepatic percutaneous drainage), they all depend, in fact, on the two basic principles of extraction and dissolution. *Extraction* requires an approach via a large biliary route. *Dissolution* involves adaptation of the chemical composition of the calculi and is often slow. Fragmentation of stones by lithotripsy can facilitate both extraction (reduction in the size of the required approach route) and dissolution (acceleration because of smaller size particles). For cholelithiasis, therefore, fragmentation by extracorporeal lithotripsy can be used to accelerate the effects of oral dissolution by bile salts.[1] Our preliminary results of a regimen of gallbladder electrohydraulic lithotripsy followed by oral administration of bile salts are presented.

MATERIAL

The treatment was performed with the Technomed Sonolith 3000 lithotripter. The shock waves were produced by an underwater spark-gap discharge between two electrodes situated at the first focal point of an ellipsoidal reflector (electrohydraulic generator). Waves thus created were reflected from the internal surface of the reflector and converged at the second focus, situated above the generator. A second generation electrohydraulic generator with a larger aperture was also used, in order to reduce the pressure and trauma to tissues situated in the beam of the shock waves. Patients were placed on a flat support mattress, such that only the dependent abdomen or back was in contact with a small water bath containing the ellipsoid reflector. Water served as a coupling agent, ensuring negligible loss of shock wave energy entering the patient's body. The ultrasound probe was attached to a multiarticulated arm. Designed with 6 degrees of freedom, the locating arm provided maximum maneuverability of the ultrasound probe. The spatial coordinates of the stone were calculated by a computer using data related to the location and direction of the probe tip as transmitted via the locating arm and data from measurements of the distance between the probe and the stone using the ultrasound scanner. The spatial coordinates of the stone were calculated several times to ensure minimum deviation. Once a set of coordinates had been validated by the operator, the computer provided displacement of the shock wave generator such that the target point coincided with the stone. During the treatment, fragmentation could be followed by ultrasonography.

PATIENTS AND METHODS

Ninety-one patients (56 women and 35 men, aged 23 to 76 years) with nonradiopaque stones were treated. Informed consent, specifying all aspects of treatment including potential risks, was obtained from all patients. Stone diameter ranged from 7 to 35 mm. Single stones were present in 44 patients and multiple stones in 47 patients (2 stones in 29 patients; 3 stones in 8 patients; and 4 to 10 stones in 10 patients). In cases in which multiple stones were treated, patients were informed that more than one lithotripsy session could be required.

For the first patients, care was taken to avoid problems resulting from fragment migration into the common bile duct and possible pancreatitis. Therefore, the first seven patients underwent endoscopic sphincterotomy at least 10 days prior to lithotripsy. The remaining 84 patients were treated without endoscopic sphincterotomy. All patients presented with symptoms attributed to cholelithiasis and normal gallbladder function as shown by an oral cholecystography.

All patients selected had normal pretreatment evaluation including chest x-ray; EKG; complete blood cell count; bleeding, clotting, partial thromboplastin, and prothrombin times; BUN; serum creatinine, amylase, bilirubin, alkaline phosphatase, and aminotransferases tests. Exclusion criteria were pacemakers, abnormal atrioventricular conduction, pregnancy, liver disease, acute or chronic cholecystitis, cholecholithiasis, bleeding abnormality, and anticoagulant therapy.

Patients received vegetable charcoal, starting 3 days before lithotripsy, to reduce intestinal gas.

Lithotripsy was followed by prolonged oral administration of both chenodeoxycholic and ursodeoxycholic acids, 7.5 mg/kg/day of each. The oral treatment, which was started 10 days before lithotripsy, lasted at least 6 months.

Two sessions of lithotripsy were required in 31 patients and 3 sessions in 5 patients. During treatment, 2 patients were placed in the supine position, 3 in the right lateral position and the others in the prone position. The first generator was used in 20 patients (1200 to 1500 shock waves per session). Pain treatment in those patients required epidural anesthesia (13 patients) or neuroleptanalgesia (7 patients). With the second generator, 71 patients required Phenoperidine 1.5 mg IV for pain treatment, and fragmentation was optimized by systematically applying 2500 shock waves to the gallbladder. Treatment time ranged from 45 to 180 minutes. Pulse, blood pressure, and temperature were recorded every 4 hours for 24 hours following the procedure. Patients were fed 1 hour after treatment.

Evaluation the day after the treatment included plain chest and abdominal x-rays; abdominal ultrasonography; BUN; serum creatinine, amylase, bilirubin, alkaline phosphatase and aminotransferases. Such evaluation was repeated every 3 months. Hospital stay ranged from 2 to 4 days.

RESULTS

Results of fragmentation are reported in Table 1. Since we defined satisfactory lithotripsy re-

TABLE 1.

Results of Fragmentation

	NUMBER OF CASES	FRAGMENTATION	FRAGMENTS <5 MM
1 stone	44	36(82%)	25(57%)
Diameter <20 mm	32	26(81%)	21(66%)
Diameter >20 mm	12	10(83%)	4(33%)
2–10 stones	47	29(62%)	16(34%)
2	29	17	9
3	8	5	3
4–10	10	7	4
Total	91	65(71%)	41(45%)

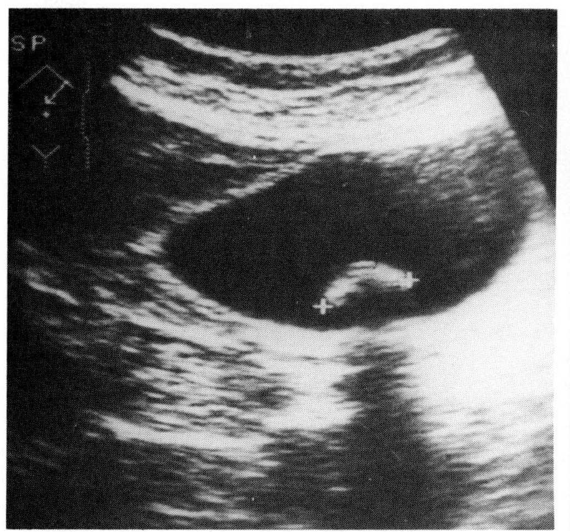

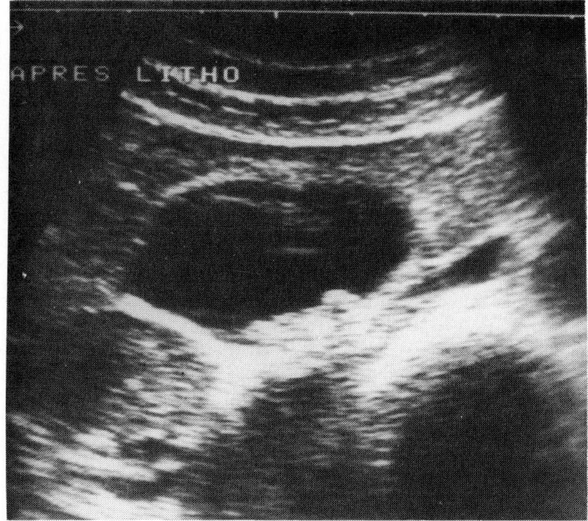

FIG 1.
A single stone (12 mm diameter) **A,** before and **B,** after fragmentation. All fragments are less than 5 mm in diameter.

sults as obtaining fragments less than 5 mm in diameter, lithotripsy was successful in 25 cases (57 percent) for single stones and in 16 cases (34 percent) for multiple stones (see Figs 1 and 2). Two side effects that were observed with the first generator but never with the second were (1) a threefold to fourfold fold increase in serum aminotransferase levels (ultrasound and CT scans in the first five patients did not reveal any hepatic abnormalities) and (2) asymptomatic thickening of the gallbladder wall (5 to 8 mm). Both of these side effects disappeared within a week after lithotripsy.

One patient experienced severe epigastric pain and hyperamylasemia 1 day after the treatment. Diagnosis of edematous pancreatitis was confirmed by CT scan, and the patient responded to medical treatment. Six patients suffered mild right hypochondrial pain the day following treatment. Transient macroscopic hematuria was ob-

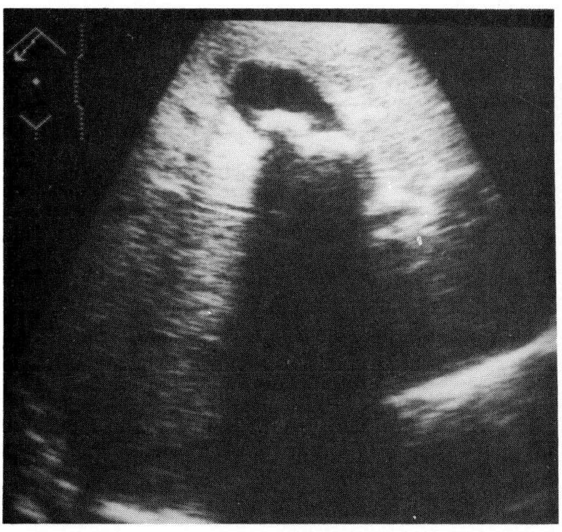

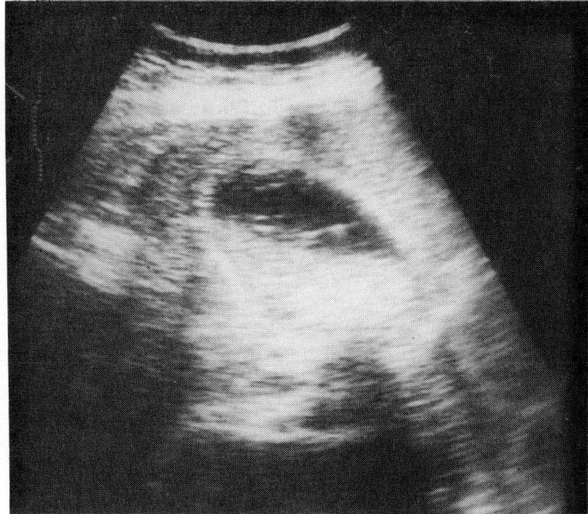

FIG 2.
Two stones (20 and 22 mm diameter) **A,** before and **B,** after fragmentation. Only sand and small fragments are present in the gallbladder after lithotripsy.

served in two patients. Two patients required cholecystectomy 10 days following lithotripsy. They were the most symptomatic patients of the group. One presented with daily biliary colic and the other with biliary colic approximately once per week. Their pain was unchanged, despite successful fragmentation in one and partial fragmentation in the other. Chronic cholecystitis was found at laparotomy.

The results of dissolution in patients who did not have endoscopic sphincterotomy are reported in Table 2. Continued follow-up will be required in these patients.

In the 7 patients who had previously undergone endoscopic sphincterotomy, dissolution was stopped after 1 year because of poor results and advanced age. Only one case had dissolved after 1 year of treatment. Ten patients presented with biliary colic during the dissolution therapy. Two patients presented with cholecystitis that required surgery, and a fragment was found to be impacted in the cystic duct in both cases.

COMMENTS

For electrohydraulic lithotripsy, we chose the prone position in most cases because it allowed the fragments to regroup in the fundus of the gallbladder after each shock wave and it avoided the shock waves hitting ribs, thereby increasing fragmentation success and reducing pain. The ultrasonic probe attached to a multi-articulated arm was found to be very helpful in stone localization because gallbladder position varies from patient to patient and stones can be hidden by ribs or intestinal gas.

Our preliminary experience indicated that gallstone lithotripsy was more difficult to perform and less successful than kidney stone lithotripsy, confirming previous in vitro studies. Improvements in the pressure waveform, as opposed to increased pressure amplitudes, may be required to improve fragmentation results. Furthermore, multiple stones appear to be more difficult to break than single stones. This may be due to the fact that the probability of fragmentation is inversely proportional to the number of stones. Diameter also influences the success of stone fragmentation. Thus, single stones less than 20 mm in diameter appear to be the best indication for lithotripsy. Since energy damping in the transmission path of the shock wave by ribs and/or intestinal gas may reduce the success rate of fragmentation, orientation of the shock wave generator to optimize shock wave transmission should be helpful.

Our experience suggests that highly symptomatic stones are not a good indication for lithotripsy. Certainly, lithotripsy does not appear to be an alternative to emergency gallbladder surgery. The development of a wide-aperture shock wave generator eliminated side effects observed with the earlier generator model. However, complications owing to possible fragment migration (pancreatitis, cholecystitis) still need to be assessed.

The follow-up in our series is too short to determine conclusively the success of this regimen. We have demonstrated only that satisfactory initial fragmentation, that is, obtaining fragments of less than 5 mm, appears to be necessary to observe significant dissolution with long-term treatment with a combination of chenodeoxycholic and ursodeoxycholic acids. In certain cases, certainly surgery provides a better solution.

In our hands, endoscopic sphincterotomy modified the effectiveness of bile salts administered for stone dissolution by slowing the dissolution process. Thus, in cases where an endoscopic sphincterotomy has been performed, removal of fragments may require procedures other than oral dissolution.

TABLE 2.

Results of Dissolution

		STONE-FREE (%)	
MONTHS	NUMBER OF PATIENTS	TOTAL	IF GOOD FRAGMENTATION
3	51	14	24
6	38	32	53
9	16	50	66

REFERENCE

1. Sackmann M, Delius M, Sauerbruch T, et al: Shock wave lithotripsy of gallbladder stones: The first 175 patients. *N Engl J Med* 1988; 318:393–397.

Biliary Lithotripsy at Baylor: The First 30 Cases—Medstone

David Vanderpool, Ronald C. Jones, J. Patrick O'Leary, J. Kent Hamilton, and Herbert S. Steinbach

"Disease is very old, and nothing
about it has changed. It is we who change, as
we recognize what was formerly imperceptible."

CHARCOT

An estimated 15 to 20 million Americans have gallstones.[1] The first cholecystectomy was performed over 100 years ago by Langenbuch.[2] It has become safe and effective, the standard treatment for cholelithiasis. With nearly 500,000 cholecystectomies being performed each year in the United States, it is the operation most frequently performed by general surgeons.[3] Nevertheless, it is a major operation, and in recent years nonoperative alternatives have been sought. The use of orally administered bile acids for the dissolution of gallstones has been disappointing because it is slow, expensive, and usually ineffective.[4] Percutaneous or endoscopic retrograde instillation of solvents in the biliary tract appears to be successful in the treatment of gallstones, but it requires invasive intubation of the biliary tract and has been associated with significant complication rates.[5–7]

Extracorporeal shock wave lithotripsy was first used to break up renal calculi in humans in 1980, at the Klinikum Grosshadern in Munich[8] and was reported by Chaussy in 1982.[9] In 1983, Brendel and Enders[10] reported fragmentation by lithotripsy of human gallstones implanted in the gallbladders of dogs. In 1986, Sauerbruch and colleagues[11] reported successful extracorporeal shock wave therapy for gallstones in nine patients. Although lithotripsy has been used in conjunction with endoscopic manipulation of hepatic and common bile duct stones,[12] the first successful treatment in the United States in a completely noninvasive manner with a combination of extracorporeal shock wave lithotripsy and bile acid therapy under an FDA–approved protocol was at Baylor University Medical Center, Dallas, January 27, 1988, by Doctors David Vanderpool, Ron Jones, Pat O'Leary, and Kent Hamilton.

MATERIALS AND METHODS

The Medstone 1050 is an American-made lithotripter that uses a spark-gap generator with a semi-ellipsoidal reflector capable of delivering pressure amplitudes of approximately 1 kilobar to the F2 focal point at 24,000 V. The point of peak pressure, F2 is the second focus of the shock wave generated by the sparkplug and reflected by the ellipsoid. Medstone uses a flat, dry table without a water bath and has both ultrasound and x-ray localization capability, making it a truly dual-purpose machine for both gallstones and kidney stones. The shock wave generator is located beneath the table, and patients are treated prone for cholelithiasis and supine for nephrolithiasis. The gallstones are localized, and the device is focused on three axes by means of computer-assisted ultrasound.

This machine is installed in a dedicated lithotripsy room in the operating suite at Baylor University Medical Center, Dallas. At Baylor, prior to the use of this treatment in humans, we successfully disrupted gallstones in vitro and implanted human gallstones in animals.

In January 1988, the United States Food and Drug Administration approved an Investigational Device Exemption protocol for the treatment of gallbladder stones in humans using the Medstone 1050 unit which was approved by the Baylor IRB.

The protocol has undergone minor modifications, and at this time, patients must have a history of biliary pain and a functioning gallbladder, demonstrated by oral cholecystography. The gallstones may not be calcified and should range in size from 4 to 20 mm. Patients must not have common duct obstruction, significant liver disease, or pancreatitis; suffer from acute cholecystitis; be older than 75 years of age; have a cardiac pacemaker; or be pregnant at the time of treatment. Currently patients are randomized to be given 10 mg/kg/day of ursodeoxycholic acid or a placebo beginning 7 to 14 days prior to the procedure and ursodeoxycholic acid for 90 days after complete clearance of all demonstrable stone fragments. No more than 2000 shocks may be administered in any one treatment, but one additional treatment may be given if there are residual fragments larger than 4 mm.

CASE REPORT.—A 37-year-old school teacher who had a history of biliary colic was demonstrated to have a 1.4-cm solitary stone in her gallbladder by abdominal ultrasound. She had normal liver chemistries, and her gallbladder functioned on oral cholecystogram. CT scan of the abdomen showed the blast path to be clear of gas. On January 27, 1988, she underwent 1637 shocks at 24 kV by the Medstone 1050, with complete disruption of the stone to sandlike particles. The gallbladder was observed with ultrasound continuously during the procedure. The localization of the gallstone was verified after each 400 shocks, and the treatment required approximately 90 minutes.

She had a small cutaneous hematoma, but did not experience pain following the procedure and did not require analgesics. A sonogram performed 36 hours following the procedure demonstrated that all stone fragments had been eliminated from the gallbladder. Laboratory values including CBC, liver function tests, serum amylase, and urinalysis were normal the next day. At 1, 2, and 3 months after the lithotripsy treatment, both oral cholecystography and ultrasonography of the gallbladder were completely normal. Administration of ursodeoxycholic acid was continued for 90 days.

An additional 29 cases have been performed through April 6, 1988. The patients' ages ranged from 26 to 62 years, with a mean age of 43. Their weights ranged from 47 to 99 kg (103 to 218 lb), with a mean weight of 72 kg (159 lb). Twenty-five of the patients were women. Ten patients had solitary stones, and 20 had two or more. Sixteen of the patients had stones 10 mm or less, while 14 had larger stones. Twenty-nine of the 30 patients had their stones broken, for a fragmentation rate of 96.6 percent. No deaths occurred and no significant complications were encountered from the lithotripsy treatments.

There were no significant changes in hemoglobin, white blood cell count, bilirubin, SGOT, SGPT, alkaline phosphatase, serum amylase, or BUN following administration of ursodiol or lithotripsy. In the immediate post-treatment period, one patient had guaiac positive stools and two patients had hematuria. None reported any pain, had a drop in hematocrit, or required treatment.

Approximately 30 percent of the patients experienced RUQ pain which we ascribe to the passage of stone particles, usually a week or more following lithotripsy, and required mild oral analgesics. The serum amylase was found to be elevated in 3 patients, but not in the immediate post-lithotripsy period. Two patients were re-admitted to the hospital for biliary pain. One of these patients was felt to have acute cholecystitis and had a twofold amylase elevation. She had experienced a similar episode 1 year prior to treatment. She resolved with IV fluids and antibiotics and now is symptom-free and has reduced her stone volume by 80 percent. No patient required surgery or ERCP because of complications of the lithotripsy treatment or from passage of stone particles.

One patient was found to have a carcinoma of the kidney on a routine post-treatment CT scan. He underwent a nephrectomy 1 week after lithotripsy. The gallbladder was removed incidentally at this procedure and showed minimal changes from the treatment.

DISCUSSION

Following the advent of extracorporeal shock wave lithotripsy for the treatment of kidney stones, it became apparent that other concretions within the body could be fractured by the application of such highly focused shock waves. It was inevitable that this technology would be applied to the biliary tract.

In the treatment group first reported by Sauerbruch and associates[11] from Europe, no deaths occurred, although a third of the patients had biliary colic and two developed pancreatitis after treatment. Sauerbruch and co-workers administered a combination of chenodeoxycholic and ursodeoxycholic acid prior to lithotripsy, and continued it until no further evidence of stone was detected. In this small series, two-thirds of the patients were free of stones within 25 weeks of lithotripsy. Their inclusion criteria for this study included patients with abdominal pain attributable to gallstones, a functioning gallbladder, and no more than three radiolucent stones with a maximum diameter of 25 mm. Subsequently they[13] have reported 175 patients who have been followed up to 2 years. The fractured gallstones were cleared in all but one patient at the time of the 2-year follow-up. At 18 months, 91 percent of the patients had become stone-free. In this study, solitary stones less than 2 cm were more likely to disrupt completely than larger solitary stones or multiple stones. Complete absence of stone fragments was obtained earlier in patients with solitary stones smaller than 20 mm than in those with larger solitary stones. The slowest to clear the debris were patients in whom multiple stones were present at the time of treatment. One patient required cholecystectomy because of failure of the stone to fracture.

A number of considerations obtain in the biliary tract that increase the complexity of such treatment. Most gallstones contain cholesterol and occur as a result of a failure of the bile to keep cholesterol dissolved in a micelar solution owing to an imbalance in the concentrations of cholesterol, bile acids, and phospholipids in the bile, as well as to factors that contribute to nucleation, gallstone growth, and impairment of gallbladder contraction.[14,15] The administration of ursodeoxycholic acid, the 7-beta epimer of chenodeoxycholic acid, facilitates cholesterol stone resorption by desaturating the bile and produces a choleretic effect,[15] which may help to flush out small stone particles.[16] Although there is a low incidence of new stone formation after cholecystectomy, shock wave therapy alone would not be expected to change the lithogenic properties of bile or reduce the risk of future stones. It is therefore reasonable to suppose that gallstones will recur after lithotripsy unless the lithogenic state of the bile can be altered. In a follow-up of 42 lithotripsy patients for up to 24 months, recurrent stone formation occurred in 1 patient at 4 months.[13] Pimstone and Mok[17] have suggested that if the saturation of the bile can be changed by long-term or intermittent bile acid therapy, or if there is a subset of patients who may be able to modify their lifestyles, it might be possible to reduce the likelihood of further gallstone formation.[17] Recurrent stones can be retreated with bile acid therapy.[13]

The lithotripter requires a dedicated room, but the Medstone 1050 unit can be used for shock wave therapy of both kidney stones and gallstones. Lithotripsy is a complex procedure requiring careful patient selection; expensive, technologically advanced equipment; and an experienced team. Cholecystectomy is an extremely efficient operation. It is safe, in most instances curative, and associated with a short hospital stay. Despite the efficacy of this procedure, shock wave therapy holds considerable appeal for many patients as it is not associated with an incision, allows the patient to return to work the following day, and is not associated with the abdominal pain that surgery produces. The recurrence rate after lithotripsy is not known.

CONCLUSION

We report 30 patients with gallbladder stones treated in the United States under an FDA-approved protocol using shock wave lithotripsy and bile acid therapy. Lithotripsy is a safe and effective technique for fragmenting gallstones. Fragments of stones are left and must be either expelled from the biliary tree or dissolved by desaturating the bile. Success of lithotripsy must be judged by the rapidity and reliability of clearance of all stone fragments from the biliary tree.

Although lithotripsy for kidney stones has established itself as an effective and safe technique, biliary lithotripsy is in its early stages of development. This emerging modality may be expected to play an important role in the future treatment of calculi in the gallbladder and biliary tree.

REFERENCES

1. Inglefinger FJ: Digestive disease as a rational problem: V. Gallstone. *Gastroenterology* 1968; 55:102–104.7.
2. Langenbuch C: Ein Fall von Exstirpation der Gallenblase wegen chronischer Cholelithiasis: Heilung. *Berl Klin Wochenschr* 1882; 19:725–727.
3. Van Landingham SB: Cholecystectomy in cirrhotic patients. *South Med J* 1984; 77:38–45.
4. Schoenfield LJ, Lachin JM, The Steering Committee and The National Cooperative Gallstone Study Group: Chenodiol (chenodeoxycholic acid) for dissolution of gallstones. The National Cooperative Gallstone Study: a Controlled trial of efficacy and safety. *Ann Intern Med* 1981; 95:257–282.
5. Thistle JL, Carlson GL, Hoffman AF, et al: Monoocatanoin, a dissolution agent for retained cholesterol bile duct stones: Physical properties and clinical application. *Gastroenterology* 1980; 78:1016–1022.
6. Allen MJ, Borody TJ, Bugliosi TF, et al: Rapid dissolution of gallstones by methyl tertbutyl ether: Preliminary observations. *N Engl J Med* 1985; 312:217–220.
7. Fromm H: Gallstone dissolution therapy. Current status and future prospects. *Gastroenterology* 1986; 91:1560–1567.
8. Extracorporeal shockwave lithotripsy. Dornier Medizentechnik GmbH. Germering FRG. 1987.
9. Chaussy C, Schmiedt E, Jocham D, et al: First clinical experience with extracorporeally induced destruction of kidney stones by shock waves. *J Urol* 1982; 127:417–420.
10. Brendel W, Enders G: Shock waves for gallstones: Animal studies. *Lancet* 1983; 1:1054.
11. Sauerbruch T, Delius M, Paumgartner G, et al: Fragmentation of gallstones by extracorporeal shock waves. *N Engl J Med* 1986; 314:818–822.
12. Brown BP, Loenig SA, Johlin FC, et al: Fragmentation of biliary tract stones by lithotripsy using local anesthesia. *Arch Surg* 1988; 123:91–93.
13. Sackmann M, Delius M, Sauerbruch T, et al: Shock-wave lithotripsy of gallbladder stones: The first 175 patients. *N Engl J Med* 1988; 318:393–397.
14. Small DM: Gallstones. *N Engl J Med* 1968; 279:588–593.
15. Bennon LJ, Grundy SM: Risk factors for the development of cholelithiasis in man (Parts I & II). *N Engl J Med* 1978; 299:1161–1167, 1221–1227.
16. Okolicsanyi L, Liruss F, Strazzabosco M, et al: The effect of drugs on bile flow and composition. An overview *Drugs* 1986; 31:430–448.
17. Pimstone NR, Mok HYI: Current status of medical treatment of gallstones. *Surg Clin North Am* 1981; 61:865–874.

Fragmentation of Bile Duct and Gallbladder Calculi by Extracorporeal Shockwaves: Initial Experience

Christoph D. Becker and H. Joachim Burhenne

Gallstone disintegration by means of shock waves generated by intracorporeal spark discharge was reported in 1975[1] and subsequently employed by some investigators using varying direct approaches.[2,3] However, biliary shock wave lithotripsy did not become a practicable method for widespread use until the advent of the extracorporeal lithotripter. The first successful clinical results with extracorporeal biliary shock wave lithotripsy have been reported by Sauerbruch and colleagues[4] in 1986. More recently, a second generation of extracorporeal lithotripters has become available that no longer require immersion of the patient in a water bath. Shock wave generators based on modified electrohydraulic,[5,6] piezoelectric,[7–9] or electromagnetic principles[10,11] require either no anesthesia at all or intravenous analgesia only. However, only preliminary results are yet available with most of these newer units,[5–10] and many questions regarding their efficacy and safety still need to be answered. At the University of British Columbia, we began to treat selected patients with bile duct calculi with an unmodified first-generation lithotripter in 1987.[12] Since December 1987, we have used a tubless second-generation lithotripter to fragment both bile duct and gallbladder calculi. Here, we discuss clinical and technical aspects of extracorporeal biliary lithotripsy based on preliminary data of 100 patients referred to the Radiology Department for this new form of treatment.

EQUIPMENT AND TECHNICAL CONSIDERATIONS

With the unmodified first-generation electrohydraulic lithotripter (HM3, Dornier, Munich, West Germany), bile duct stones were disintegrated with the patient in a supine or semioblique position and immersed in a water bath, quite similar to the treatment of urinary calculi with this unit; biplane fluoroscopy was used for targeting.[13]

The second-generation extracorporeal lithotripter employed an electromagnetic principle[11] for shock wave generation, and did not require immersion of the patient in a water bath. Coupling of the shock waves with the patient was achieved by means of a water cushion. The device, also designed originally for renal lithotripsy (Lithostar, Siemens, Erlangen, West Germany), consisted of an x-ray table with two overhead x-ray tubes and two high-resolution digital image intensifiers. Two shock wave generators (right and left) were integrated in the table, and their foci aligned with the intersecting geometry of the biplanar fluoroscopy. A motor drive permitted table-top movements in two horizontal and all the vertical axes for positioning of the target in the focus of the shock waves. The focal length of the shock wave generators was 11.5 cm, which was originally optimized for kidney stones. Most proximal bile duct stones, intrahepatic stones, and cystic duct and gallbladder stones were situated too far anteriorally to be treated in the supine position. Virtually all patients were, therefore, treated in a prone or semi-oblique position. Bile duct calculi were targeted by means of direct cholangiography; radiographic targeting of radiolucent gallbladder calculi was achieved by means of oral cholecystography. Imaging was performed with a 1024 image matrix combined with a digital image processor, and it was also possible to obtain conventional bucky radiographs. Because targeting of gallbladder calculi is preferably performed by means of ultrasound rather than by fluoroscopy, an additional overhead shock wave module has recently been added as a modification to the second-generation device that allows ultrasound-guided treatment of gallbladder calculi. Ideally, equipment for biliary lithotripsy should include availability of both ultrasound and x-ray targeting to provide optimal versatility for treatment of gallbladder and bile duct calculi.

INDICATIONS FOR EXTRACORPOREAL LITHOTRIPSY AND PRELIMINARY RESULTS

BILE DUCT CALCULI

Extracorporeal lithotripsy was used in 28 patients as an adjunct to other nonoperative techniques to remove gallstones that were unusually large or impacted in an inaccessible portion of the biliary tract, so that fragmentation with subsequent fragment removal was not feasible by established means of nonoperative intervention (Fig 1).[14] The most common indications included failed endoscopic stone removal after retrograde sphincterotomy (n = 11), unsuccessful removal of retained biliary calculi via the T-tube tract after cholecystectomy (n = 7), or retained calculi in the cystic duct or gallbladder neck after cholecystostomy (n = 7). Because all bile duct calculi were radiolucent, opacification of the bile ducts by means of direct cholangiography was required. Depending on the interventional procedures preceding lithotripsy, the bile ducts were opacified by varying approaches, that is, through an endoscopically inserted nasobiliary catheter, via a surgical T-tube tract, or through a cholecystostomy catheter.[12] A transhepatic catheter was used for bile duct opacification in three cases in which endoscopic sphincterotomy and bile duct catheterization had failed. Repeat injections of contrast material through these catheters allowed visualization of the radiolucent bile duct calculi for positioning in the focus of the shock wave generator.

With the first-generation unit, all nine patients were treated with epidural anesthesia. An average of approximately 2300 shockwaves were administered. Minor side effects were noted in four patients, including transient fever, mild hemobilia, or hematuria.[12] Lithotripsy of bile duct calculi with the second-generation unit was done on 19 patients, and required more than twice as many shock waves than did the first-generation unit. On the other hand, administration of the second-generation shock waves to these usually frail, elderly, and hospitalized patients required either no pain control at all or intravenous neuroleptanalgesia (fentanyl/diazepam) only; general or epidural anesthesia were not necessary. Except for mild or moderate petechiae or slight superficial bleeding or occasional cutaneous hematomas at the shock wave entry site, no other relevant side effects were noted. Better radiographic imaging was considered an advantage of

FIG 1.
Nonsurgical removal of two retained calculi impacted in a cystic duct remnant after surgery. **A,** Opacification of the bile ducts via the T-tube tract demonstrates two calculi in a low-inserting cystic duct remnant. These calculi were impacted and, owing to their size and location, removal through the T-tube tract was not feasible in this case. **B,** Both calculi have been fragmented by extracorporeal shockwave lithotripsy. **C,** The fragments were consecutively moved distally, engaged in a wire basket, and extracted percutaneously. **D,** Completion cholangiogram prior to catheter removal demonstrates complete clearance of fragments. (Fig 1A, B, and D reproduced, with permission, from Becker CD, Fache JS, Gibney RG, et al: Treatment of retained cystic duct stones using extracorporeal shockwave lithotripsy. *AJR* 1987; 1121–1122. Used by permission.)

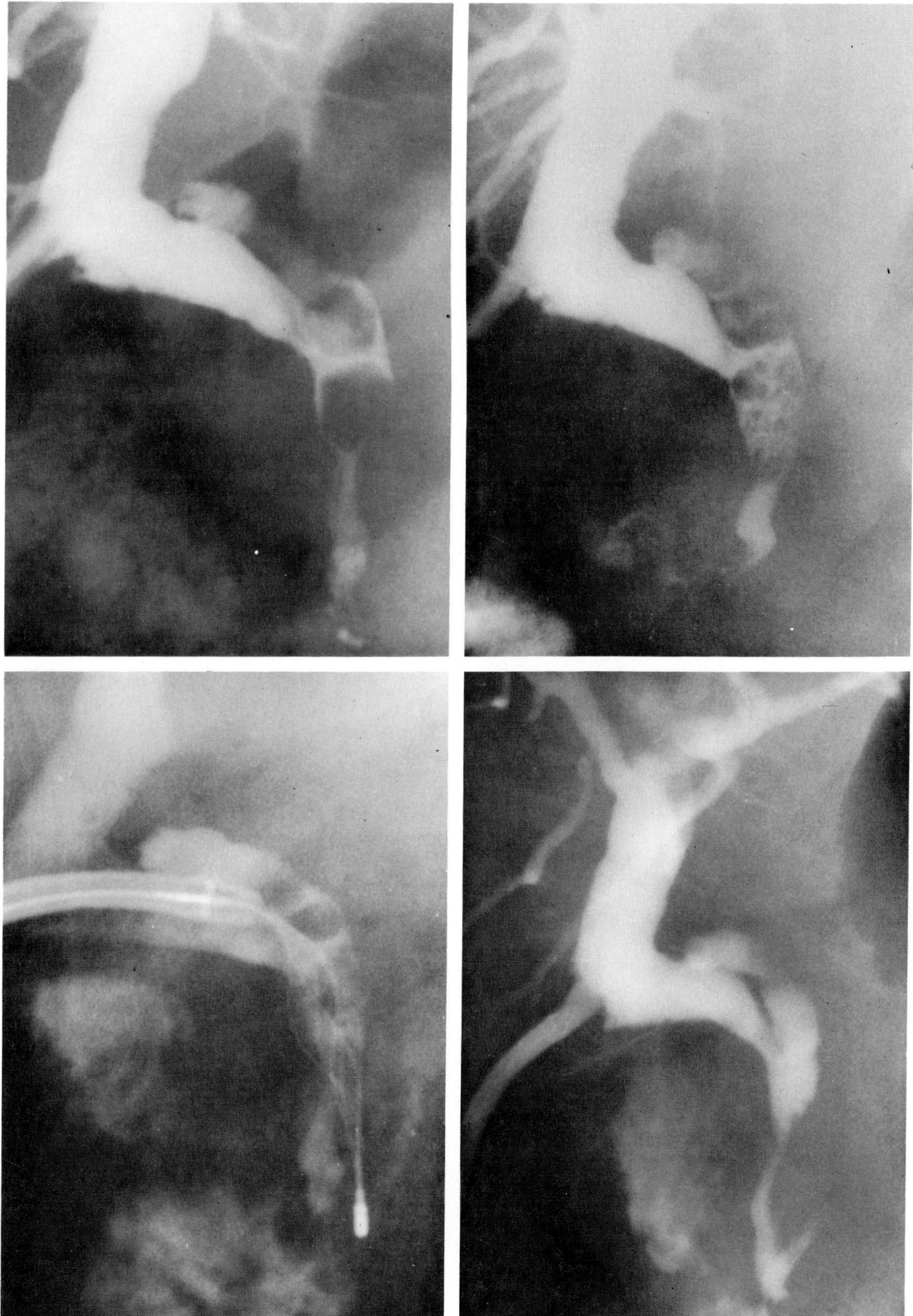

the second-generation device. On the other hand, treatment on the table in the prone position was cumbersome for elderly and debilitated patients who were unable to cooperate or had respiratory difficulties.

Because most patients had large and/or multiple calculi, more than half of them required more than one treatment session. In the beginning, we insisted on complete stone fragmentation. Later, we discontinued the treatment when coarse fragmentation had been achieved to such a degree that fragment extraction by other interventional procedures such as endoscopic retrograde or percutaneous stone extraction became feasible. Fragmentation and/or disimpaction of bile duct calculi by extracorporeal shock wave lithotripsy was achieved in 20 of 28 patients (71 percent). In six cases, the fragments passed spontaneously into the duodenum via a spincterotomy; the other patients required additional interventional radiologic or endoscopic procedures after successful ESL for fragment extraction. If stone fragmentation was not achieved after approximately 2 to 3 sessions, treatment was discontinued. Failures occurred with both the first-generation and the second-generation unit, and were considered to be due to unusually large size or impaction of calculi.[12]

GALLBLADDER CALCULI

Patients with symptomatic cholecystolithiasis who were referred for lithotripsy by their primary physicians were evaluated for eligibility by clinical members of an interdisciplinary "biliary lithotripsy committee," which consists of gastroenterologists, surgeons, radiologists, and pathologists of the University of British Columbia. Preliminary diagnostic workup and post-treatment follow-up was organized by a "biliary lithotripsy clinic" and included clinical, laboratory, sonographic, and radiographic examinations. Selection criteria included, besides full informed consent, normal clotting parameters, normal liver and pancreatic function tests, no more than six calculi on ultrasound, and a gallbladder contracting at least by 20 percent upon a fatty meal on ultrasound. To achieve gallbladder opacification for x-ray targeting by oral cholecystography, 6 grams of iopanoic acid (Telepaque, Winthrop, Aurora, Ontario) and 3 grams of sodium ipodate (Oragrafin, Squibb, Montreal) were given over 2 days prior to lithotripsy. This regimen results in the lowest proportion of gallbladder nonvisualization.[15,16] Seventy-two patients with cholecystolithiasis were referred to the radiology department for lithotripsy. In 62 patients (86 percent), the gallbladder calculi were properly visualized in both fluoroscopic planes. In 10 patients (14 percent), the gallstones could not be sufficiently visualized to allow targeting, either because gallbladder opacification was too faint or because the quality of the fluoroscopic image in the oblique second x-ray plane was unsatisfactory. Two patients were found to have more than six calculi and did therefore not fulfill the protocol requirements. Thus, a total of 60 cholecystolithiasis patients underwent lithotripsy according to the above protocol, including 41 patients with single calculi (mean diameter 17.5 mm, range 0.5 to 3.5 mm) and 19 patients with two to five stones (diameter of the largest stone: 30 mm). Treatment was done on an outpatient basis in all cases. Fifty-six patients (94 percent) were treated either without analgesia or with transcutaneous electric nerve stimulation (TENS) only. Only four patients (6 percent) required intravenous analgesia with fentanyl/diazepam. A typical treatment session consisted of 4000 shock waves and was administered in the prone position. Shock wave administration was discontinued if complete stone disintegration occurred prior to this and the resulting fragments were no longer targetable. Radiographic targeting of calculi or fragments with a diameter of 10 mm or larger was usually straightforward (Fig 2*B*), whereas calculi or fragments in the range of 5 to 9 mm were often more difficult to localize, particularly in the oblique fluoroscopic plane. Small fragments were quite easily obscured by the contrast material in the gallbladder (Fig 2*C*) or by adjacent bowel gas, and also tended to move during shock wave application. In some instances, intravenous injection of 2 to 3 ml cholecystokinin (Kinevac, Squibb) resulted in sufficient gallbladder contraction to facilitate targeting of small calculi or fragments. Although the effect of treatment was often visible on fluoroscopy or post-procedural bucky films (Fig 2), follow-up was done by ultrasound 2 days after each treatment session. During the same visit, follow-up laboratory tests (AST, amylase, alkaline phosphatase) were obtained.

After the initial lithotripsy session, there was evidence of gallstone fragmentation on ultrasound in comparison to the baseline scans in 51 patients (85 percent). We found, however, that determination of the exact size of small asymmetrical fragments on ultrasound was fraught with some technical difficulty. Limitations in lateral resolution, differences in focusing of varying ultrasound systems, and the inability to distinguish between a large size fragment and a conglomeration of multiple small fragments were some of the encountered problems. We are presently evaluating the accuracy of ultrasound to determine fragment size. It is our first impression that overestimation of fragment size is more common than underestimation. Gallstone fragmentation was considered satisfactory if the size of the largest remaining fragment was 4 mm or less. This was achieved in the initial lithotripsy session in 33 percent of patients with single calculi 20 mm or less in diameter, and in 22 percent of the patients of the entire series. Thus, additional treatment sessions were or will be required in 67 percent and 78 percent of patients, respectively.

Because of the necessity of repeat treatment and an average follow-up period of only a few months, conclusions regarding the overall success of treatment cannot yet be drawn. To date, only four patients have been seen at follow-up ultrasound who cleared their gallbladder completely from fragments; two of these as soon as 2 days after lithotripsy (Fig 2). Side effects can, so far, be considered minor. Only three patients developed significant subcutaneous hematomas. Chest x-ray examinations obtained in each patient before and after lithotripsy have not revealed any traumatic pulmonary tissue changes. On follow-up, several patients experienced right-upper-quadrant pain, which was described as being similar to their previous symptoms. Complications attributable to gallstone lithotripsy have, to date, been observed in two patients of this series (3 percent). In one patient, acute cholecystitis owing to cystic duct obstruction was managed conservatively and subsided. The other patient developed moderate acute pancreatitis owing to fragment passage and underwent cholecystectomy with common bile duct revision to prevent further complications from fragment passage.

INITIAL IMPRESSION AND FURTHER CONSIDERATIONS

Extracorporeal lithotripsy of *bile duct calculi* is a useful adjunct in combination with nonoperative, that is, radiologic or endoscopic, stone removal. The absence of complications and successful fragmentation of calculi in over two-thirds of our small series suggests that an attempt of this treatment is warranted in patients who would otherwise have to undergo surgery. Because bile duct calculi are best visualized by direct cholangiography, a lithotripter used for this purpose should include the option of x-ray targeting.

Fluoroscopic targeting of *gallbladder stones* was done only in a preliminary phase, and is expected to become obsolete with the advent of ultrasonic targeting, which will obviate premedication (oral cholecystography) on the day of treatment as well as radiation exposure to the patient for targeting. Ultrasound targeting is also expected to facilitate destruction of small calculi and fragments. Because application of second-generation shock waves did usually not require anesthesia, fragmentation of gallbladder calculi was feasible on an ambulatory basis. This may outweigh the fact that the majority of patients required or will require more than one treatment session to achieve a fragment size of 4 mm or less. Technical improvements and further experience will probably increase the initial fragmentation rate.

It remains to be seen on long-term follow-up how many patients can pass their fragments spontaneously and what overall complication rate will result from fragment passage. Because disintegration of large ($\geq$ 20 mm) and multiple calculi results in a considerable fragment bur-

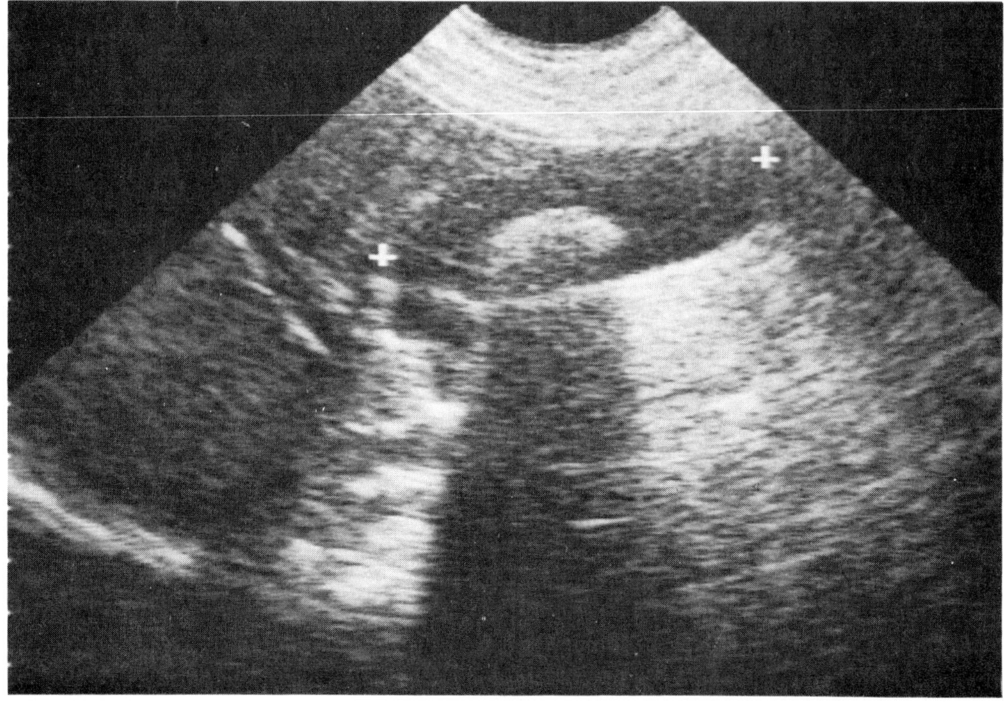

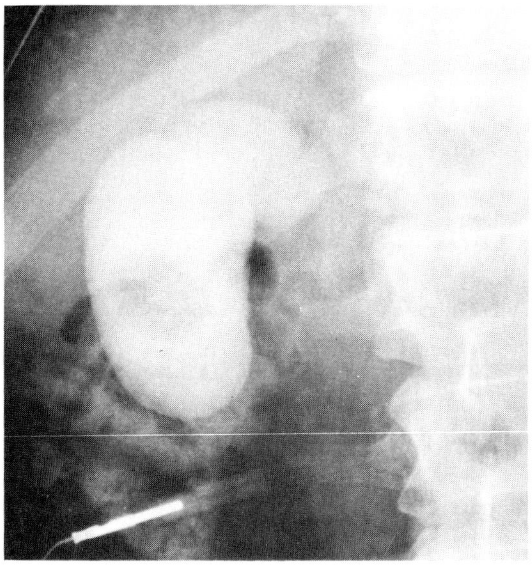

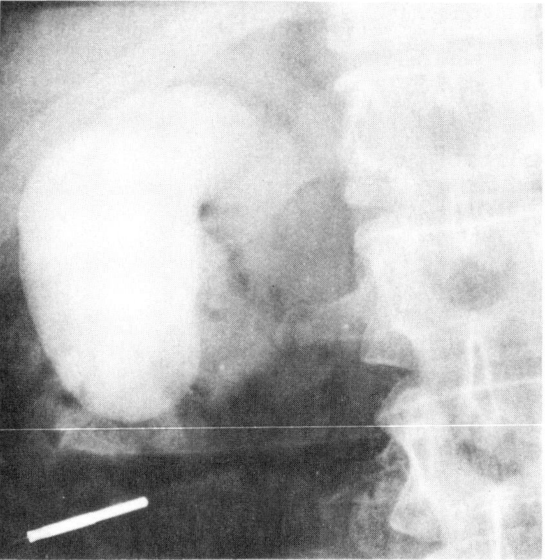

FIG 2.
Shock wave lithotripsy for cholecystolithiasis. **A,** Preliminary ultrasound study and **B,** oral cholecystography demonstrate a single gallbladder calculus measuring 25 × 17 mm. **C,** After 2000 shock waves, the calculus has been disintegrated into multiple small fragments. **D,** Ultrasound follow-up 2 days after lithotripsy demonstrates that there are several residual, irregular fragments larger than 6 mm. Another lithotripsy session was performed. **E,** Two days following repeat lithotripsy, no residual fragments were found. Rapid spontaneous fragment clearance, as seen in this patient, was, however, not the rule.

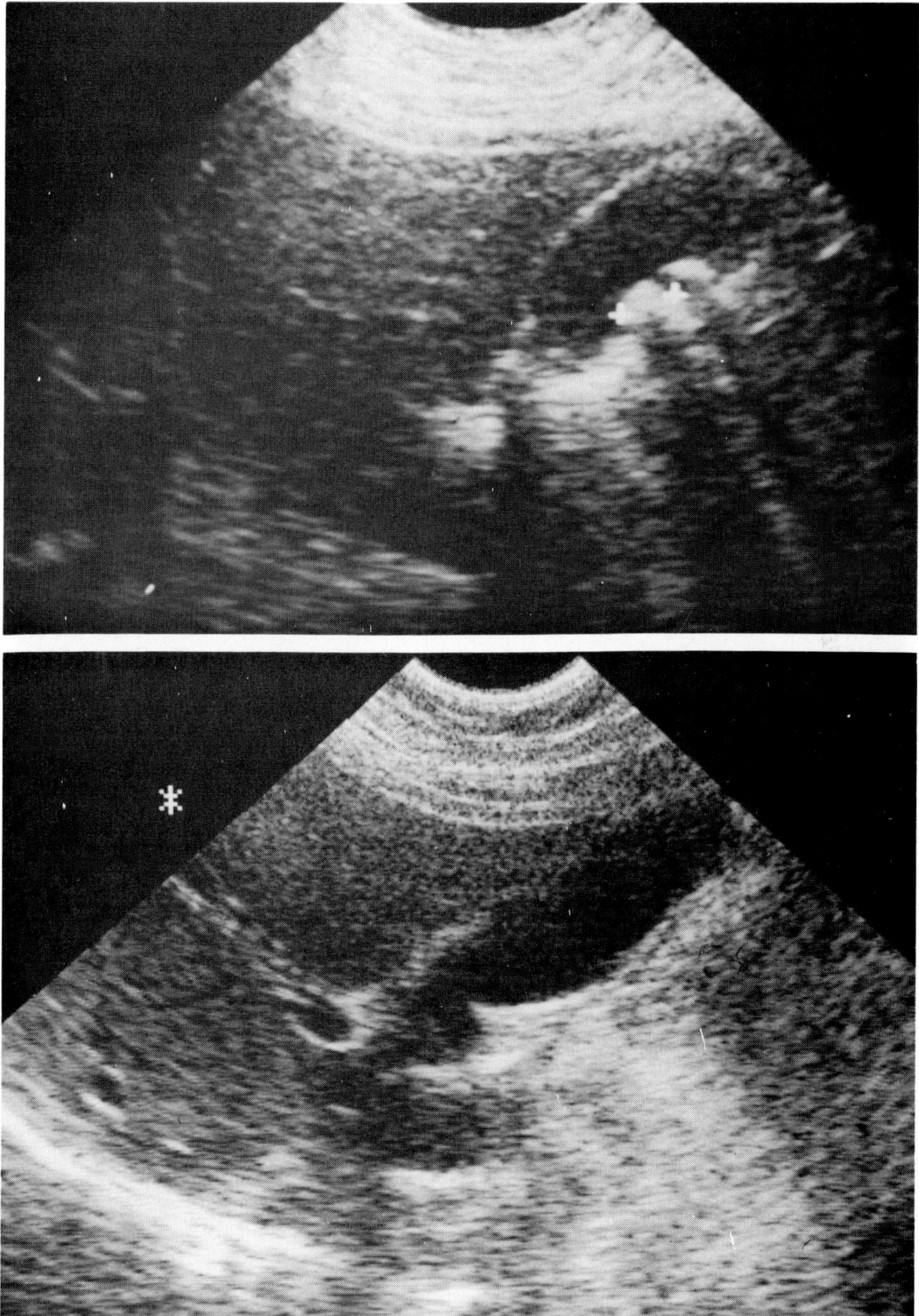

den, rapid clearance of the gallbladder, although seen occasionally, cannot be expected in the majority of these instances. The first long-term results of ESL indicate that, even with adjuvant oral cholecystolitholysis with chenodeoxycholic/ursodeoxycholic acid, 6 to 12 months are often required to render the gallbladder free of residual fragments.[6] During this entire period, potential complications owing to fragment passage cannot be ruled out. The protocol at this institution does, so far, not include adjuvant bile acid therapy to dissolve fragments. Instead, direct contact dissolution by means of methyl-tert-butyl ether (MTBE) is presently considered as an adjuvant to achieve clearance of the gallbladder from stone fragments. This powerful cholesterol dissolving agent[17] might offer the quickest solution of the fragment problem to patients with a large fragment burden. MTBE is instilled directly into the gallbladder via a percutaneous gallbladder catheter. Because fragmentation by ESL greatly increases the surface area and, thus, the solubility of cholesterol calculi, dissolution may become feasible in only a few hours. First reported results of direct contact dissolution of gallstones following biliary lithotripsy, even in patients with partially calcified calculi, have been encouraging,[18] but more experience with this form of treatment is required to determine its role.

REFERENCES

1. Burhenne HJ: Electrohydrolytic fragmentation of retained common duct stones. *Radiology* 1975; 117:721–722.
2. Martin EC, Wolff M, Neff RA, et al: Use of the electrohydraulic lithotriptor in the biliary tree of dogs. *Radiology* 1981; 139:215–217.
3. Lear JL, Ring EA, Macoviak JA, et al: Percutaneous transhepatic electrohydraulic lithotripsy. *Radiology* 1984; 150:589–590.
4. Sauerbruch T, Delius M, Paumgartner G, et al: Fragmentation of gallstones by extracorporeal shock waves. *N Engl J Med* 1986; 314:818–822.
5. Ponchon T, Martin X, Mestas JL, et al: Extracorporeal lithotripsy of gallstones. *Lancet* 1987; 2:448.
6. Sackmann M, Delius M, Sauerbruch T, et al: Shock-wave lithotripsy of gallbladder stones: The first 175 patients. *N Engl J Med* 1988; 318:393–397.
7. Ell C, Kerzel W, Heyder N, et al: Piezoelectric lithotripsy of gallstones (letter). *Lancet* 1987; 2:1149.
8. Ryan PC, Darzi A, Kiely E. Piezoelectric lithotripsy (letter). *Lancet* 1988; 1:296.
9. Hood KA, Keightley A, Dowling RH, et al: Piezo-ceramic lithotripsy of gallbladder stones: Initial experience in 38 patients. *Lancet* 1988; 1:1322–1324.
10. Staritz M, Floth A, Rambow D, et al: Shock-wave lithotripsy of gallstones with second-generation device without conventional water-bath (letter). *Lancet* 1987; 1:155.
11. Reichenberger H, Naser G: Electromagnetic acoustic source for the generation of shock waves in lithotripsy. Siemens Forsch.-u. Entwickl.-Ber. Bd 15 1(1986), Nr.4, Springer Verlag, pp 187–194.
12. Burhenne HJ, Fache JS, Gibney RG, et al: Biliary lithotripsy by shock waves: Integral part of nonsurgical intervention. *AJR* 1988; 150:1279–1283.
13. Chaussy C, Schmiedt E, Jocham D, et al: First clinical experience with extracorporeally induced destruction of kidney stones by shockwaves. *J Urol* 1982; 127:417–420.
14. Becker CD, Fache JS, Gibney RG, et al: Treatment of retained cystic duct stones using extracorporeal shockwave lithotripsy. *AJR* 1987; 148:1121–1122.
15. Burhenne HJ, Obata WA: Single-visit oral cholecystography. *N Engl J Med* 1975; 292:627.
16. Burhenne HJ, Morris DC, Graeb DA: Single visit oral cholecystography for inpatients. *Radiology* 1981; 140:505.
17. Allen MJ, Borody TJ, Bugliosi TF, et al: Rapid dissolution of gallstones by methyl tert-butyl ether: Preliminary observations. *N Engl J Med* 1985; 312:217–220.
18. Peine CJ, Petersen BT, Williams HJ, et al: Fragmentation and dissolution of calcified cholesterol gallstones using ESWL and MTBE in humans. *Hepatology* 1987; 7:1113.

Results of the Gallstone Lithotripsy in 212 Patients Using the EDAP LT.01

J. P. Delmont, M. Magnier, H. Mosnier, J. Moreaus, M. Guivarc'h, S. Sokolowsky, R. Capdeville, and D. Branche

Extracorporeal shock wave lithotripsy (ESL) is an established treatment for renal stones. The recent publication in 1986 of its application in the treatment of biliary stones[1] prompted us to purchase a lithotripter. At that time there were only three machines on the market: two using an electrohydraulic source (Dornier and Technomed) and a third using a piezoelectric device (EDAP) to create shock waves. We chose the piezoelectric system for the following reasons:

1. The urologists were satisfied with its performance in dealing with renal stones.
2. It was cheaper than the other systems.
3. It was easier to install (e.g., it does not require degased water) and less time-consuming in its management.
4. It offers a painless treatment, and the patient does not require any premedication or anesthetic.
5. The manufacturers claim that it produces a finer (powderlike) disintegration than the other systems.

It was evident to us, based on these advantages, that it would be possible to develop a new nonsurgical ambulatory treatment for gallstones. We accept that cholecystectomy is an excellent and definitive treatment for gallstones with a low mortality and morbidity rate. But ESL, despite its limitations relating to the possibility of recurrence of stones could be a competitive alternative treatment to cholecystectomy, especially considering its potential for ambulatory treatment.

This report is the collective experience of four French centers listed in Table 1. Several of these centers had prior experience with its use in animal models[2, 3] and have confirmed the observations of Amouretti and colleagues[4] that, at low frequency, shock waves do not cause tissue damage. Our clinical experience is from January 1, 1987, to May 30, 1988. We feel from this experience that we can confidently predict the capabilities of this second-generation lithotripter.

METHODS

MACHINE

The EDAP LT-01 lithotripter is the same model used in urology. In the centers included in this report, the machine served a dual purpose in treating both renal and gallbladder stones.

Generation of Shock Waves

The piezoelectric system has principles similar to those of sound wave formation in a diagnostic ultrasound system. An applied voltage causes the vibration of small ceramic plates, producing shock waves. These waves are different from ultrasound waves in that they are not

TABLE 1.

Participating Centers

Clinique du Vert-Galant (Tremblay-Les-Gonesse) M. Magnier, D. Branche	77 patients
Clinique Medico-Chirurgicale Foch (Paris) M. Guivarc'h, H. Mosnier	48 patients
Clinique Medico-Chirurgicale Porte de Choisy (Paris) J. Moreaux, R. Capdeville	35 patients
Hôpital Universitaire de Nice J. Delmont, S. Sokolowsky, F.X. Caroli-Bosc	52 patients

continuous and sinusoidal but are isolated and peak, with a rapid rise time (approximately 0.5 microsecond). The maximum pressure recorded in vitro (as it is impossible to measure it in vivo) is about 0.5 kilobar, and is half the amount generated by the elctrohydraulic systems. It is possible to regulate this with the control panel to alter the power setting from 0 to 100 percent and the frequency of the wave from 1.25 to 1.60 per second. The shock waves generated by this system are of shorter duration and more stable, with minimal or no low frequency waves unlike those of the electrohydraulic systems. Furthermore, each semiconductor generator is contained in an individual drawer, which allows easy maintenance (Figs. 1 and 2).

Transmission and Focusing of the Shock Waves

The shock wave is transmitted in water, as its acoustic impedance is close to that of human tissue. To avoid the inconvenience of having the patient totally immersed in water, a water-filled cushion that contains the piezoelectric source is applied to the right upper quadrant of the abdo-

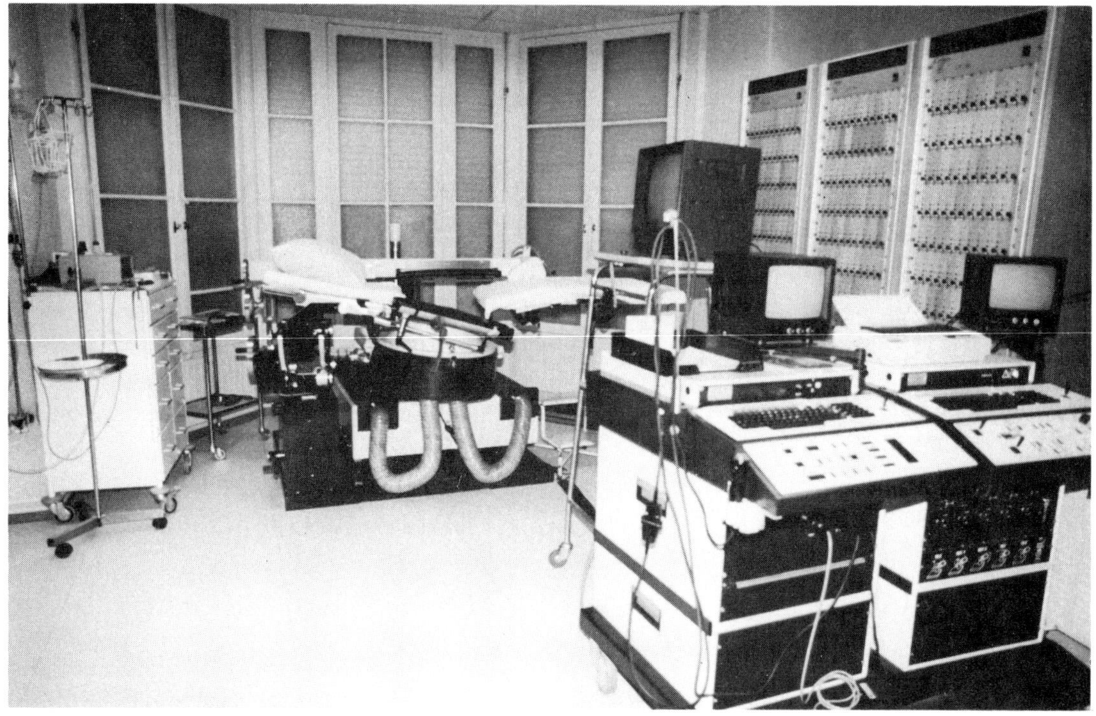

FIG 1.
EDAP LT-01 lithotripter.

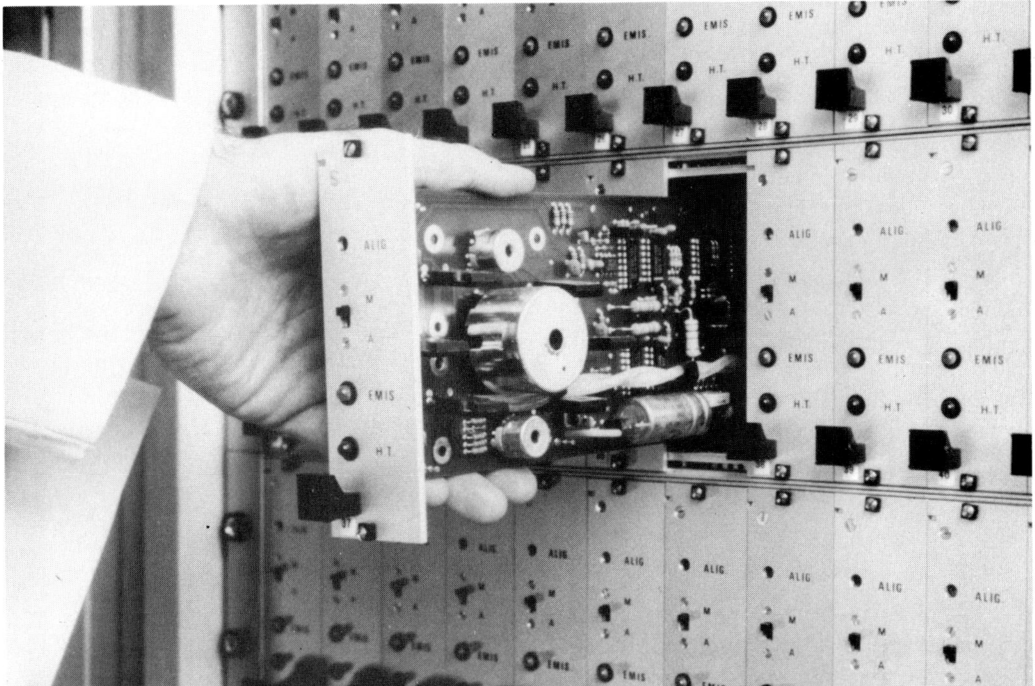

FIG 2.
Individual drawer for each piezo element allows easy maintenance.

men. An ultrasound gel is applied between the cushion and the skin to create better contact. Air (lungs and intestinal gas) should be avoided because air does not have the same acoustic impedance as tissue and could result in damage to these organs. The shock waves are focused by the convergence of the synchronous emission of 320 piezoelectric plates in a hemispherical mosaic. The shock waves follow a bi-conical trajectory (Fig 3). The focus point is tiny (5 mm)

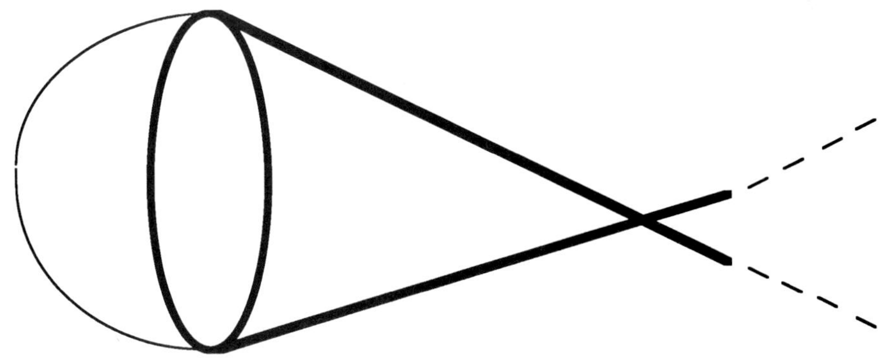

FIG 3.
Hemispherical piezo mosaic array produces shock waves that follow a bi-conical trajectory.

and is far smaller than the focus point of the other systems (see infra).

Localization of Stones

The stones are localized by real-time ultrasonography. Although not ideal for many ureteral and common bile duct stones, ultrasonography is particularly suited for gallstones. The ultrasound probe is housed in the water-filled cushion at the geometric center of the generating hemisphere. This allows continuous visualization of the gallstone and aiming of the shock waves at the stone. The operator can focus the shock waves, if the patient moves during the session, either by moving the table on which the patient lies or by moving the water-filled cushion.

PATIENTS

Patients with intrahepatic or common bile duct stones were excluded from this study. All of the patients were symptomatic and surgically fit for an operation if a complication arose. Inclusion criteria were:

1. Functioning gallbladder as determined by an oral cholecystogram.
2. Number of gallstones: less than five.
3. The dimension of the largest stone < 3 cm.

Calcified gallstones were not a contraindication.

Sixty-seven men and 145 women were included, with an age range from 8 to 86 years (median: 54.4 years). All of the patients gave their written informed consent.

Patients who had complicated biliary stone disease or other associated medical conditions were excluded by abnormal results on the routine laboratory tests listed in Table 2. None of the patients had a coagulopathy, although some were taking warfarin which was stopped and replaced by subcutaneous heparin every 6 hours. One injection was omitted and the treatment resumed 6 hours after the session.

TABLE 2

Pre- and Post-Procedure Laboratory Monitoring

Biology:	Coagulation: platelets, prothrombin time, etc.
	Liver function tests: ASAT, ALAT, bilirubin, alkaline phosphatases
	Pancreatic enzymes
	Microscopic hematuria
	RBC, WBC, ESR
Imaging:	Ultrasound before, the day after, and monthly

PROTOCOL OF LITHOTRIPSY

Patient Position

The patient lies prone or in a slightly prone right oblique position so that there is a minimum distance between the water-filled cushion and the gallbladder. Gallstones gravitate to the fundus of the gallbladder in this position.

Duration of Sessions

The sessions varied between 25 to 95 minutes (median 54 minutes).

Frequency of Shock Wave

Three centers elected not to administer any anesthetic or analgesic, and used 1.25 or 2.5 shocks per second. The fourth center (Clinique Vert-Galant) often used a higher frequency, up to 10 shocks per second, under premedication (fentanyl or propofol IV).

Number of Sessions

The patients underwent a second session if the stones were not fragmented or if the fragments were too large. The second session was carried out 3 days after the first one or 1 month later.

FOLLOW-UP

Patients were hospitalized for 3 days following treatment, and the tests listed in Table 2 were repeated. All the patients were given the same adjuvant dissolving agents as described by Sauerbruch and associates, that is, chenodeoxycholic and ursodeoxycholic acid 8 mg/kg body weight 8 days before treatment and continued for 3 months after complete dissolution, as with chemo-ursotherapy.[5] The main reason for selecting a combination of two bile acid agents was to follow the same schema as that of Paumgartner and colleagues.[6]

Patients had a repeat ultrasound the day after and 30 days after ESL treatment, and then every subsequent 3 months.

RESULTS

Fragmentation and dissolution must be distinguished because, theoretically, the stone can be transformed into a fine powder and can pass through the cystic duct. Randomized controlled trials are in progress to determine if migration or dissolution occurs with ESL. This study does not address this problem. However, two of our patients with calcified stones were followed up: plain abdominal x-ray showed complete disappearance of these stones. In these cases it is very doubtful that adjuvant dissolving agents had any effect.

FRAGMENTATION OF GALLSTONES

Two hundred and twelve patients with gallstones were treated with ESL. In six of these patients gallstones could not be visualized because of obesity, interposition of the right colonic flexure in front of the liver, and previous abdominal surgical scars. In eight elderly patients, treatment could not be completed because of positional back pain. Therefore, we evaluated fragmentation of gallstones in 198 patients and observed fragmentation in 171 (86.36 percent).

DISSOLUTION OF GALLSTONES

The overall dissolution rate to date is 21.7 percent, that is, 43 out of 198 patients. Only three of the four centers have classified their results according to the size and number of the stones. Concerning 155 patients to date, results are:

- Solitary stones <20 mm: 22/69 (31.8%)
- Solitary stones >20 mm: 3/16 (18.8%)
- Multiple stones 7/70 (10.0%)

So far, only two of the four centers have data giving results according to the time of follow-up. Table 3 shows these data.

SIDE EFFECTS

Twenty-one patients complained of minor symptoms such as abdominal pain, nausea, and sweating during the treatment. These symptoms resolved when treatment was stopped a brief moment and recommenced.

Twenty patients had moderate abdominal pain in the 24 hours following the treatment. These symptoms subsided spontaneously and did not require any medication.

Five patients had biliary colic; six had elevation of alkaline phosphatase (maximum 118 u. for a normal up to 90 u.); nine had mild hyperamylasemia without pain (maximum twice the normal); one had an isolated elevated transaminase (normal × 4) without any clinical symptoms 48 hours after treatment which settled to a normal value within 1 week.

No side effect was observed when the frequency used was 1.25 shocks per second. Hematuria (macroscopic or microscopic) or cutaneous petachia were not observed in any of the patients.

Thirteen patients have undergone cholecystectomies: 9 for psychological reasons (continuance of pains); 2 for acute pain (but without fever and with WBC normal); 2 for acute cholecystitis (one at the 2d day, the other at the 45th day).

TABLE 3.

Dissolution (81 Evaluable Patients) Over Time

	SIZE			TOTAL NO.
DURATION	20 MM	20 MM	MULTIPLE	OF GALLSTONES
0–2 months	11/28	1/7	2/46	14/81
2–4 months	7/21	1/5	2/35	10/61
4–8 months	5/13	1/3	2/23	8/39
8–12 months	4/7	1/2	2/9	7/18 (39%)

DISCUSSION

This report describes the use of piezoelectric lithotripsy with the EDAP LT-01 machine for the treatment of gallstones, from several French centers. Our results suggest that this machine offers a nonsurgical *ambulatory* treatment for gallstones; the efficacy of this treatment depends on *patient selection*.

In 212 patients, there was only one complication requiring surgery 2 days after the session. But it was at the beginning of the trials and 20 shocks per second were used in this particular patient. The pathology of the surgically removed gallbladders did not show any lesions clearly imputable to the ESL. Thus, there is an overall complication rate of 0.47 percent without acute pancreatitis requiring endoscopic sphincterotomy.

None of the patients required bed rest following treatment. The initial protocol design obliged us to keep the patient hospitalized for 3 days. Now patients return home 1 hour after treatment. The minor ailments recorded (nausea, pain) no longer occur when low frequency shock waves (1.25 to 2.5 maximum) are employed.

None of the patients develped skin petechia or macroscopic or microscopic hematuria. These complications are still encountered using the new Dornier MPL 9000 machine which also does not require anesthesia.* It is worth noting that abdominal petechiae were also observed in 10 percent of cases using the other lithotripter with a piezoelectric source.[7] These may not be of great significance but do point to certain risk potentials not observed with EDAP LT-01 machines. What could account for this difference? Three factors can be suggested:

1. The power pressure of the Dornier machine is 1 kilobar, whereas it is only around 500 atmospheres in the EDAP.

2. The focus point of 5 mm of the EDAP is the smallest of all the machines available on the market.

3. The shock waves of EDAP system are the shortest with a minimum of low frequency waves.

The noninvasive nature of this treatment permits retreatments (within 2 to 3 days, whereas the electrohydraulic machines require a wait of 2 to 3 months). However, the need for subsequent treatment is less using the Dornier machine. We conclude that the EDAP LT-01 is effective as an ambulatory nonsurgical treatment for gallstones.

Our results when compared with those recently published by the Munich group[6] are inferior in both fragmentation and dissolution. However, their *patient selection* was quite different than ours. Furthermore, another German center using the same Dornier machine obtained results similar to ours,[8] using the same patient selection criteria. It would be a pity if some patients were denied the benefit of this treatment even if the success rate is not as impressive as in the case of the solitary stone less than 20 mm (which accounted for 83 percent of Sackmann and colleagues' patients).

Extracorporeal shock wave lithotripsy by the EDAP LT-01 machine has been shown to induce fine, powderlike fragmentation of renal stones in vitro,[9] but so far we have not been able to confirm this for biliary stones. However, we are not too disappointed, as the rapid evacuation of the residue of a whole stone could result in the equivalent of "steine strasse" as described by German urologists at the uretero-vesical junction. This could result in an obstruction of the sphincter of Oddi, inducing jaundice or acute pancreatitis. This would be far from the ideal of a simple noninvasive ambulatory treatment competitive with cholecystectomy. One of our patients had a cholecystectomy on the same day at his own request (disappointment with the treatment failure), and cavitation of the stone (pitting) was evident.

PLACE OF ESL IN GALLSTONE TREATMENT

The most important question is to ascertain if ESL will modify the current therapeutic schema of managing gallstones (Table 4). In the patient with asymptomatic, or silent, stones, ESL does not change the noninterventional management

---

T. Sauerbruch: Personal communication (Nice, June 1988).

TABLE 4.

Current Management of Gallstones (Before ESL)

1. Complicated gallstones (infection, migration)	Surgery
2. Silent gallstones (dyspepsia)	Observation
3. Symptomatic gallstones (biliary colic)	Surgery or observation (depending on operative risk and patient preference

required because of the problem of recurrence and the necessity and cost of adjuvant bile acid dissolving agents. However, if more potent effective dissolving agents are developed, as some recent reports suggest,[10, 11, 12] it would be feasible to treat silent stones. Perhaps eventually it would be logical to screen certain high-risk populations and treat them by ESL. Finally, because a large size and number of gallstones and a nonfunctioning gallbladder indicate late stages of gallstone disease,[13] early detection and treatment could prevent this evolution.

In symptomatic gallstones characterized by biliary colic, there is a choice of either immediate surgery or expectant treatment. Will ESL have a role in that case? This role is minor if it must be reserved for patients with a solitary stone of less than 20 mm diameter. We feel we should enlarge the selection criteria proposed by our colleagues in Munich. Even though our results are not that favorable, there is no doubt that in some patients surgery can be avoided.

In conclusion, our study of 212 patients shows piezo-lithotripsy to be a safe alternative to the surgical treatment of gallstones. As the prevalence and incidence of the disease are very high in Western Europe,[14] this appears to us a result of paramount importance. We may already imagine a change of the classical management of gallstone disease for a new one, as proposed in Table 5.

REFERENCES

1. Sauerbruch T, Delius M, Paumgartner G, et al: Fragmentation of gallstones by extracorporeal shockwaves. *N Engl J Med* 1986; 314:818–822.
2. Branche D, Magnier M: Lithotritie biliaire: expérience du Centre du lithotripteur de Paris-Nord. *Gastroenterol Clin Biol* 1988; 12:189.
3. Capdeville R, Barrat F, Andre J, et al: La lithotritie extra-corporelle dans la lithiase vésiculaire. Etudes expérimentales et premières applications cliniques. *Gastroenterol Clin Biol* 1988; 12:12.
4. Amouretti M, Perissat J, Arnoux R, et al: Etude sur un modèle de lithiase biliaire expérimentale du chien des effets secondaires tissulaires de la lithotritie extra-corporelle par ondes de choc. *Gastroenterol Clin Biol* 1988; 12:11.
5. Delmont J, Rampal P, Math M, et al: Traitement de la lithiase biliaire par l'acide ursodesoxycholique. *Sem Hôp Paris* 1980; 56:1613–1616.
6. Sackmann M, Delius M, Sauerbruch T, et al:

TABLE 5.
Proposed Management of Gallstone Disease

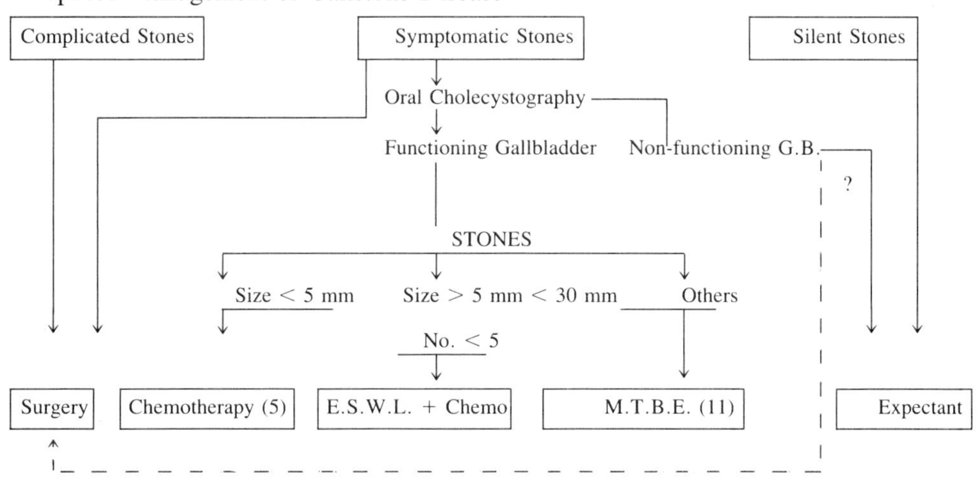

Shockwave lithotripsy of gallbladder stones: The first 175 patients. *N Engl J Med* 1988; 318:393–397.

7. Hood K, Keightley A, Dowling R, et al: Piezoceramic lithotripsy of gallbladder stones: Initial experience in 38 patients. *Lancet* 1988; 1:1322–1324.
8. Greiner L, Wenzel H, Jakobeit C: Combination of extracorporeal shock-wave fragmentation and bile acid dissolution treatment of gallstones: Further data and experience. *Dtsch Med Wochenschr* 1987; 112:1893–1896.
9. Moreaux J. Lithotritie expérimentale. Revue Française de Gastroentérologie 1988; 238:805.
10. Pitt H, McFadden D, Gadacz T: Agents for gallstone dissolution. *Am J Surg* 1987; 153:233–246.
11. Fromm H, Malavolti M: Dissolving gallstones, in Stollerman G (ed): *Advances in Internal Medicine,* vol 33. Chicago, Year Book Medical Publisher, 1988, pp 409–430.
12. Carey M, Cahalane M: Whither biliary sludge? *Gastroenterology* (in press).
13. Jorgensen T: Cholecystolithiasis in a Danish community: Design of a cross-sectional and longitudinal study, in Capocaccia L, Ricci G, Angelico F, et al (eds): *Epidemiology and Prevention of Gallstones Diseases.* Lancaster, MTP Press, 1984.
14. Barbara L, Sama C, Labate AM, et al: A population study on the prevalence of gallstone disease: The Sirmione study. *Hepatology* 1987; 7:913–917.

Piezoelectric Lithotripsy of Gallstones: Experimental Studies and Preliminary Clinical Results

C. Ell, W. Kerzel, N. Heyder, E. Günter, and W. Domschke

Nonsurgical procedures for the treatment of cholecystolithiasis must be measured against the effectiveness of cholecystectomy and its low morbidity and mortality rates. In contrast to oral chemolitholysis alone, extracorporeal shock wave lithotripsy in combination with chemolitholytic after treatment appears to be a promising alternative to cholecystectomy in selected patients.[1,2]

For noninvasive alternative procedures to cholecystectomy, however, apart from adequate effectiveness, freedom from pain is a requirement that must be met. This is particularly so when partial success on initial treatment, or recurrent stones, make repeat lithotripsy necessary. Piezoelectric lithotripsy has now been proven to be both successful and pain-free in the treatment of kidney stones.[4] We summarize our preliminary in vitro experiments concerning the feasibility of gallstone lithotripsy by means of piezoelectric shock waves, tissue reactions caused by piezoelectric shock waves, and our initial clinical experience in 31 patients (January though May 1988).

MATERIALS AND METHODS

The equipment we employed for our experimental work was a piezoelectric lithotripter manufactured by Wolf, Inc., Federal Republic of Germany (Piezolith 2200). For the clinical treatments we used the Piezolith 2300 (Fig 1). The main difference between the Piezolith 2200 and the 2300 is the new dual scanner location system (Fig 2). The shock waves are produced by a self-focusing piezoelectric acoustic generator that has a bowl-shaped configuration and bears a mosaic of more than 3000 ceramic elements on its concave surface.

For transmission of the shock wave, the "bowl" is filled with degassed water warmed to body temperature. The patient is placed in the prone position, the skin over the region of the gallbladder being immersed in the water contained within the bowl. The stones are localized ultrasonographically in two planes with the aid of one of the two real-time ultrasonic B scanners arranged in the longitudinal axis of the shock wave generator.

The pulse sequence can be adjusted in four steps between 1 and 2:5 Hz, and the pulse energy can be selected from among four different settings. Depending upon the pulse energy selected, the pressure effective at the shock wave focus varies between 600 and 1200 bar.

GALLSTONE LITHOTRIPSY IN VITRO [5,6]

A total of 177 surgically removed gallbladder stones were submitted to piezoelectric shock

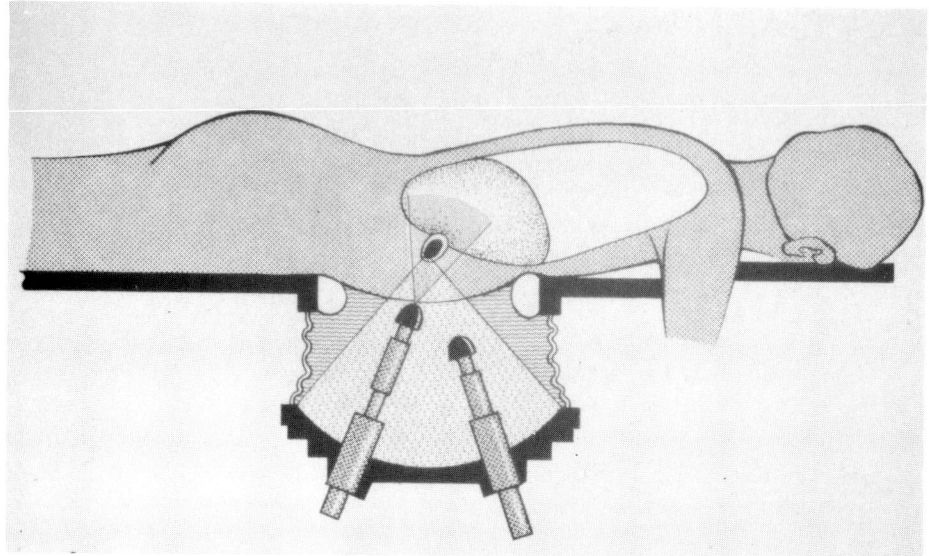

FIG 1.
Piezolith 2300 with patient in prone position for gallstone lithotripsy

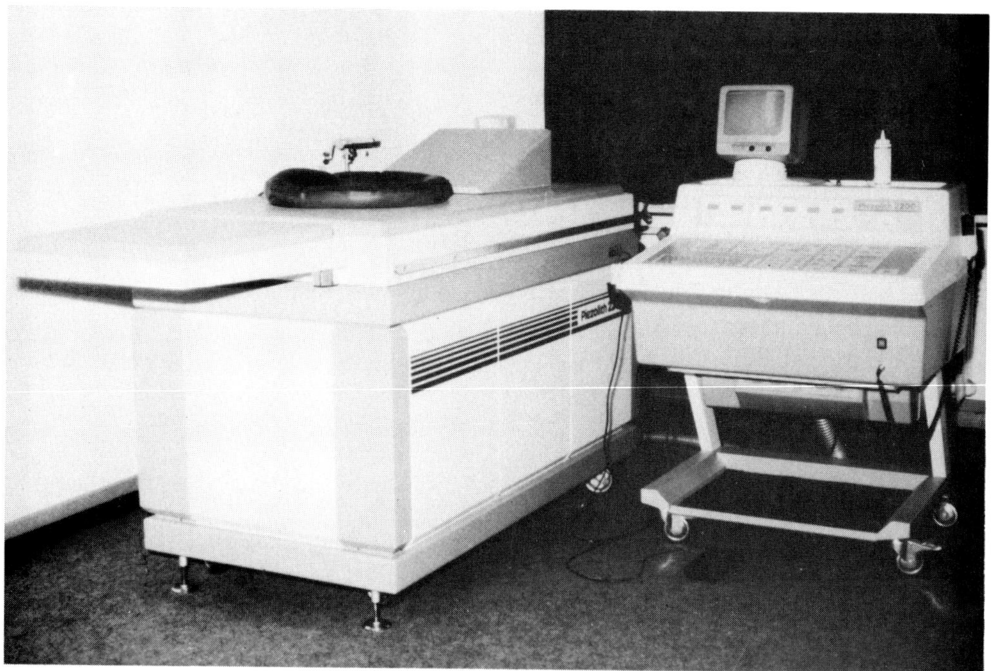

FIG 2.
Piezoelectric lithotripsy system: self-focusing bowl shaped shockwave generator with the coaxial dual ultrasound transducer for targeting the gallstone.

wave treatment. Prior to shock wave application, the diameter, weight, volume, CT density, and NMR signal intensity of the stones were determined. Shock waves were applied under standardized conditions (intensity setting 4, frequency 2 Hz) to the gallstones previously positioned in the center of focus of the shock waves. The application was terminated when the size of the residual fragments was 4 mm or less or a maximum of 4000 discharges had been applied. The chemical composition of 85 stones was investigated by x-ray diffractometry and or infrared spectrometry.

The following results were achieved: All the stones were successfully fragmented; calculi with the maximum diameter of 17 mm, a maximum weight of 1800 mg, and a maximum volume of 2 cc, were regularly disintegrated into fragments <4 mm. The number of shock waves required correlated most closely with volume, weight and, to a somewhat lesser degree, diameter. No correlation was found between the chemical composition of the calculi and the number of pulses needed for fragmentation.

TISSUE REACTIONS IN VITRO AND IN ANIMALS[7]

Piezoelectric shock wave discharges (100 to 4000) were applied to surgically removed, stone-containing human gallbladders. In acute and chronic experiments on mongrel dogs, between 500 and 3000 shock waves were applied to the gallbladder, liver, spleen, lungs, and bowel. Prior to and after shockwave application, CT, MRT, and laboratory tests were performed.

The results can be summarized as follows: shock wave application to the human gallbladders resulted in disintegration of the stones with no macroscopically or microscopically detectable tissue changes. In acute animal experiments, small hematomas were observed at organ surfaces (e.g., capsule of the liver, bed of the gallbladder) and also inside the organs. Perforations or intra-abdominal or pleural bleeding did not occur. In chronic experiments, no macroscopic, and only slight microscopic, residual lesions were observed at 3 weeks after shock wave applications. In almost all cases, the lesions were detected by CT, MRT, and ultrasonography, while laboratory tests were negative.

GALLSTONE LITHOTRIPSY IN HUMANS

The inclusion and exclusion criteria for this study corresponded to those employed by the Munich group.[2] The application of shock waves was carried out under standardized conditions (pulse intensity stage 4, pulse sequence stage 3). Lithotripsy was terminated when, ultrasonographically, no obvious individual fragments with an acoustical shadow were recognizable, or after a maximum of 3000 discharges.

For 7 days prior to lithotripsy, and up to 3 months after complete freedom from stones, each patient received 7.5 mg/kg body weight of ursodesoxycholic acid and chenodesoxycholic acid, respectively. These drugs were administered in a single dose at bedtime.

In 31 patients, a total of 51 therapy sessions were carried out (16 patients were treated once only, 10 patients twice, and 5 patients 3 times). In none of the cases was anesthesia or any analgesic or sedative premedication or medication during treatment required. All the calculi were fragmented at the first lithotripsy session. The average maximum fragment size after initial therapy was 4.7 mm (± 3.3 SD), after 2 months 2.6 mm (± 1.9 SD).

The maximum fragment diameter after the first lithotripsy session was less than 50 percent of the initial stone diameter in 90 percent of the patients (n = 28), between 50 and 75 percent in 2 patients (6.4 percent), and between 75 and 100 percent of the original diameter in a single case. A median of 2080 (500 to 3000) discharges were applied at the first lithotripsy session, 1730 (1000 to 3000) at the second session, and 1520 (1000 to 3000) at the third session. In 21 out of the 31 patients, follow-up examinations were carried out after 1 or 2 months (14 patients). Seven out of the 21 patients (33.3 percent) complained of colic-like upper abdominal pain that responded to enterally administered

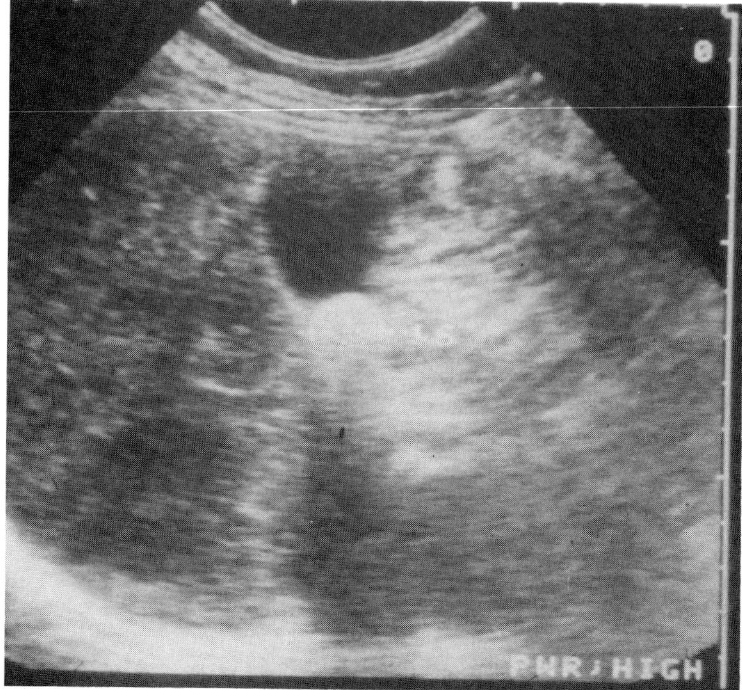

FIG 3.
A solitary radiolucent gallbladder stone prior to lithotripsy.

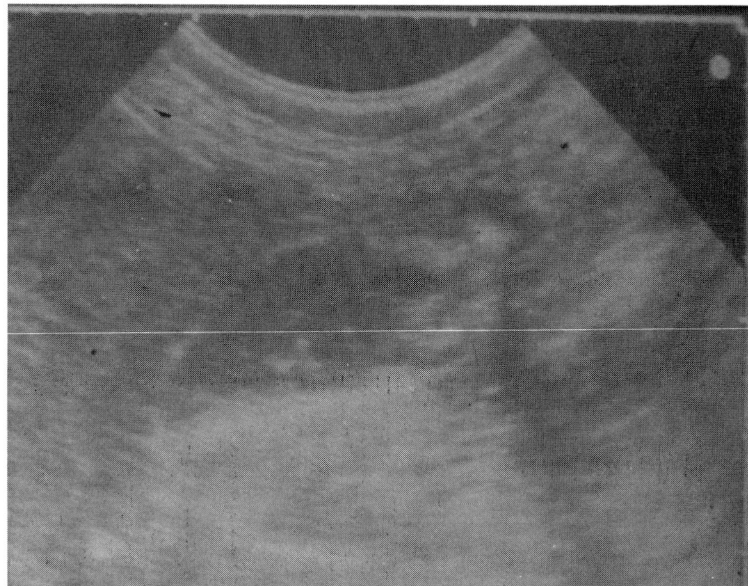

FIG 4.
The same radiolucent gallbladder stone immediately after lithotripsy.

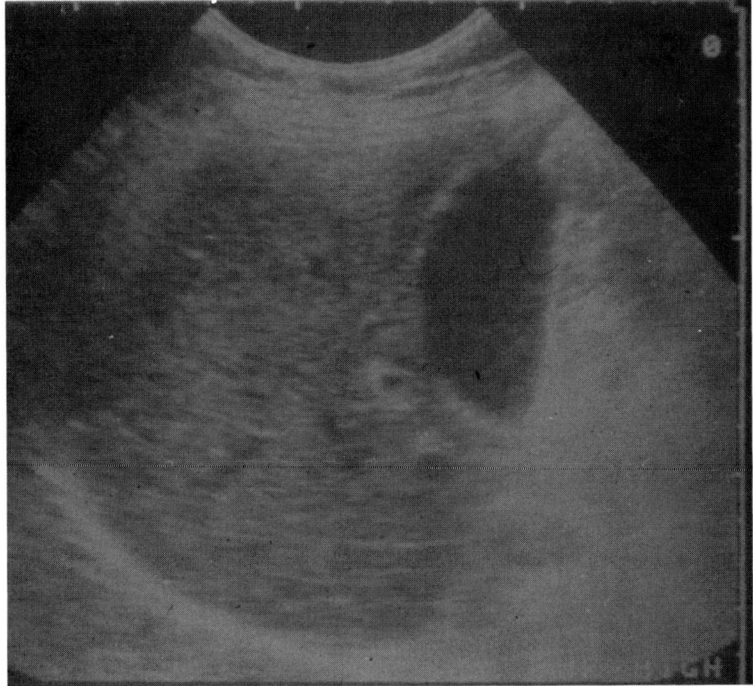

FIG 5.
Two months later, the gallbladder is completely free of stone fragments.

spasmo-analgesics. In none of the cases was emergency intravenous spasmo-analgesic treatment or hospitalization necessary. In 5 out of 21 patients (23.8 percent) ultrasonography revealed freedom from stones (Figs 3 to 5). In 14 patients, a considerable reduction in the size and number of stone fragments was observed. In 2 patients, a largish conglomerate of fragments with an acoustic shadow had developed. These two patients, and three others with residual calculi >5 mm, were submitted to a third lithotripsy session.

DISCUSSION

The painlessness of piezoelectric shock waves, even in the case of organs with visceral innervation, is, indeed, a decisive clinical advantage vis-á-vis spark discharge and electromagnetic techniques of shock wave generation. This advantage can, however, be of importance only when fragmentation efficiency and the stone-free rate achieved with the piezoelectric mechanism are comparable.

If our preliminary results are compared with published data using spark discharge systems,[2,3,8] fragmentation potential would appear to be equal. While Greiner and associates[3] reported maximum fragment diameters of less than 50 percent of the original stone diameter in only 59.4 percent of their patients, in the recently published Munich study,[2] the mean maximum fragment size after lithotripsy, at 2.8 + 1.8 mm (mean ± SD), was somewhat smaller than in our patients.

Although reliable information on the long-term results of piezoelectric lithotripsy is not yet available, we have already demonstrated freedom from stones in about one quarter (23.8 percent) of our patients submitted to follow-up ultrasonography 1 to 2 months following lithotripsy (n = 21).[1] This parallels results reported using spark discharge systems.[2,3]

Even though initial clinical experience with piezoelectric gallstone lithotripsy suggests that this type of shock wave application is free from significant side effects in the internal organs, and despite the painlessness of the procedure, the application of shock waves without proper precautions would not seem justified. Thus, the not insignificant tissue lesions found in animal models with all extracorporeal procedures should prompt us to keep the number of shock waves applied to produce therapeutically adequate fragmentation as small as possible, by accurate focusing and constant ultrasound monitoring during treatment.

In summary, based on our preliminary experience with piezoelectric lithotripsy of gallbladder stones, it may be expected that, analogous to kidney stone lithotripsy, piezoelectric gallstone lithotripsy will prove an effective and, in particular, pain-free procedure that will decisively influence the further development of extracorporeal lithotripsy.

REFERENCES

1. Sauerbruch T, Delius M, Paumgartner G, et al: Fragmentation of gallstones by extracorporeal shock waves. *N Engl J Med* 1986; 314:818–822.
2. Sackmann M, Delius M, Sauerbruch T, et al: Shock wave lithotripsy of gallbladder stones: The first 175 patients. *N Engl J Med* 1988; 318:393–397.
3. Greiner L, Wenzel H, Jakobei C: Stoßwellen-Lithotripsie von Gallenblasensteinen. *Dtsch Med Wochenschr* 1987; 112:239.
4. Philip T, Whitfield HN, Kellett MJ: Painless lithotripsy: Experience with 100 patients. *Lancet* 1988; 1:41.
5. Ell C, Kerzel W, Heyder N: Piezoelectric Lithotripsy. *Lancet* 1987; 2:1149.
6. Ell C, Kerzel W, Langer H, et al: Fragmentation of biliary calculi by means of extracorporeally generated piezoelectric shock wave. *Dig Dis Sci*, in press.
7. Ell D, Kerzel W, Langer H, et al: Tissue reactions under piezoelectric shock wave application for the fragmentation of biliary calculi. *Gut*, in press.
8. Ponchon T, Martin X, Mestas JL, et al: Extracorporeal lithotripsy of gallstones. *Lancet* 1987; 1:448.

Experiences with a PiezoCeramic System

R. H. Dowling, K. Hood, U. Rajagopal,
A. Keightley, and C. Mallinson

During the past year, we have been using a piezoceramic system (the Wolf Piezolith 2200/2300) to treat over 40 symptomatic patients with radiolucent gallbladder stones. Our initial results have already been published.[1] Since then, the number of patients treated has increased (modestly), but the overall pattern of results has not changed appreciably. For this reason, our results in the 40 patients treated over the first year are summarized here only briefly.

PATIENT AND GALLSTONE CHARACTERISTICS

As in most other ESL protocols for gallbladder stones, our aim was to treat only symptomatic patients with 1 to 3 radiolucent (by plain x-ray and OCG) stones with a minimum diameter of 10 mm in "functioning" gallbladders. In theory, we did not have an upper limit of gallstone size. In practice, the maximum stone diameter proved to be 30 mm, with a median of 15 mm.

There were 15 men and 25 women, aged 27 to 73 years (median age: 49). Although all the patients had radiolucent stones, in 73 percent we checked the conventional x-ray findings (plain abdominal x-ray and OCG) with localized CT scanning of the gallbladder. Twenty-five had CT–lucent stones [arbitrarily <100 Hounsfield Units (HU)]; and although all the stones were radiolucent by conventional methods, in two patients, they proved to be CT–dense (>100 HU) and in two other individuals, the stones had CT–dense rims. Forty percent (16 of 40) of the patients had multiple stones—a larger percentage than in some other series.

AIMS

Although we too have already seen stone-free patients after ESL plus oral bile acids, we are not yet in a position to report final results of complete gallstone dissolution/disappearance. At this stage, therefore, our aims are to describe only the fragmentation efficacy, safety, and side effects of piezoceramic lithotripsy using the Wolf Piezolith 2200/2300.

PROTOCOL

It takes 1 to 4 weeks after starting oral CDCA treatment before biliary bile acid and bile lipid composition can reach a new steady state. If the same delay applies to UDCA treatment or to the combination of CDCA and UDCA, logically patients undergoing ESL for gallbladder stones should be pretreated with oral bile acids for up to 1 month before lithotripsy. (This recommendation assumes that after ESL, the majority of gallstone fragments remain within the gallbladder and must be dissolved with oral bile acids, rather than pass spontaneously). Indeed, although most of our patients did receive oral bile acids for 1 to 4 weeks before lithotripsy, there were occasional violations of the protocol.

The patients were fasted overnight in the belief that gallstone localization and fragmentation are easier in a distended, than in a partially contracted, gallbladder. However, this reasoning has never been systematically tested.

With the piezoelectric system, the patients required no sedation, analgesia, or anesthesia despite being given 2000 to 5500 shocks per treatment session (mean 4182 ± SD 806). This relatively large number of shocks was based on clinical experience gained by ourselves while treating patients with gallbladder stones, and by our colleagues in urologic surgery who have used the same machine to treat renal stones in over 500 patients. Initially, we gave 2000 to 3000 shocks per treatment, but found that large numbers of discharges were needed to achieve effective fragmentation and that the increased number of shocks caused no clinical or laboratory evidence of complications.

The percentage of patients with multiple stones (16 of 40, or 40 percent) was larger than that in some other reports. As a result, independent of the variable of different types of lithotriper and the total numbers of shocks given, the number of ESL treatments necessary to fragment all the stones was almost certainly larger than that which would have been required had we selected only patients with solitary stones.

PATIENT MONITORING: SAFETY AND SIDE-EFFECTS

Until recently, with very few exceptions, patients were admitted overnight to monitor vital signs, to look for evidence of microscopic hematuria, and to carry out routine hematologic and biochemical screening tests before and at 4 and 24 hours after ESL. Based on the Munich experience, we anticipated that a significant number of patients would experience post-lithotripsy biliary pain—and possibly even pancreatitis as a result of some of the fragments passing through the cystic duct and down the common bile duct. In the event, no patient developed immediate post-lithotripsy pain or pancreatitis.

Two patients developed transient microscopic hematuria. In one, this may have been due to a proven urinary tract infection that antedated the ESL. The second also had mild transient abnormalities of liver function that returned to normal within 48 hours. The only clinically evident immediate complication of the lithotripsy was the development of cutaneous petechiae in the shock wave path, in thin patients (n = 4).

Many patients were unaware of any sensation during ESL. However, some noted a pricking sensation in the target area—particularly at the start of treatment—while others found that it was uncomfortable to lie prone with the right arm extended above the head, for the 40 to 50 minutes of treatment. In women with large breasts, local pressure of the padded ring around the water bath also caused some discomfort, even when the breast was elevated.

PATIENT MONITORING: FRAGMENTATION EFFICACY

Fragmentation was assessed in several ways:

1. Crudely, with the integral, in-line ultrasound transducer during treatment.

2. By definitive ultrasound in the radiology department, 24 hours after lithotripsy.

3. By OCG. Initially, the cholecystograms were carried out 24 to 48 hours after ESL. However, on 7 of 15 occasions, the OCG was unsatisfactory because of transient, poor, or nonvisualization of the gallbladder suggesting reversible damage to the gallbladder mucosa. In all seven patients, normal opacification of the gallbladder had returned when the OCG was repeated 2 to 3 weeks later. For this reason, we now defer post-lithotripsy cholecystography until this time. We do not yet know if it is necessary or helpful to check fragmentation efficacy by both cholecystography *and* ultrasonography.

4. In a separate, but related study, by examining the contents of gallbladders removed during elective cholecystectomy at different times, for example, 24 or 48 hours after lithotripsy with various numbers of shocks. This approach, which was approved by the Hospital Ethical Committee, is being used in patients who do not

fulfill the selection criteria for ESL plus oral bile acid treatment. It is also being used in those who opt for surgery but consent to undergo lithotripsy before their operation, not only to study fragmentation efficacy but also to monitor for induced tissue damage.

5. As part of a study in which CT–density (Hounsfield Units) of the stones, measured before cholecystectomy, is being correlated with (a) stone composition, (b) stone dissolvability, and (c) stone fragmentability—all measured in vitro after surgery.

We suspect that piezoceramic lithotripsy is less powerful than underwater spark-discharge systems in fragmenting stones. If so, the advantage of a pain-free system must be set against the disadvantage of one that requires more shocks and more treatment sessions and that may leave the patient with fewer and larger gallstone fragments than those reported using alternative machines. We are not convinced, however, that it is possible to determine fragment size accurately using either ultrasonography or cholecystography. This is particularly true when more than one stone is present or when multiple small fragments cluster around and mask a larger particle—the so-called "cloud effect." We would question, therefore, the reliability of claims that ESL yields fragments with a mean size of 2.8 or 4.7 mm diameter implying a degree of precision that seems inappropriate. Prospective validation studies in volunteer patients undergoing lithotripsy before elective cholecystectomy are needed to relate estimates of fragment size in vivo to accurate measurements of their size when retrieved from the gallbladder at the time of surgery.

RESULTS

Thirty-five of the 40 patients (87.5 percent) achieved partial (n = 13) or complete (n = 22) gallstone fragmentation. By complete fragmentation, we mean that none of the gallstone particles measured more than 5 mm. Partial fragmentation indicates either that the treatment is not yet complete because, for example, one stone has been fragmented but the second (or third) requires further ESL (eight patients,) or that despite stone disruption, one or more fragments measuring >5 mm in diameter remain (five patients). Extracorporeal shock wave lithotripsy failed to fragment stones in two patients despite two and four treatments, respectively, with a total number of 9000 and 16,500 shocks. One patient defaulted after an uncomplicated, but only partially successful, treatment session. In two other patients, attempts to administer ESL were abandoned because, with the original unmodified machine (Piezolith 2200), it was not possible to localize the stone(s) within the target area. However, with the simple modifications of a thicker "mattress" on the treatment table and a more mobile piezoceramic dish capable of greater vertical travel, these problems have now largely been overcome.

Thus, although we failed in 5 patients on an "intention to treat" basis, the ESL itself failed in only 2 of 40 patients. Put another way, the efficacy of lithotripsy in fragmenting stones was 95 percent. It remains to be seen what percentage of patients will achieve a stone-free gallbladder as a result of either spontaneous passage of the fragments or their dissolution with adjuvant bile acids.

CONCLUSIONS

Whether ESL is an adjuvant to oral bile acid treatment or vice versa is a semantic argument; but in the opinion of the authors, lithotripsy shares many of the advantages and many of the limitations of oral bile acid treatment alone. Extracorporeal shock wave lithotripsy is likely to prove successful only if based on knowledge learned about oral bile acid treatment over the past 18 years. Nonetheless, lithotripsy is an exciting new tool that expands the number of management options open to the patient with gallstones. It almost certainly renders a higher percentage of patients gallstone-free than oral bile acid treatment alone, and it accelerates the rate at which this can be achieved. Despite this, all the nonsurgical approaches involving dissolution of gallstones apply only to a minority of gallstone patients. For the foreseeable future, therefore, most gallstone patients requiring active treatment will come to cholecystectomy. With the other new approaches, however, surgery for cholecystolithiasis no longer holds a therapeutic monopoly, and its one-time unassailable position is now being slowly eroded.

ACKNOWLEDGMENTS

We are grateful to the Special Trustees of Guy's Hospital; the New Moorgate Trust; Roussel UCLAF, Paris; and the St. Martin's Group of Hospitals for their financial support. We also wish to thank the nursing staff of the lithotripsy suite at the London Bridge Hospital; and Mrs. Ann Hollington for her help in preparing the manuscript.

REFERENCE

1. Hood K, Keightley A, Dowling RH, et al: Piezoceramic lithotripsy of gallbladder stones: Initial experience in 38 patients. *Lancet* 1988; 1:1322–1324.

Biliary Lithotripsy: A Uroradiological Perspective

Bruce L. McClennan

Given the remarkable success of extracorporeal shock wave lithotripsy (ESL) in the kidney and ureter,[1–4] numerous manufacturers and investigators have applied both existing and prototype technology to the treatment of biliary tract calculi.[5–7] Initial satisfactory fragmentation of gallstones and biliary ductal stones, with eventual passage, extraction, and/or dissolution or both, in selected patients has sparked considerable research and the development of machines designed to perform biliary tract ESL. Although the goals of a stone-free and symptom-free patient are the same, there are obvious parallels and some paradoxes when the two procedures are compared and contrasted. In the majority of patients, renal ESL is the only therapy necessary for the treatment of symptomatic renal and ureteral calculi, with little or no preprocedure or postprocedure intervention required for successful stone passage.[2,8] Certainly, this is the case for solitary renal or ureteral calculi less than 1 to 1.5 cm in size.[2,8] Calyceal calculi, ureteral calculi, and large or branched stones (greater than 2 cm in diameter) or hard stones (cystine, uric acid, or calcium monohydrate) require more treatments, stent placements, and/or adjunct procedures, such as percutaneous nephrostomy or ureterorenoscopy for eventual stone clearance.[9,10] Stone remnant rates vary depending upon the above-described stone characteristics or locations as well as with the size and number of stones treated.[11,12] The eventual success and integration into clinical service of biliary ESL will depend on similar factors as well as on an understanding of some fundamental differences in anatomy and physiology between the kidney and the biliary system. A strict scientific approach to this exciting new technology will be required, and it is to be hoped that rapid and widespread implementation of the technique will not precede proper evaluation.[13–15] In order to compare and contrast biliary and renal lithotripsy, an understanding of morphology, physiology, pathogenesis of stone formation, the evolution of therapy, and competing technologies is in order.

MORPHOLOGY/PHYSIOLOGY

The entry of bile and presumably biliary concretions or calculi into the intestine is a complex coordination of hepatic bile production; gallbladder storage and contraction; cystic duct, common bile duct, and pancreatic duct function; intestinal wall motility; and interdigestive motor activity (stomach and small intestine) and sphincter of Oddi activity.[16] The biliary tree has many more anatomical components, and therefore more potential sites for obstruction, than the urinary tract. Urinary excretion into the collecting system from the distal collecting ducts into the calyces via the duct of Bellini depends on the complex but well-understood function of the nephron. Urine peristalsis begins at the infundibulocalyceal junction, propelling urine distally through the renal pelvis, into the ureter, and through the ureteral-vesicle junction into the bladder. The ureteral vesicle junction is not a true sphincter as is the sphincter of Oddi and its surrounding papilla of Vater, which includes both the terminus of the common bile duct and the pancreatic duct.[16] While duplications and anatomical variants occur in both the biliary tree and urinary tract, the passage of a renal or ureteral calculus less than 4 to 5 mm in size is relatively unencumbered, albeit painful, by comparison to a gallstone or ductal calculus of similar size. Anatomical and physiological differences between the formation and flow of bile and urine are fundamental to the understanding of the potential efficacy of ESL in the treatment of biliary calculus disease. Bile formation is much slower than urine; a lower volume is produced each day, and it flows into the intestines at a much slower rate than urine flows into the bladder.[17] Furthermore, compared with the gallbladder, the kidney is a complex excretory-endocrine organ that receives a significant amount (25 percent) of the cardiac output. The kidney is a critical organ for the regulation of body fluid and electrolyte balance, whereas the gallbladder performs largely a reservoir or storage function for bile, which is produced in the liver. The biliary tree, however, unlike the ureter, is a complicated conduit system for the transport of bile and pancreatic enzymes into the digestive tract. Bile formation is critical to digestive function, including intestinal lipid absorption, endogenous waste production (bilirubin), and cholesterol metabolism.[17] Urine is a body waste product, and the consequences of at least unilateral urinary stone formation are less morbid to the target organ and body economy than the failure of bile formation, cholestasis, and obstruction by biliary calculi.

CALCULUS DISEASE

Precise prevalence data for gallstones in the general population are not available, but estimates of 10 to 20 percent exist for gallstone disease in developed countries.[18,19] However, renal calculi occur only in 2 to 3 percent of the population during a lifetime.[20,21] Patients with "silent" gallstones are usually asymptomatic.[20,21] The majority of gallstones are cholesterol stones (70 to 80 percent),[18] the rest being pigment stones (approximately 20 percent).[18] Mixed or pure cholesterol stones exist, with measurable pigment ranging from 40 to 95 percent (mean = 60 percent).[18] The rest of the components are mucoprotein, water, and protein. Calcium, bilirubinate, phosphate, and carbonate are common ions in pigmented stones. All types of gallstones may calcify, with the more frequent calcified pigment stones (radiographically) having central calcifications. For cholesterol stones, calcification is less frequent and may be either central or peripheral.[18] The pattern of calcification is important to detect with conventional radiography or CT, because ESL treatment and dissolution therapy is best directed at noncalcified biliary stones. Renal calculi rarely occur in pure form like cholesterol gallstones. They are made up of mucoproteinaceous matrix with crystalline aggregates of varying nature.[20,21] Most are dihydrate or monohydrate calcium oxylate stones, with calcium phosphate (apatite) and magnesium ammonium phosphate (struvite) being common as well. Urate stones are uncommon; and cystine, xanthine, or pure matrix stones are rare. The causes of gallstones and renal stones are complex and to some extent, unknown, but significant determinates for gallstone formation are discussed elsewhere in these proceedings.[18,20,21]

The hardness of renal calculi varies, with cystine, urate, and calcium monohydrate being among the hardest calculi and, therefore, among the most difficult to fragment. Noncalcified, cholesterol biliary calculi appear to fragment better[5,6] than those with any degree of calcification, although insufficient experience exists to date with ESL in a large number of biliary calculi with varied composition.[22-24] The size and number of renal or ureteral calculi and their location directly relate to degree of initial stone fragmentation and eventual passage. Additionally, the presence of obstruction affects eventual fragment clearance. The presence of urinary tract infection and stasis are other factors that bear on patient selection for renal ESL, and active infection is a contraindication. Likewise, with biliary ESL, since initial trials have been only on symptomatic patients, the role of positive signs and symptoms in terms of patient selection and outcome is still evolving.[5,6] Renal ESL has evolved beyond the treatment of merely symptomatic patients who would originally have been considered to be surgical candidates or candidates for percutaneous nephrolithotomy to a point today where smaller and less symptomatic urinary tract calculi are being treated, with the goal being avoidance of eventual symptomatology. Further refinement in criteria for patient selection, stone composition, and stone location will occur in the field of biliary lithotripsy as experience is gained. Early reports suggest that successful fragmentation of gallstones *does* depend on stone composition and density of surface calcification.[22]

EVOLUTION OF THERAPY

Growth and development of ESL of the urinary tract and now of the biliary tree have paralleled and often overshadowed those of competing technologies designed to nonoperatively relieve the organ system of its stone burden.[25–30] Rapid refinement and dissemination of percutaneous techniques for access to the kidney enabled development of the field of percutaneous nephrolithotomy (PCNL), coupling the skills and experience of interventional radiologists with endoscopic techniques developed by the urologic surgeon. Continued perfection of PCNL and endoscopic techniques has spawned the burgeoning field of *Endourology*.[9,10,31] Comparatively, percutaneous access to the biliary tree and gallbladder has recently appeared on the clinical scene,[32,33] enabling a variety of catheters, drainage tubes, electrodes and endoscopic instruments to be placed within the biliary system.[32–35] It took only 4 short years from 1980 to 1984 for the first water bath ESL unit to undergo metamorphosis from prototype device to production model for clinical human use.[1,3] The first water bath kidney lithotripter was installed in the United States at Methodist Hospital in Indianapolis, Indiana in early 1984.[11] Researchers at Klinikum Grosshadern, Ludwig-Maximilian University, Munich, combined their talents with engineers at Dornier Medical Systems to develop the first prototype kidney lithotripter, with which Chaussey and Schmiedt treated 200 patients by 1982.[3] These pioneering scientists discovered that an optimal shock wave for stone destruction was a pressure wave with a steep onset (less than 1 nanosecond), a slow decay time and a minimal tensile character.[3] Confirmation of the German experience with successful ESL for kidney stone treatment came in 1982 when the United States cooperative study of the first six sites (n = 2112 patients) reported a 77.4 percent stone-free rate at 3 months in patients who had a single kidney stone.[2] The best success was achieved with stones 1 cm or less in diameter, and only 0.6 percent of patients required open surgery to resolve stone problems.[2] Today, over 150 water bath ESL units exist in the United States, plus a growing number of non–water bath units in clinical trials. Two of the early reports of successful biliary tract ESL[5,6] are but harbingers of more clinical trials designed to duplicate the success already achieved with renal ESL in the same or perhaps shorter time frame. However, notable differences exist between the two modalities as well as their competitors (e.g., chemical dissolution, percutaneous or endoscopic access, and organ ablation). No good chemolytic agents exist for common variety renal calculi, whereas excellent results have been achieved with chemolysis in the biliary tree using both oral (chemodeoxycholic or ursodeoxycholic acid) and contact dissolution agents (monooctinoin and methyl tert-butyl ether [MTBE]).[25–28,31] Although sodium bicarbonate dissolves uric acid calculi, hemiacidrin dissolves struvite stones, and acetylcysteine dissolves cystine stones, these account for only a small percentage of symptomatic urinary tract calculi.[31] Most cholesterol gallstones will dissolve with MTBE, thereby making chemical dissolution a viable alternative to biliary ESL.[30] The adjunctive use of contact dissolution or oral medication in patients with gallstones places biliary ESL in a much less "stand-alone" category than renal ESL. The majority of patients with renal calculus disease are eligible for treatment with renal lithotripsy in spite of the considerable and widespread expertise with percutaneous techniques and endoscopy. Only distal or lower ureteral calculi are preferentially fragmented or removed under direct vision, using flexible deflectable endoscopes and electrohydraulic (EHL) or laser lithotripsy probes.[35,36] The long-term complications to the kidney, ureter, and urethra of direct visual stone fragmentation or extraction are unknown; but careful technique and adequate stenting have made complications uncommon. There is no renal corollary to gallbladder ablation, which although in its infancy as a clinical technique, shows some promise.[35] Only unsalvageable stone-laden kidneys are surgically removed today. Therefore, an unanswered question exists as to the future of the diseased or previously stone-laden gallbladder once biliary ESL has been performed. Additionally, it can only be speculated what impact direct endoscopic and percutaneous biliary stone fragmentation and removal will have on the number of patients undergoing extracorporeal shock wave therapy for biliary calculi.[35–38]

LITHOTRIPSY: RENAL VERSUS BILIARY

Comparison of an established technique such as renal and ureteral ESL, which has been used on more than 500,000 patients worldwide, with biliary ESL is formidable but, nonetheless, worthwhile. Many similarities exist, yet the stark distinctions can be better appreciated and pitfalls avoided by a careful comparison. Areas for correlation and review include patient selection; stone characteristics; imaging and intervention; procedural and technical aspects; results, short-term and long-term (i.e., stone-free rates); and complications.

PATIENT SELECTION

Rather broad guidelines exist for renal ESL as a result of the intense competition for patients among some ESL centers and the commonly held belief that ESL is nearly noninvasive with acceptably low incidence of serious side effects.[39,40] There are individual machine limitations in terms of patient height and weight, and there are requirements for anesthesia, which may preclude treatment of some patients, particularly in the spark-gap, water bath machines. Significant cardiac disease, that is, arrhythmias or pacemakers, also precludes treatment in water bath lithotripters and is a relative contraindication to treatment on other spark-gap energy devices. Furthermore, pregnancy, urinary tract infection, and bleeding diatheses remain ubiquitous contraindications. Non–water bath systems, for example EMAS* (Lithostar) or piezoelectric (PZE) devices do not have many of these patient limitations. However, the oversized patient will remain a treatment challenge on any device, and there is growing experience with treating pediatric patients successfully on several lithotripsy units.[41] Both symptomatic and nonsymptomatic patients with kidney and ureteral calculi are treated routinely today, and ESL monotherapy for large staghorn calculi is becoming more widespread.[42] Although there is every reason to expect that patient eligibility criteria for gallstone ESL will expand, a strict patient selection process is the rule in published reports to date. Only 6 percent of patients with symptomatic gallstones and 10 percent of symptomatic patients with common duct stones may be eligible.[5] The largest series to date found only 28 percent of its referred patients with symptomatic gallstone disease eligible for ESL.[6] The best success for ESL alone seems to be with common bile duct stones with or without sphincterotomy and small or solitary gallbladder calculi.[5,6,37,43] Cystic duct stones or intrahepatic duct stones, unlike ureteral calculi, present technical difficulties in terms of access and focusing.[37,43] Asymptomatic or so-called silent gallstones are not yet considered suitable for biliary ESL, but in all likelihood they will soon be treated, given the precedent set by renal ESL. Still most—60 to 70 percent—of all patients with renal calculi will pass their stones without the need for *any* intervention. Such statistics are not yet available for patients with biliary calculus disease. Surgery in the form of cholecystec-

---

*Electromagnetic acoustic source.

tomy is still the gold standard treatment for symptomatic patients with gallstone disease.

STONE CHARACTERISTICS

The most optimal results with renal ESL are for solitary renal pelvic calculi less than 1 to 1.5 cm in size and composed of calcium oxylate dihydrate or calcium phosphate.[1–4] The success rates for initial fragmentation decrease and the need for multiple treatments increases with increasing stone size and hardness.[1–4,44] Virtually all urinary tract calculi are calcified to some degree, and even urate, xanthine, cystine, and struvite stones may be minimally radiopaque or have calcific shells or rims. As the size and number of urinary tract calculi increase, the retreatment rate increases and the stone-free rates at any given follow-up interval decrease. Stone location is critical to the ultimate success of renal lithotripsy, and any obstruction requires prior alleviation or ureteral stent placement. Stones in calyceal diverticula, in excluded calyces, or proximal to ureteropelvic junction or ureteral narrowings require adjuvant intervention, either percutaneous nephrostomy or retrograde stent placement. Although some investigators treat first and stent, splint, or drain later, the pre-ESL and post-ESL intervention rates are higher when obstruction is present.[1–4] Total stone burden is also a determining factor when renal ESL is used adjunctively to chemical dissolution or irrigation, either for uric acid stones using sodium bicarbonate or for struvite stones using hemiacidrin.

Similar to the early trials with renal ESL, the most optimal treatment results for biliary ESL have been achieved with low gallstone burden or ductal stones of a pure cholesterol variety.[5,6] Only lately have calcified biliary stones or pigmented stones been attempted with ESL; and early results, at least in vitro, suggest that some clinical success can be anticipated with these types of calculi as well.[22] Whether significant amounts of calcification (hard gallstones) will present the same impediment to successful ESL that exists for calcium monohydrate or cystine renal calculi is still unknown.[44] Any obstruction, real or potential, to the gallbladder, common duct, or intrahepatic or cystic duct must be relieved prior to or shortly after biliary ESL. However, the requirement of some early trials for endoscopic sphincterotomy in all cases appears to be unnecessary with current biliary ESL techniques. Preliminary knowledge of the various stone characteristics is critical for lithotripsy in either the urinary tract or biliary system, but less so with renal ESL because most urinary tract calculi can be fragmented. However, in the biliary tree, adjunctive therapies, either oral or contact dissolution, may be necessary; there is therefore a more critical need for careful pre-ESL stone evaluation.[45]

IMAGING AND INTERVENTION

Radiological imaging tests are critical to the entire ESL process. Correctly performed and interpreted, urography, sonography, or CT scanning is a major part of the renal ESL patient evaluation process. Treatment with ESL of "nonstones," for example, rib ends, aneurysms, phleboliths, neoplasms, can and should be avoided. Radionuclide imaging is also of value pre- and post-ESL for assessment of renal function. Patient selection and targeting require a thorough knowledge of the imaging chain, whether TV fluoroscopy or real-time high-resolution ultrasound. Opacification, either intravenously or retrograde with radiopaque contrast material, is often required to target poorly calcified renal or ureteral calculi. The same armamentaria of imaging tests, both cross-sectional and functional, are required to assess size, number, location, hardness, and composition of biliary calculi and hepatic or gallbladder function prior to ESL. Interventional and/or endoscopic expertise is also required for stent and drainage tube placement for renal ESL, and some of these procedures require radiographic and fluoroscopic capabilities.

In addition to the pre-ESL requirements for imaging evaluation, intercurrent imaging, by either real-time ultrasound or fluoroscopy, is critical to the technical success of these procedures. Targeting problems are unique to different ESL systems, but consistent location and surveillance during treatment using radiography, fluoroscopy and now ultrasound are mandatory for urinary tract ESL. The targeting and intertreatment stone focusing is even more difficult when using ultrasound for renal ESL, and similar difficulties are encountered using ultrasound for biliary ESL, particularly given the resolution of real-time ultrasound and the prone positioning requirements for some patients. Large patients will attenuate the sound beam or will be hard to bring into the focal zone for ESL, thereby requiring treatment with alternative techniques such as intracorporeal shock wave lithotripsy. As the trend toward low or no anesthesia ESL continues in the kidney with increase in the number of shock waves and number of treatments to obtain optimal fragmentation, the same experience can be expected with biliary lithotripsy. Manufacturers continue to lower the energy of the individual shock wave devices to achieve so-called painless ESL.[4,46] This will increase the pressure on the initial imaging evaluation to correctly predict both suitable patient and suitable stone for treatment.

Post–renal ESL interventional procedures all require imaging, usually radiograpy or fluoroscopy, for ureterorenoscopy and percutaneous nephrostomy, but the incidence of such procedures remains low, between 2 to 10 percent in most practices. Post-ESL ultrasound, CT, or MRI are performed only on symptomatic patients or for guidance during the performance of an interventional procedure. Routine pre- and post-ESL ultrasound has been largely abandoned, since mild degrees of hydronephrosis do not correlate with patient symptoms or requirements for intervention. Most patients who develop ureteral "steinstrasse" post-ESL will pass their stones without intervention, but ureteral obstruction increases with increasing size and number of stones treated. The incidence and consequences of cystic duct or common bile duct "steinstrasse" are unknown, but judging from initial reports, appear to be low or inconsequential. Patients with large stone burdens have yet to be treated and followed long enough to know if biliary "steinstrasse" will be a significant problem. Intravenous urography has been the mainstay for the post-ESL evaluation, but noninvasive imaging tests such as ultrasound, CT, MR and radionuclide studies may be the major imaging tests used for optimal patient follow-up after biliary ESL, with ultrasound playing a major triage role.

TREATMENT METHODOLOGY AND RESULTS

The trend in renal ESL is rapidly away from water bath lithotripsy with its significant anesthesia requirements owing to the higher energy of the shock wave toward non–water bath, lower energy (EMAS or PZE), anesthesia-free ESL performed on an outpatient basis.[4] Treatment time increases slightly with lower energy shock wave units, but patient complications decrease with the same goal, that being a successfully fragmented renal or ureteral calculus.[4,46,47] These same trends have been duplicated in the early-generation biliary lithotripters, which use little or no radiography and fluoroscopy since ultrasound guidance is a major design feature. No water bath is required but a water path, water cushion, or water-filled contact device couples the shock wave generator to the patient. Patient positioning, for example, prone, supine or lateral, will depend on the type of shock wave generator and/or integrated table design of the biliary lithotripter. Requirements for anesthesia will vary with the type of shock wave used; and low or no anesthesia lithotripsy in the kidney is a reality, with marked success achieved using transcutaneous electrical nerve stimulation (TENS) and the Lithostar unit for renal ESL.[47] Targeting will require avoidance of lung, bowel, and bony structures, no matter which form of shock wave energy is used. The trade-offs to such advances as respiratory gating, lower energy shock waves, and smaller focal zones will be increased treatment time and number of treatments. Strict adherence to the basic principles of adequate coupling and optimal targeting will assure that the shock wave hits only the stone, minimizing local tissue damage. The endpoint for renal or biliary ESL, however, is the same: a fragmented stone of a particle size small enough to pass (2 to 4 mm or less in the kidney) or dissolve and a stone-free patient at a particular follow-up interval. More than one treatment and adjunctive use of chenodeoxycholic or ursodeoxycholic acid will depend on gallstone characteristics, location, and number. The smaller the fragments created, the better the overall results for renal lithotripsy; thus a similar goal exists for biliary lithotripsy, as the success of chemical dissolution is related to stone surface area. The initial fragment size affects the overall efficacy of renal ESL and the stone-free rates at follow-up periods between 3 months and 1 year. Stone recurrence or retention rates are high depending on initial stone location, particularly for lower calyceal stones. A 50 percent retained fragment rate was reported for all locations of kidney stones by Miles and associates[12] from the University of Florida at Gainesville.[12] The follow-up interval and the number of patients followed vary from institution to institution. Newman and colleagues[11] at Methodist Hospital in Indianapolis, Indiana, report only 54 percent of patients available at the 3-month follow-up interval; overall stone-free rates were 65 percent. This increased to 73 percent at 1 year for a smaller follow-up group.[11] Likewise, the follow-up period was short in the largest published series for gallstone ESL, with only 25 of 175 patients followed at 3 months.[6] The follow-up of renal ESL patients has raised other issues related to complications of the treatment. Hypertension requiring medication has been reported in 8 to 9 percent of patients undergoing water bath ESL,[40,48,49] and some loss of renal function as measured by radionuclide study has been associated with simultaneous bilateral water bath renal ESL treatment.[49] Pulmonary emboli, deep venous thrombosis, myocardial infarction, cerebral vascular accident, urosepsis, renal and perirenal hemorrhage, and required blood transfusion have all been noted or reported from large series of patients undergoing water bath ESL. Liver, lung, and pancreas injury, cholangitis, cholecystitis, and, of course, biliary colic have all been noted in animal and patient biliary ESL investigations.[2,50 55] Long-term complications of biliary ESL are still unknown, but stone recurrence rates after surgical cholecystectomy and oral dissolution therapy alone are known and can be anticipated to be similar for biliary ESL in the absence of intervention or oral dissolution therapy. The major question relates to the long-term effects of ESL on the gallbladder left in situ. Answers will be forthcoming only after considerable follow-up and research into techniques for gallbladder ablation. Reported complications for biliary ESL are few to date, with an apparent low morbidity, including emergency surgery and no reported mortality.[5,6]

THE RADIOLOGIST'S ROLE

The role of the imaging specialist or interventionalist in ESL in general and renal ESL specifically is evolving as newer generation units are developed and tested. The original lock on lithotripsy obtained by urologists has given way to a more reasoned approach with shared expertise and resources for the ultimate benefit of the patient.[56,57] Radiologists experienced in the interpretation of common or complex imaging studies, radiation protection, quality assurance, and quality control of medical imaging equipment, and those with special skills for passage of catheters and guidewires, have helped advance the field of renal lithotripsy to a position where it is the optimal method for treatment of patients with symptomatic kidney stones. With the entry of over 10 manufacturers to the renal lithotripsy marketplace, further improvements and better utilization of the technology will occur. Whether biliary ESL will be hailed as "an authentic modern miracle" by the Department of Health and Human Services, and truly lower the cost of medical care for patients with gallstones as was predicted for renal ESL, remains to be seen.[15,58] However, the team approach combining the skills and expertise of radiologists with surgeons and gastroenterologists is much more the rule than the exception as biliary lithotripsy is introduced.[38,59] Referral patterns and working relationships between angio-interventional radiologists, surgeons, and gastroenterologists already exist, and most percutaneous biliary intervention is performed by radiologists in the United States.[19,32,38] Cooperative efforts between gastroenterologists and radiologists in the performance of endoscopic studies (e.g., ERCP, gallbladder ultrasound, and upper gastrointestinal fluoroscopy), make biliary lithotripsy a logical extension of this diagnostic and treatment relationship between the specialties. Certainly parallel developments in endoscopic and percutaneous techniques to access the biliary tree will occur with, perhaps, encroachment on the number of patients eligible for biliary lithotripsy; this has already occurred for urinary tract, where ureterorenoscopy is a common technique for treatment of lower ureteral calculi. But, "beware the bearer of early results" may be coined as a caution, since there are many precedents in modern medicine where a panacea has been promised but never delivered. Drawing retrospectively on the many uroradiological similies to biliary lithotripsy, a plea must be made for good science and proper scientific evaluation of this exciting, yet emergent technology. As the many unknowns of this "slam bang" technology, such as a proper energy source and a proper imaging chain, are unraveled, the indications for treatment will broaden appropriately, increasing patient eligibility (with a resultant increase in workload for many specialists), particularly if the uroradiologic precedents are any example. The workload and patient load of many radiology departments and hospitals have already dramatically increased with renal lithotripsy. Furthermore, the team approach to biliary lithotripsy should provide enlightenment to the medical and surgical care of patients with gallstone disease, rather than the sense of encroachment on any one specialty's procedures, and ideally a rapprochement between disciplines and physicians separated or excluded from early clinical utilization of renal ESL.

REFERENCES

1. Chaussy CG, Schmiedt E: Extracorporeal shock wave lithotripsy (ESWL) for kidney stones: An alternative to surgery? *Urol Radiol* 1984; 6:80–87.
2. Drach GW, Dretler S, Fair W, et al: Report of the United States Cooperative study of extracorporeal shock wave lithotripsy. *J Urol* 1986; 135:1127.
3. Fuchs GJ, Chaussy CG: Extracorporeal shock-wave lithotripsy: An update. *Endourology* 1987; 2:1.
4. Wilbert DM, Reichenberger H, Noske E, et al: New generation shock wave lithotripsy. *J Urol* 1987; 138:563.
5. Sauerbruch T, Delius M, Paumgartner G, et al: Fragmentation of gallstones by extracorporeal shock waves. *N Engl J Med* 1986; 314:818.
6. Sackmann M, Delius M, Sauerbruch T, et al: Shock-wave lithotripsy of gallbladder stones: The first 175 patients. *N Engl J Med* 1988; 318:393.
7. Burhenne HJ, Fache JS, Gibney RG, et al: Biliary lithotripsy by extracorporeal shock waves: Integral part of nonsurgical intervention. *AJR* 1988; 150:1279.
8. Riehle RA, Fair WR, Vaughan ED: Extracorporeal shock-wave lithotripsy for upper urinary tract calculi: One year's experience at a single center. *JAMA* 1986; 255:2043.
9. Erturk E, Lange PH, Hulbert JC: Percutaneous and extracorporeal management of urolithiasis. *Invest Radiol* 1987; 22:995.
10. Bush WH, Gibbons RP, Lewis GP, et al: Impact of extracorporeal shock wave lithotripsy on percutaneous stone procedures. *AJR* 1986; 147:89.
11. Newman DM, Lingeman JE, Mertz JHO, et al: Extracorporeal shock-wave lithotripsy. *Urol Clin North Am* 1987; 14:63.
12. Miles SG, Kaude JV, Newman RC, et al: Extracorporeal shock-wave lithotripsy: Prevalence of renal stones 3–21 months after treatment. *AJR* 1988; 150:307.
13. Petitti DB: Competing technologies: Implications for the costs and complexity of medical care. *N Engl J Med* 1986; 315:1480.
14. Mulley AG, Carlson KJ, Dretler SP: Extracorporeal shock-wave lithotripsy: Slam-bang effects, silent side effects? *AJR* 1988; 150:316.
15. Mulley AG: Shock-wave lithotripsy: Assessing a slam-bang technology. *N Engl J Med* 1986; 314:845.
16. Becker JM, Moody FG: Sphincter of Oddi and biliary motility, in Condon RE, DeCosse JJ (eds): *Surgical Care II*. Philadelphia, Lea & Febiger, 1985.
17. Scharschmidt BF: Bile formation and gallbladder and bile duct function, in Sleisenger MH, Fordtran JS (eds): *Gastrointestinal Disease*. Philadelphia, Saunders, 1983, pp 1346–1355.
18. Holzbach RT: Pathogenesis and medical treatment of gallstones, in Sleisenger MH, Fordtran JS (eds): *Gastrointestinal Disease*. Philadelphia, Saunders, 1983, pp 1356–1373.
19. Burhenne HJ: The promise of extracorporeal shock-wave lithotripsy for the treatment of gallstones. *AJR* 1987; 149:233.

20. Van Arsdalen KN: Pathogenesis of renal calculi. *Urol Radiol* 1984; 6:65.
21. Goldwasser B, Weinerth JL, Carson CC: Calcium stone disease: An overview. *J Urol* 1986; 135:1.
22. Petersen BT, Thistle JL: Comparison of shock wave lithotriptors for fragmentation of human gallstones in vitro and assessment of variables influencing efficacy. Presented at the American Gastroenterological Association, New Orleans, Louisiana, May 15–18, 1988 (in preparation).
23. Michaels EK, Fowler JE: Inadvertent fracture of gallstones during extracorporeal shock wave lithotripsy. *J Urol* 1986; 136:1285.
24. Becker CD, Fache S, Gibner RG, et al: Treatment of retained cystic duct stones using extracorporeal shockwave lithotripsy. *AJR* 1987; 148:1121.
25. Schoenfield LJ, Lachin JM, et al: Chenodiol (chenodeoxycholic acid) for dissolution of gallstones: The National Cooperative Gallstone Study—a controlled trial of efficacy and safety. *Ann Intern Med* 1981; 95:257.
26. Bachrach WH, Hofmann AF: Ursodeoxycholic acid in the treatment of cholesterol cholelithiasis. *Dig Dis Sci* 1982; 27:737.
27. Thistle JL, Carlson GL, Hofmann AF, et al: Monooctanoin, a dissolution agent for retained cholesterol bile duct stones: Physical properties and clinical application. *Gastroenterology* 1980; 78:1016.
28. Allen MJ, Borody TJ, Bugliosi TF, et al: Rapid dissolution of gallstones by methyl tert-butyl ether: Preliminary observations. *N Engl J Med* 1985; 312:217.
29. Neubrand M, Sauerbruch T, Stellaard F, et al: In vitro cholesterol gallstone dissolution after fragmentation with shock waves. *Digestion* 1986; 34:51.
30. Pitt HA, McFadden DW, Gadacz TR: Agents for gallstone dissolution. *Am J Surg* 1987; 153:233.
31. Clayman RV, Castaneda-Zuniga W: *Techniques in Endourology: A Guide to the Percutaneous Removal of Renal and Ureteral Calculi*. Dallas, Heritage Press, 1984.
32. vanSonnenberg E, Hofmann AF: Horizons in gallstone therapy: 1988. *AJR* 1988; 150:43.
33. Wholey MH, Smoot S: Choledocholithiasis: Percutaneous pulverization with a high-speed rotational catheter. *AJR* 1988; 150:129.
34. Becker CD, Quenville NF, Burhenne HJ: Long-term occlusion of the porcine cystic duct by means of endoluminal radio-frequency electrocoagulation. *Radiology* 1988; 167:63.
35. Becker GJ, Kopecky KK: Can the newer interventional procedures replace cholecystectomy for cholecystolithiasis? The potential role of percutaneous cystic duct ablation. *Radiology* 1988; 167:275.
36. Jenkins AD: Laser lithotripsy. *J Urol* 1986; 139:1076.
37. Becker CD, Fache JS, Gibney RG, et al: Choledocholithiasis: Treatment with extracorporeal shock wave lithotripsy. *Radiology* 1987; 165:407.
38. Ferrucci JT: Biliary lithotripsy: What will the issues be? *AJR* 1987; 149:227.
39. Goldsmith MF: Stones are crushed and many patients elated by results of new ESWL therapy. *JAMA* 1986; 256:437.
40. Williams CM, Kaude JV, Newman RC, et al: Extracorporeal shock-wave lithotripsy: Long-term complications. *AJR* 1988; 150:311.
41. Kramolowsky EV, Willoughby BL, Loening SA: Extracorporeal shock wave lithotripsy in children. *J Urol* 1987; 137:939.
42. Winfield HN, Clayman RV, Weyman PJ: Monotherapy of renal calculi: Comparative study between percutaneous nephrolithotomy and extracorporeal shock wave lithotripsy. *J Urol* 1988; 139:895.
43. Meyer WW, Hottenrott CH: Lithotripsien intrahepatischer Gallensteine. *Dtsch med Wsch* 1986; 111:1280.
44. Dretler SP: Stone fragility: A new therapeutic distinction. *J Urol* 1986; 139:1124.
45. Baron RL: CT/MR imaging characteristics of gallstones. Proceedings of the First International Symposium on Biliary Lithotripsy, July 11–13, 1988, Boston, Massachusetts.
46. Graff A, Schmidt J, Pastor D, et al: New generator for low pressure lithotripsy with Dornier HM3: Preliminary experience of 2 centers. *J Urol* 1988; 139:904.
47. Fernandez J, Clayman RV, McClennan BL, et al: Transcutaneous electrical nerve stimulator: An approach to anesthesia free shockwave lithotripsy with the Lithostar unit. *J Endourol* (in press).
48. Lingeman JE, Evans AP, Wood JR, et al: The biological effects of shockwaves and the risk of hypertension following ESWL. *J Urol* 1988; 139:291A.
49. Thomas R, Sloane B, Roberts J: Effect of extracorporeal shockwave lithotripsy on renal function. *J Urol* 1988; 139:323A.
50. Krongrad A, Kirschenbaum A, Saltzman B: Case report: Biliary obstruction complicating extracorporeal shock wave lithotripsy. *J Urol* 1988; 139:344.
51. Karawi MAA, Mohamed ARE-S, El-Etaibi KE, et al: Extracorporeal shock-wave lithotripsy (ESWL)-induced erosions in upper gastrointestinal tract: Prospective study in 40 patients. *Urology* 1987; 30:224.

52. Delius M, Enders G, Heine G, et al: Biological effects of shock waves: Lung hemorrhage by shock waves in dogs—pressure dependence. *Ultrasound Med Biol* 1987; 13:61.
53. Rubin JI, Arger PH, Pollack HM, et al: Kidney changes after extracorporeal shock wave lithotripsy: CT evaluation. *Radiology* 1987; 162:21.
54. Papanicolaou N, Stafford SA, Pfister RC, et al: Significant renal hemorrhage following extracorporeal shock wave lithotripsy: Imaging and clinical features. *Radiology* 1987; 163:661.
55. Roth RA, Beckmann CF: Complications of extracorporeal shock wave lithotripsy and percutaneous nephrolithotomy. *Urol Clin North Am* 1988; 15:155.
56. Barth KH, Pahira JJ, Elliott LP: Extracorporeal shockwave lithotripsy: Role of the radiologist. *Radiology* 1985; 155:835.
57. Pollack HM, Banner MP: Extracorporeal shock wave lithotripsy and the radiologist. *AJR* 1986; 147:94.
58. Hofmann AF: Bile, bile acids, and gallstones: Will new knowledge bring new power? *AJR* 1988; 151:5.
59. Goldsmith MF: Biliary, as well as urinary, calculi become the targets of new, improved shock wave lithotripsy. *JAMA* 1987; 258:1282.

An Introduction to Bile Formation and Physiology

James M. Richter

Bile formation begins in the liver, where the components are formed by hepatocytes and secreted into intrahepatic canaliculi by active transport and are followed by passively transported water. Eighty-two percent of hepatic bile is an isotonic fluid with an electrolyte composition similar to that of plasma, totaling about 600 milliliters daily. Other components in bile include bile acids, phospholipids and lecithin, and cholesterol (Table 1). Cholesterol, which is the principal component of most gallstones, comprises only about 1 percent of hepatic bile.

The organic components of bile are particularly important. Cholesterol is largely insoluble in an aqueous milieu and is dependent on other organic constituents for solubilization. Bile acids are amphophiles which are soluble in water and, with lecithin, the principal phospholipid, form micelles that hold cholesterol in solution. Physiologic concentrations of bile salts solubilize some cholesterol, but the addition of lecithin increases cholesterol solubilization fourfold. Cholesterol is solubilized in the gallbladder and in the bile by the formation of micelles with the polar groups of the bile acids and lecithin in an aqueous environment.

TABLE 1.

Hepatic Bile Composition

Isotonic fluid (electrolytes similar to plasma)	82%
Bile acids	12%
Pospholipids (including lecithin)	5%
Cholesterol	1%

At steady states, 0.3 to 0.6 grams of primary bile acids are synthesized in the liver daily. They are principally cholic acid and chenodeoxycholic acid. After conjugation with glycine and taurine to taurocholic and glycocholic acids, they are secreted into the intrahepatic canaliculi. Secondary bile acids are bacterial metabolites formed in the intestine; the major ones are deoxycholic acid and lithocholic acid. Ursodeoxycholic acid is a minor secondary bile acid.

After secretion from the liver and passage down the biliary tree into the intestine, both conjugated and unconjugated bile acids are passively absorbed throughout the intestine. More important, conjugated bile acids are actively reabsorbed in the distal ileum. In aggregate, the intestine reabsorbs about 95 percent of these bile acids, about 3 to 4 grams daily, leading to a daily loss of fecal bile acids of about 0.3 to 0.6 grams. These reabsorbed secondary bile acids are then extracted from the portal circulation by the liver. This action tends to suppress the formation of further primary bile acid through homeostatic feedback. Again there is a total bile pool of 3 to 4 grams per day, which recirculates approximately 5 to 10 times daily. If the bile acid pool is increased by oral chenodeoxycholic acid, hepatic bile acid formation decreases. Ursodeoxycholic acid does not inhibit endogenous bile acid formation significantly.

Decreased bile acid formation or impaired intestinal absorption may reduce the bile acid pool and its recirculation. This may be due to the effects of cholestyramine combining with bile acids to form a product that cannot be absorbed, thereby increasing the excretion of bile acids and inhibiting the digestion of dietary cholesterol. Other causes include ileal disease, resection or bypass of the intestines, and delayed gallbladder emptying.

After hepatic bile is formed, it passes into the gallbladder. In the fasting state, the gallbladder stores approximately 50 milliliters of bile. In the normal gallbladder, bile is concentrated approximately eightfold by active reabsorption of electrolytes and osmotic reabsorption of water. There is also some passive reabsorption of organic constituents of gallbladder bile, principally cholesterol. The clinical importance of this reabsorption is uncertain.

During fasting, the gallbladder sequesters bile, reabsorbing fluid and interrupting the enterohepatic flow. Therefore, potentially less bile acids are entering the gallbladder and the balance of phospholipids, bile acids, and cholesterol may be changed. This is one of the physiologic circumstances in which gallbladder bile may become supersaturated with cholesterol and cholesterol crystallization may occur. During the eating process, fatty acids and amino acids enter the duodenum and stimulate the secretion of cholecystokinin. This relaxes the sphincter of Oddi in the normal state, causing contraction of the gallbladder and restoring the intrahepatic circulation of the bile salts.

The cholesterol *Saturation Index* is defined as the relative degree of cholesterol saturation in the bile as determined by the chemical composition. A cholesterol saturation index of "one" is complete saturation; greater than one is supersaturation, which occurs in many normal individuals during fasting. Supersaturation does not inherently indicate abnormal bile, because in many individuals there are periods during the fasting and eating cycles when gallbladder bile is supersaturated by crystallization and stone formation does not occur. Many additional factors are necessary for or contribute to stone formation.

TABLE 2.
Mechanism of Abnormal (Lithogenic) Bile

Diminished bile acid synthesis
Diminished bile acid reabsorption
Excess cholesterol secretion
Gallbladder factors
Combinations

Factors that promote the formation of supersaturated bile are diminished bile acid synthesis, diminished reabsorption of bile acid, excess cholesterol secretion, factors affecting the function of the gallbladder, and combinations of these factors, (Table 2). Clinically, these correlate with overproduction of cholesterol owing to obesity, diabetes, clofibrate, hyperlipidemia, increased dietary fat, and the decreased catabolism of cholesterol. The resultant cholesterol stones are the most common of all gallstones and are the focus of the most recent advances in clinical treatment for gallstone disease.

Pigment stones, however, account for about 20 percent of gallstones and are of significant clinical concern. Their formation is much different from that of cholesterol stones. Normally bilirubin in bile is conjugated and highly soluble. Unconjugated bilirubin, however, is insoluble and may precipitate as a calcium salt forming bile pigment stones. Generally, factors that decrease bilirubin in conjugation may lead to the formation of pigment stones. Pigment stones may result from intrabiliary deconjugation of bile pigment owing to stasis or chronic infection in the biliary tree. Hemolytic diseases increasse bile pigment production, and age or cirrhosis may diminish the ability of the liver to conjugate pigment and may lead to pigment stone formation.

Composition and Classification of Gallstones

Edwin L. Prien, JR.

The analysis and classification of gallstones have lagged behind those of urinary stones, and for good reasons. Gallstones present special analytic problems among biologic concretions as they contain major amounts of noncrystalline bile pigment, which has been difficult to study. In fact, pigment has been ignored entirely in some classifications of gallstone composition. The presence of pigment obscures important tinctorial characteristics of crystalline components on both gross inspection and microscopical examination.

ANALYTICAL METHODS

Table 1 lists the common analytic methods with their advantages, disadvantages, and sensitivities. Simple inspection of "morphologic description" is surprisingly effective, especially with a little practice. Cholesterol stones are white or tan, and pigment stones are dark brown or black. However, pigment is so intensely dark that it is easy to overestimate the amount present. Also calcium salts are not apparent by this method.

TABLE 1.

Methods of Analysis

	ADVANTAGES	DISADVANTAGES	SENSITIVITY
Inspection (morphological)	Simple; "works"	Overestimates pigment; can't see calcium	—
Radiograph	Widely available	Can't see cholesterol; can't see pigment	—
Chemical	"Historical"	Insoluble residue; alters compounds; elements, radicals	—
Polarization microscopy	Rapid; structural detail; small samples	variable specificity; subjective; requires crystallinity; pigment obscures;	(0.1%)
X-ray diffractometry (XRD)	Very specific	Larger samples; time-consuming; requires crystallinity; very expensive	5–10%
Infrared spectroscopy IR (dispersive)	Specific; tiny samples; no crystallinity; quantitative	Mixtures of similar compounds a problem; expensive	5–10%
Fourier Transform Infrared spectroscopy (FTIR)	Same as above; very sensitive	Very expensive	0.5–1.0%

The plain radiograph is widely available and can be or some help but only in defining the presence or absence of significant amounts of calcium salts. Both cholesterol and pigment are radiolucent and not appreciated without contrast.

Chemical analsis by "wet" chemical techniques has been used from the beginning but is mainly of historical interest. A major limitation is the poor solubility of stone components. In pigment stones as much as 66 percent of the dry weight remains insoluble and therefore unanalyzed. Also chemical methods measure mainly elements or radicals while providing no information on their pairing to form compounds or the crystalline phases that define the solution chemistry.

Modern crystallographic methods have greatly simplified and improved calculus analysis. Polarization microscopy, x-ray diffraction, and, more recently, infrared spectroscopy have proved very useful especially when employed in concert. Furthermore, these three methodologies utilize the same starting material, namely, crushed but otherwise unaltered stone.

Polarization microscopy allows rapid analysis of small samples. Although it can have great sensitivity, pigment in gallstones tends to conceal the tinctorial qualities of crystals and may obscure other optical properties and constants.

X-ray diffraction measures the interplanar spacings between like atoms in the crystalline array and provides a unique result for every crystalline substance. Since most pigment is calcium bilirubinate or its polymer, and since it is mostly noncrystalline, it does not register. For this reason stone classifications based on x-ray diffraction have not been widely accepted.

For gallstones, infrared spectroscopy is the most useful. The specimen is irradiated with a spectrum of infrared wavelengths that induce the molecular bonds to vibrate at characteristic frequencies. The result is a kind of chemical (rather than crystallographic) analysis. It can deal with small samples and can be quantitative. Most important, crystallinity is not required. However, the commonly available instruments (dispersive instruments) suffer from suboptimal sensitivity in the study of mixtures. With some luck analyses can be guided by visual inspection, polarization microscopy, or even plain radiograph to isolate minor components for direct study. But if the component is dispersed though-out the stone below the 10 percent level, it will not be detected.

Fourier transform infrared spectroscopy (FTIR) is evolving rapidly as the methodology of choice. It is quite expensive but, depending on the machine, is capable of significantly increased sensitivity.

GALLSTONE COMPONENTS

In Table 2 the common gallstone components are listed in order of decreasing abundance. Also comment is made as to the radiodensity of each component as it would appear on the clinical radiograph. Cholesterol monohydrate or, if stored in air, the anhydrous form, is most abundant, being either white or tan with generally obvious crystallinity. Pigment is amorphous and either brown and soft or black and brittle. In spite of the fact that it is composed of calcium bilirubinate and its polymers, its radiodensity is minimally increased over that of cholesterol and it remains radiolucent on clinical radiographs. This difference is apparent, however, in Hounsfield units obtained with computerized axial tomography.[1] Calcium carbonate in any of its three polymorphic crystalline forms is radio-

TABLE 2.
Gallstone Components

	OPAQUE/LUCENT
Cholesterol monohydrate (anhydrous)	L
Pigment:calcium bilirubinate (brown)	L
bilirubinate polymers (black)	L
Calcium carbonate:vaterite	O
calcite	O
aragonite	O
Calcium phosphate: apatite	O
Calcium palmitate	L
Others: bilirubin	L
bile pigments	L
protein	L
glycoprotein	L

dense, as is calcium phosphate in its typically complex biologic phase known as hydroxy- or carbonate-apatite. Calcium palmitate is a newly appreciated species especially in the West and will be commented on later. It would be considered radiolucent.

The substance that has caused the most confusion is calcium bilirubinate. In fact, its attributes read like a riddle.

1. All gallstones contain pigment especially and importantly in the center of the stone. And yet, because pigment is poorly soluble and noncrystalline, it has been largely ignored.

2. Most of this universally occurring pigment is calcium bilirubinate. Yet, the gallstone category termed "calcium bilirubinate" (and more recently, "brown pigment" stones) was thought to exist only in the Orient.

3. Unlike calcium carbonate and calcium phosphate it is a calcium salt that is not radiodense and its occurrence is not confined to calcium-containing calculi.

It has been regularly noted that many gallstones contain all of the above listed components (except for calcium palmitate). This has led to the perception that all gallstones are fundamentally the same. As recently as 1964 Bogren[2] reviewed his considerable experience and wrote:

> All biliary calculi are essentially built up the same way. There is pigment at the centre and the remainder of the stone contains cholesterol monohydrate, pigment and inorganic calcium salts in different proportions and with varying distribution from stone to stone. The pure pigment stone may seem to be a special type of gall stone, but it might equally well be regarded as derived from a central (pigment) nucleus . . . . There is consequently no reason to seek to classify gall stones, since they have all probably the same aetiology, and since there does not seem to be any real qualitative difference between them.

GALLSTONE CLASSIFICATION

With refined quantitative techniques utilizing primarily infrared spectroscopy, it has become clear that gallstones fall nicely into two or three major categories, based on composition. The nomenclature, which has recently been revised, defines these types as cholesterol, black pigment, and brown pigment. Each type may be further subdivided according to the presence or absence of the radiopaque calcium salts, calcium carbonate and calcium phosphate. Table 3 is a composite of analytic results from the very active group at the University of Pennsylvania Medical School. Although cholesterol and black pigment stones contain entirely the same constituents, it can readily be appreciated that for two of the components, cholesterol and pigment, there is no overlap between the two categories. Cholesterol stones contain very little pigment, and black pigment stones contain little cholesterol. There are few if any calculi with intermediate composition. Calcium carbonate and calcium phosphate occur in both groups, although more often and in greater amounts in black pigment stones. By clinical radiographs 93 percent of cholesterol stones are lucent, while only 50 percent of pigment stones are calcified.[6] Consequently, classification of cholesterol and pigment stones by the criterion of radiodensity will result in a 17 percent overall misclassification.

So while qualitatively similar, the two major stone types may be differentiated by quantitative analysis. Since these two categories are morphologically and chemically distinct, the presumption is that they are etiologically distinct as well. However, in an interesting study of stone centers the University of Pennsylvania group made some provocative observations.[7] As expected calcium bilirubinate was found in the centers of cholesterol calculi. There was, however, a relative absence of calcium carbonate and calcium phosphate, suggesting that cholesterol stones are not formed on otherwise typical pigment stones as a center. Surprisingly, there was more cholesterol in the centers of pigment stones than in the peripheries. These observations raise the possibility that there is some process or substance present at the time of formation or nucleation of these dissimilar stone types which binds both cholesterol and pigment. Mucin resulting from gallbladder hypersecretion and being a component of biliary sludge is one candidate for this function.[8] Perhaps Bogren was correct. The fundamental etiology may be the same.

The third stone category is that of brown pig-

TABLE 3.

Composition and Type of Gallstone*

	GALLBLADDER			COMMON DUCT
	CHOLESTEROL, USA (n = 31)	BLACK PIGMENT, USA (n = 25)	BROWN PIGMENT, JAPAN (n = 16)	BROWN PIGMENT, USA (n = 22)
Cholesterol	85.2 ±1.9 (60–109)	2.1 ± 1.0 (0–25)	10.9 ±1.8 (1.9–27.8)	10.1 ±1.8 (0.6–35.0)
Pigment	0.49 ± 0.07 (0–1.4)	34.4 ± 3.1 (9.8–80)	62.8 ±6.8 (27.8–78.7)	52.7 ±5.2 (7.3–85.8)
Carbonate	0.53 ±0.4 (0–8.6)	6.7 ± 1.9 (0–35)	0 0	1.7 (one = 37.7)
Phosphate	0.95 ±0.3 (0–7.8)	7.7 ± 2.1 (0–32)	0.1 ± 0.06 (0–0.8)	0.4 ±0.1 (0–2.7)
Palmitate	0 0	0 0	25.4 ±4.1 (11.7–66.8)	16.5 ±1.9 (5.0–35.3)
Total calcium	1.53 ±0.6 (0–6)	9.4 ± 1.3 (1.7–25)	5.9 ±0.3 (3.2–8.4)	3.4 ±0.7 (1.7–18.6)
Total measured	89.4 ±1.5 (75–110)	63.7 ± 3.6 (36–98)	105 ±3.9 (69–142)	82.5 ±4.3 (43.7–100)

*Values are percentage initial dry weight expressed as mean ± SEM with range in parentheses. Adapted from references 3–5.

ment stones, which appears to be an important though less common stone disease. This entity known also as bile pigment-calcium, calcium bilirubinate, and "earthy" stone disease was thought to exist almost exclusively in the Orient in the presence of bile infected with bacteria and parasites. So common was such biliary infection, especially after World War II, that brown pigment stone disease accounted for 60 percent of all gallstones in Japan.[9] The current incidence is closer to 20 percent. The hallmark of this event is the signal presence of calcium palmitate thought to be derived from the breakdown of phospholipid lecithin by bacterial phospholipases. The stones themselves are described as soft and brown with yellowish concentric laminations representing calcium palmitate. However, a word of caution is in order here. Black pigment stones can appear brown and may have tan striations or laminations of cholesterol.

The evidence is mounting that infection precedes the stones and is not simply secondary to them. In 1988 the University of Pennsylvania group reported a study of 56 sets of common bile duct calculi collected over a 10-year period from patients in the United States.[5] Forty-three percent of the stones were cholesterol; 18 percent were black pigment stones; and 39 percent were brown pigment stones. Many of the biliary stones were doubtlessly primary (and conventional) gallbladder stones missed at cholecystectomy; therefore, special attention was paid to stones removed 21 months or longer post-cholecystectomy. Of these, 59 percent were brown pigment stones. The conclusion seems inescapable that although brown pigment stones represent only about 1 percent of gallbladder calculi, they constitute the majority of primary biliary stones and presumably result from biliary infection. The finding of calcium palmitate in gallstones would appear to carry the same significance as the finding of struvite (magnesium ammonium phosphate) in urinary calculi. A particular infection is present and is etiologically important. However, in these stones calcium palmitate is not the major component and could often be missed with analytic techniques of suboptimal sensitivity.

We now have three major categories of gallstone composition as defined by quantitative analysis. In the United States 75 percent of gallbladder stones are cholesterol, 24 percent are black pigment, and about 1 percent are brown pigment. In the biliary tree brown pigment stones probably constitute the majority of primary biliary calculi. Although cholesterol and black pigment stones may have different etiologies, it is possible that they may have the same fundamental etiology being preciptated about centers of similar composition. The composition of the bulk of the stone would then be governed by differing physicochemical characteristics of the patient's bile. Brown pigment stones are likely the result of biliary infection which may be a sequela of cholecystectomy.

REFERENCES

1. Hickman MS, Schwesinger WH, Bova JD, et al: Computed tomographic analysis of gallstones. *Arch Surg* 1986; 121:289–291.
2. Bogren H: The composition and structure of human gall stones. *Acta Radiol [Suppl] (Stockh)* 1964; 226:7–74.
3. Trotman BW, Morris TA, Sanchez HM, et al: Pigment versus cholesterol cholelithiasis: Identification and quantification by infrared spectroscopy. *Gastroenterology* 1977; 72:495–498.
4. Soloway RD, Trotman BW, Maddrey WC, et al: Pigment gallstone composition in patients with hemolysis or infection/stasis. *Dig Dis Sci* 1986; 31:454–460.
5. Malet PF, Dabezies MA, Huang G, et al: Quantitative infrared spectroscopy of common bile duct gallstones. *Gastroenterology* 1988; 94:1217–1221.
6. Trotman BW, Petrella EJ, Soloway RD, et al: Evaluation of radiographic lucency or opaqueness of gallstones as a means of identifying cholesterol or pigment stones. *Gastroenterology* 1975; 68: 1563–1566.
7. Malet PF, Williamson CE, Trotman BW, et al: Composition of pigmented centers of cholesterol gallstones. *Hepatology* 1986; 6:477–481.
8. Lee SP, Nicholls JF: Nature and composition of biliary sludge. *Gastroenterology* 1986; 90:677–686.
9. Trotman BW, Soloway RD: Pigment gallstone disease: Summary of the National Institutes of Health—International Workshop. *Hepatology* 1982; 2:879–884.

Epidemiology of Gallstone Disease

E. Roda, A. M. Morselli Labate, C. Sama, D. Festi, and L. Barbara

INTRODUCTION

The epidemiology of gallstones has been debated for many years in the medical literature. However, the overall impression of an increasing incidence of the disease and the conventional wisdom as to risk factors are mainly based on data from clinical observation, necroscopy series, or surgical records.

Because reliable epidemiological studies provide important information regarding the etiology, risk factors, and natural history of cardiovascular disease, in the last few years gastroenterologists have focused their attention on the epidemiology of gallstones. Two additional facts have further supported this renewed interest in gallstones: the spread of ultrasound techniques and the availability of new therapeutic nonsurgical approaches, such as litholytic bile acids, local solvents, and lithotripsy.

Decisions about whether to administer therapy (cholecystectomy, medical dissolution, lithotripsy) should be based in part on estimates of prognosis or natural history. In practice, however, which patients, when, and how to treat are matters of heated controversy.

Only prospective studies in large population groups can give a real insight into the problem, mainly because a large proportion of gallstones remains asymptomatic and ignored, but these studies necessitate simple and noninvasive techniques for detecting gallstones.

Ultrasonography, besides having high sensitivity and specificity compared with the traditional x-ray procedures, is simple, safe, and noninvasive.

In recent years many ultrasound studies on the epidemiology of gallstones have been undertaken, especially after the publication of two Italian studies: the GREPCO[1, 2] and the Sirmione[3] studies. The first is a study based on a selected occupational group in Rome (male and female civil servants); the second studied a free-living population of a town in the north of Italy.

For the Sirmione study, we selected all subjects aged 18 to 65 of both sexes living in the town of Sirmione, which is located on Lake Garda. The study was planned as a longitudinal 5-year examination of the population of Sirmione; 70.6 percent of the selected population participated.

Owing to the results of these two studies, in 1985 a group of Italian researchers under the supervision of the Italian National Institute of Health initiated a multicenter study (MICol: Multicenter Italian Study of Cholelithiasis) composed of 18 peripheral units in different parts of Italy (including us), in order to determine the prevalence, associated factors, and natural history of gallstone disease.

PREVALENCE AND INCIDENCE OF GALLSTONE DISEASES

Autopsy studies[4–6] had the great merit of indicating racial and geographical differences in the prevalence of gallstones (Fig 1). Prevalence seems to be higher in Europe and the Americas

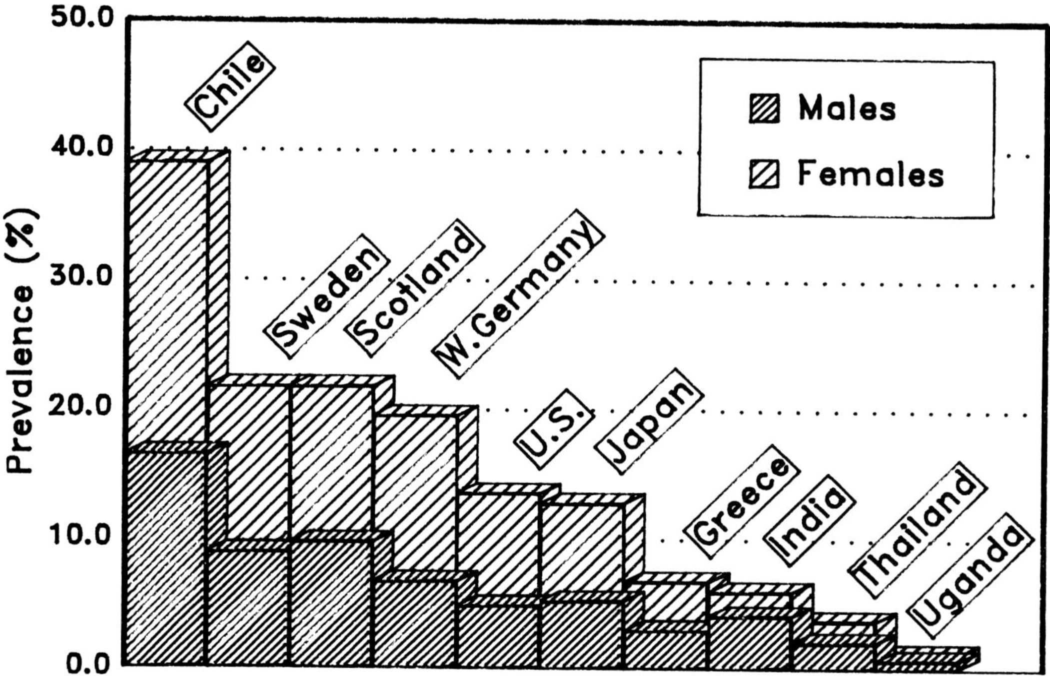

FIG 1.
National differences in the prevalence of gallstone disease observed in autopsy studies.

and lower in Eastern countries and Africa. Studies on the American Indians have shown a very high prevalence (more than 70 percent over the age of 50 years), which is probably the highest prevalence detected in the world.[7]

Apart from these studies, two major reports on the epidemiology of gallstones were published in the pre-echographic era: the Framingham[8] and the Bainton[9] studies.

The Framingham study reported "clinical prevalence," that is, cases obtained from clinical practice. The bias of this, and other similar studies,[10, 11] is to underestimate the prevalence of gallstone disease because of the large proportion of asymptomatic cases not seeking medical care. In the Framingham study, the overall prevalence was 3.9 percent, and the incidence, calculated over 10 years, was 4.5 percent.

Bainton and colleagues performed oral cholecystography on a weighted sample of the population of an industrial town in South Wales. Reported prevalence of gallstone disease was 9.2 percent.

The first study, published in the echographic era was the GREPCO[1] study based on a population of female civil servants in Rome. The reported prevalence of gallstone disease in 1082 women aged 20 to 64 was 9.4 percent. Later the same group of researchers published a study on a population of male civil servants in Rome, in which the prevalence was 8.2 percent.[2]

In 1982 we started the Sirmione study, which showed an overall prevalence of gallstone disease at entry of 11 percent.[3] Preliminary results of the MICol study indicates a prevalence of 19 percent.

Five years later in Sirmione we were able to obtain the first data on incidence of gallstone disease, which showed a figure of 3 percent in 5 years (unpublished personal data).

RISK FACTORS IN GALLSTONE DISEASE

Prevention of cholelithiasis, still at a very early stage, depends largely on a clear understanding of events concerning pathogenesis and risk factors. Although many factors have been considered in recent years, the current literature on the epidemiology of gallstone disease makes it very difficult to support clinical impressions with statistics.

However, most of these risk factors are supported by prevalence data or clinical studies. Risk factors for pigment stones are mainly related to the concomitant pathological condition, and risk factors for cholesterol gallstones are more related to metabolic conditions. We will now consider the major putative risk factors for gallstones in the West, where cholesterol gallstones predominate.

AGE

Both prevalence and incidence of gallstone disease seem to increase with age. These impressions have been supported in the past by autopsy[5, 12] and clinical studies[13] and have been confirmed by the Framingham study.[8]

The South Wales study[9] failed to find a positive correlation between gallstones and age. This is probably due to the fact that the age span considered in this study (45 to 69 years) was not wide enough to allow a sufficient distribution of subjects in different age groups.

Both the GREPCO[1] and the Sirmione[3] studies showed that the prevalence of gallstone disease increased steadily with age in both sexes. Moreover, in the Sirmione study (unpublished personal observation) the 5-year incidence rate was about four times higher in the age span 40 to 69 years than in younger subjects. Interestingly (Fig 2) the cut-off point between relatively low and high incidence rates seems to be 40 years; incidence seems to be fairly stable from the middle age to elderly.

SEX

Autopsy studies[4] have shown in the past that, at least in the West, females have a higher frequency of gallstones.

However, the male-female ratio seems to have changed from the very first reports, which showed figures of 1:4–6, to recent years, when the ratio has been 1:2 or less.[8, 9, 13]

This trend has been confirmed by the prevalence study in Sirmione, where a significantly higher prevalence of gallstone disease in females was observed in all age groups, with a female-male ratio of 2:1.

The causes of this difference are not fully understood at present. Pregnancy and sex hormones could be involved by altering biliary secretion and/or gallbladder motility.

An astonishing result comes from the 5-year incidence in Sirmione. In fact, the incidence was slightly, but not significantly, higher in males than in females (Fig 2). If this result is confirmed by the 10-year incidence study, we could hypothize that once again sex-related differences are changing in the present era, as has been observed for other diseases (heart disease, lung cancer, etc.)

PREGNANCY

Pregnancy is thought by many investigators to promote gallstone formation. In both the GREPCO[1] and Sirmione[3] studies, the prevalence of gallstones increased with the number of pregnancies. Furthermore, both studies demonstrated that the increase in the relative risk due to pregnancy is higher among younger than among older women.

This finding has been confirmed in Sirmione as far as the incidence is concerned. In fact, no new cases of gallstone disease have been observed in women with no pregnancies in 1982 versus 3.3 percent in pregnant women (unpublished personal observation).

Pregnancy could influence gallstone formation in several ways. Composition of bile may be altered adversely by hormonal changes during pregnancy. Recent studies[14] have shown sluggish gallbladder emptying during the third trimester of pregnancy. This could induce gallstone formation by altering bile acid enterohepatic circulation and promoting retention of cholesterol crystals, the prerequisite for gallstone formation. In addition, rapid weight variations during and after pregnancy can influence biliary lipid secretion.

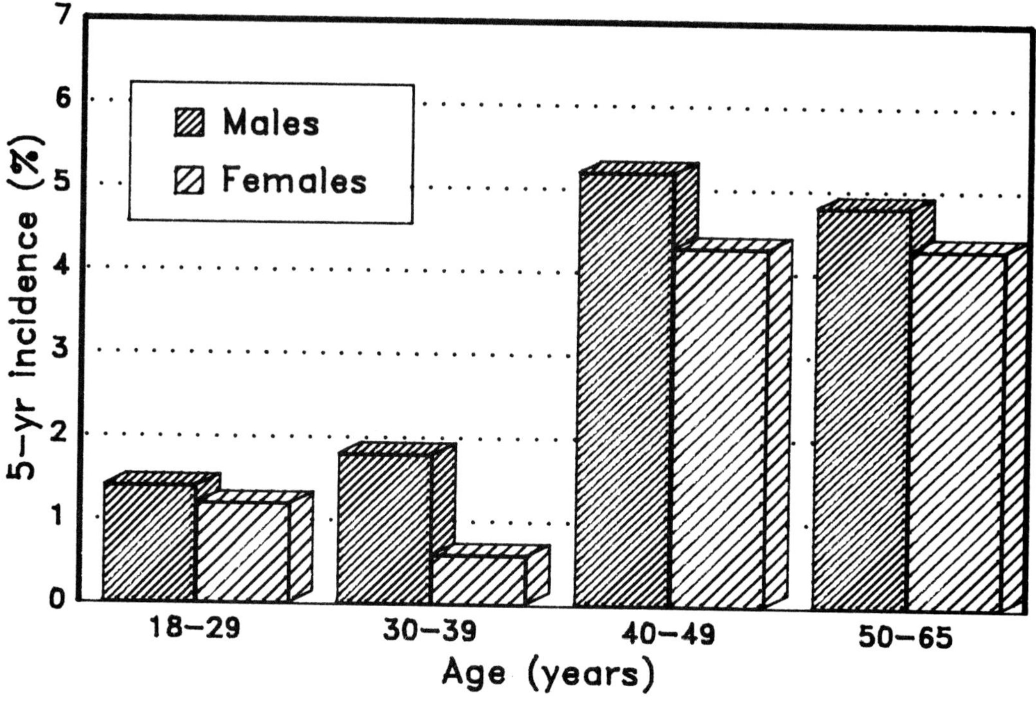

FIG 2.
Sex and age distribution of 5-year incidence of gallstone disease in the Sirmione study.

OBESITY

Many clinical and epidemiological studies indicate that cholesterol gallstones are more common in obese subjects. For instance, the Framingham study[8] has shown a positive correlation between gallstones and obesity. In agreement with previous reports, obesity is associated with a higher frequency of gallstones in both the GREPCO[1] and the Sirmione studies[3]. In the Sirmione study, we have also found that gallstone incidence is about three times higher in obese than in nonobese subjects (unpublished personal data). Moreover, the Sirmione study showed that the risk of developing gallstones for currently obese subjects is higher in the lower age groups.

The link between obesity and gallstones is supersaturated bile. Obesity raises the saturation of bile by increasing biliary secretion of cholesterol, the latter depending probably on a higher synthesis of cholesterol in obese subjects.

SERUM LIPIDS

In the West, serum cholesterol levels do not seem to be higher in gallstone sufferers than in normal subjects. This has been confirmed by both the Framingham[8] and the Sirmione[3] studies. Moreover, in the GREPCO study,[15] cholesterol serum levels were found to be inversely related with the prevalence of gallstones, confirming the early observation in Pima Indians,[7] where a high prevalence of gallstones was associated with low cholesterol serum levels. Hypertriglyceridemia was found to be associated with a higher frequency of gallstones in the prevalence study in Sirmione. However, this finding was not confirmed by the incidence study.

CHARACTERISTICS OF THE STONES AND SYMPTOMS

No conclusive data yet exist regarding the possible relationship between the physicochemical properties of gallstones and the natural history of gallstone disease. In particular, it is not known whether any inherent characteristics of stones predispose them to cause symptoms. Data from surgical series[16, 17] indicate that large solitary stones and multiple small stones more frequently provoke biliary symptoms and complications, such as acute cholecystitis and gallbladder cancer.

Different information derives from the study of Mok and co-workers.[18] Studying the chronology of gallstones with profiles of ^{14}C incorporated into human organs from the $^{14}CO_2$ in the atmosphere resulting from nuclear bomb tests as a growth indicator, these authors did not find any difference between symptomatic and asymptomatic subjects in terms of growth period and yearly growth rate.

Floating stones and multiple stones were found to be closely related to the development of biliary symptoms in the National Cooperative Gallstone Study, a double-masked, placebo-controlled, therapeutic trial of chenodeoxycholic acid for gallstone dissolution.[19]

This result was obtained in the placebo group (305 patients with radiolucent gallstones in functioning gallbladders), during an ancillary study aimed at evaluating the natural history of gallstone disease.

The predictive value of gallbladder function with respect to clinical outcome was investigated by McSherry and co-workers[20] in an evaluation of the natural history of both symptomatic and asymptomatic gallstone patients. These authors concluded that patients with nonvisualization of the gallbladder present a higher frequency of symptoms and are more likely to have, at surgery, acute cholecystitis than patients with a visualized gallbladder.

The epidemiologic studies on the general population have provided the first data on the x-ray characteristics of gallbladder and stones in unselected series of cases. In the GREPCO study,[21] the occurrence of biliary colic in the 5 years previous to the study or an awareness of having gallstones was not related to the x-ray appearance of gallstones.

In the Sirmione study, multiple stones of whatever size were significantly related to the presence of specific biliary symptoms; no correlation was found between symptoms and type of the stones (unpublished personal data).

NATURAL HISTORY OF GALLSTONES

Over the past decade, several therapeutic alternatives to cholecystectomy for the treatment of gallstone disease have become available, oral bile acid treatment with chenodeoxycholic and ursodeoxycholic acids,[22] and more recently innovative techniques such as local solvents[23] and extracorporeal lithotripsy.[24]

Moreover, epidemiologic studies on large population samples[1-3] have confirmed that about 80 percent of gallstones are asymptomatic. These studies have underscored the need to define more precisely the natural history of untreated gallstones in order to better define the risk-benefit ratio of different treatments. Reports concerning untreated gallstones have been infrequent and sometimes difficult to compare with each other.

In the past, many texts have indicated that up to 50 percent of persons with silent gallstones will develop biliary symptoms or complications and that complications make gallstones symptomatic. Several studies carried out in the last 40 years have tried to define the natural history of gallstones. Unfortunately, many of the studies failed to fulfill the criteria for a correct natural history study.

In many instances, dyspeptic symptoms were grouped together with specific biliary symptoms when defining the population at risk and the rate of appearance of symptoms. We and others[3] have demonstrated that dyspeptic symptoms are not related to the presence of gallstones. As a second point, most studies on the natural history of gallstones have grouped together truly symptomatic gallstone patients, subjects with infrequent or mild symptoms, and asymptomatic subjects. The natural history of the disease is perhaps different in these categories of gallstone subjects. Nevertheless, it seems that the natural history of asymptomatic stones is fairly benign. In a study published by Gracie and Ransohoff on a group of faculty members at the University of Michigan, the incidence rate of biliary symptoms in 10 to 20 years was 18 percent.[25] However, persistence or recurrence of symptoms has been observed in about 50 percent of symptomatic patients.[20, 26–29]

In Sirmione we conducted a follow-up study for the 132 subjects who had gallstones in their gallbladder in 1982. At this time 103 were asymptomatic. After 5 years, 3 of the 132 gallstone subjects had died (2 asymptomatic) and 18 had failed to complete the follow-up (12 asymptomatic).

In the group of 89 asymptomatic subjects who completed the follow-up, 15 developed biliary symptoms but no complications. Of the group of 22 subjects who were symptomatic in 1982, 10 needed a cholecystectomy and 12 still have gallstones. Interestingly, 9 of them did not suffer from biliary symptoms during the 5 years of follow-up. In this study, therefore, the rate of development of biliary symptoms over 5 years in a previously asymptomatic subject was 16.8 percent. This figure is somewhat higher than that of Gracie and Ransohoff but has to be controlled during the next years of follow-up. In fact, of the 15 subjects who developed symptoms, 11 did so during the first 2 years of follow-up.

CLINICAL LESSON FROM EPIDEMIOLOGY

Together with G. Paumgartner, D. L. Carr-Locke, and J. L. Thistle, we have developed an algorithm for the therapy of gallbladder stones (Fig 3) for presentation to the September 1988 International Congress of Gastroenterology in Rome. The large series of numbers, derived from epidemiologic studies, may be useful in clinical practice in order to answer the question

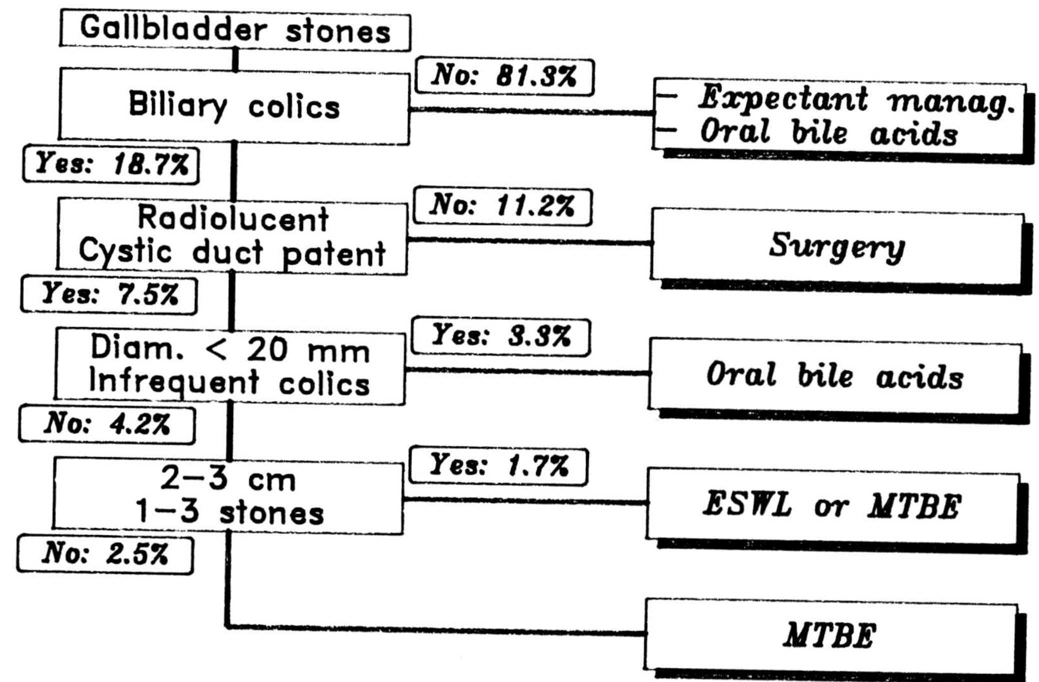

FIG 3.
Algorithm for therapy of gallbladder stones.

of how many patients are available for each possible treatment. Using the Sirmione and MICol (Bologna experience only) studies, we have completed the algorithm with quantitative data.

The algorithm shows that patients with gallbladder stones without biliary colic are suitable for expectant management and/or for oral bile acid treatment. If biliary colic is present the stones are radiopaque, or the gallbladder is not visualized at x-ray examination, surgery is the treatment of choice. If the stones are radiolucent with a diameter smaller than 2 cm and the colics are mild and infrequent, oral bile acid therapy may be considered. In all the other situations, ESL or MTBE must be considered.

In order to answer these questions we need:

A. Data about the presence of symptoms:
   - 18.7 percent of gallstone patients are symptomatic.

B. Data about the stones:
   - 40 percent of the stones are radiolucent, 29 percent are radiopaque, and 31 percent occur in a nonfunctioning gallbladder.
   - 44 percent of the stones are less than 2 cm in diameter.
   - 23 percent of the patients have stones between 2 and 3 cm in diameter and no more than 3 stones in the gallbladder.
   - 33 percent of the patients have large and numerous stones.

Using these data we estimate (Fig 3) that 81 percent of the patients are suitable for expectant management and/or bile acid therapy, 11 percent for surgery, and the remaining for oral bile acid treatment, ESL, and MTBE.

If the data on the prevalence of gallstone disease obtained in the Sirmione study are applied to the Italian general population, the number of gallstone patients in our country should be 2,241,000. Of these gallstone subjects, 419,000 would be symptomatic, 251,000 would be suitable for surgery, and 168,000 would be suitable for other nonsurgical treatments, such as contact dissolution using MTBE or ESL.

The data in the algorithm are based on the assumption that every case is identified by the physician. Even if we are now able to predict how many patients in Italy have gallstones, we still cannot apply these data to any individual patient because of the high frequency of asymptomatic stones, which results in many patients being completely unaware that they have gallstones. Furthermore, even some of the symptomatic subjects are unaware that their symptoms indicate gallstone disease. Therefore, the evaluation of a management approach and its socioeconomic implications must be based on calculations made on documented cases of gallstone disease.

The expanded application of ultrasound in diagnosis and epidemiologic studies on the general population will allow the identification of asymptomatic and symptomatic gallstone patients.

Finally, controlled trials or decision analysis approaches using the scientific method can be used to define the optimal management approach to gallstone disease. When that occurs, such debates will be eliminated, patient care will improve, and the physician and the patient will experience less indecision.

REFERENCES

1. GREPCO: Prevalence of gallstone disease in an Italian adult female population. *Am J Epidemiol* 1984; 119:796–805.
2. GREPCO: The epidemiology of gallstone disease in Rome, Italy. Part I. Prevalence data in men. *Hepatology* 1988 (in press).
3. Barbara L, Sama C, Morselli Labate AM, et al: A population study on the prevalence of gallstone disease: The Sirmione study. *Hepatology* 1987; 7:914–917.
4. Torvik A, Hoivik B: Gallstone in an autopsy series. *Acta Chir Scand* 1960; 120:168–174.
5. Zahor S, Sternby NH, Kagan A, et al: Frequency of cholelithiasis in Prague and Malmö: An autopsy study. *Scand J Gastroenterol* 1974; 9:3–7.
6. Brett M, Barker DJP: The world distribution of gallstones. *Int J Epidemiol* 1976; 5:335–341.
7. Sampliner RE, Bennet PH, Courres LJ, et al: Gallbladder disease in Pima Indians: Demonstration of high prevalence and early onset by cholecystography. *N Engl J Med* 1970; 283:1358–1364.
8. Friedman GD, Kamel WB, Dawber TR: The epidemiology of gallbladder disease: Observation in the Framingham study. *J Chron Dis* 1966; 19:273–292.
9. Bainton D, Davies GT, Evans KT, et al: Gallbladder disease: Prevalence in a South Wales industrial town. *N Engl J Med* 1976; 294:1147–1149.

10. Diehl AK, Rosenthal M, Hazuda HP, et al: Socioeconomic status and the prevalence of clinical gallbladder disease. *J Chron Dis* 1985; 38:1019–1026.

11. Hanis CL, Ferrell RE, Tulloch ER, et al: Gallbladder disease epidemiology in Mexican Americans in Starr County, Texas. *Am J Epidemiol* 1985; 122:820–829.

12. Newman HF, Northrup JD: The autopsy incidence of gallstones. *Int Astr Surg* 1949; 109:1–13.

13. Holland C, Heaton KW: Increasing frequency of gallbladder operations in the Bristol area. *Br Med J* 1972; 3:672–675.

14. Braverman DZ, Johnson ML, Kern F. Jr: Effect of pregnancy and contraceptive steroids on gallbladder function. *N Engl J Med* 1980; 302:362–364.

15. Angelico F, GREPCO: Factor associated in the gallstone disease: Observations in the GREPCO study, in Capocaccia L, Ricci G, Angelico F, Angelico M, Attili AF (eds): *Epidemiology and Prevention of Gallstone Disease*. Lancaster (UK), MPT Press, 1984, pp 185–192.

16. Schein CJ, Elliot SH, Rosenblatt MA: The significance of calculous size in determining the indication for elective cholecystectomy. *Gastroenterology* 1955; 29:377–380.

17. Diehl AK, Beral V: Cholecystectomy rates and changing mortality from gallbladder cancer. *Lancet* 1981; 2:187–190.

18. Mok HYI, Druffel ERM, Rampone WM: Chronology of cholelithiasis. Dating gallstones from atmospheric radiocarbon produced by nuclear bomb explosion. *N Engl J Med* 1986; 314:1075–1077.

19. Thistle JL, Cleary PA, Lachin JM, et al: The natural history of cholelithiasis: The National Cooperative Gallstone Study. *Ann Intern Med* 1984; 101:171–175.

20. McSherry CK, Ferstenberg H, Carlhoun F, et al: The natural history of diagnosed gallstone disease in symptomatic patients. *Ann Surg* 1985; 202:59–63.

21. GREPCO: Radiological appearance of gallstones and its relationship with biliary symptoms and awareness of having gallstones. Observations during epidemiological studies. *Dig Dis Sci* 1987; 32:349–353.

22. Roda E, Bazzoli F, Morselli Labate AM, et al: Ursodeoxycholic acid vs. chenodeoxycholic acid as cholesterol dissolving agents: A comparative randomized study. *Hepatology* 1982; 2:804–810.

23. Allen MJ, Borody TJ, Bugliosi TF, et al: Rapid dissolution of gallstones in humans using methyl tert-butyl ether. *N Engl J Med* 1985; 312:217–220.

24. Sauerbruch T, Delius M, Paumgartner G, et al.: Fragmentation of gallstones by extracorporeal shock waves. *N Engl J Med* 1986; 314:818–822.

25. Gracie WA, Ransohoff DF: The natural history of silent gallstones. *N Engl J Med* 1982; 307:798–800.

26. Wenckert A, Robertson B: The natural course of gallstone disease: Eleven year review of 781 nonoperated cases. *Gastroenterology* 1966; 50:376–381.

27. Newman HF, Northup JD, Rosenblum M, et al: Complications of cholelithiasis. *Am J Gastroenterol* 1968; 50:476–496.

28. Comfort MW, Gray HK, Wilson JM: The silent gallstone: A ten to twenty year follow-up study of 112 cases. *Ann Surg* 1948; 128:931–937.

29. Lund J: Surgical indication in cholelithiasis: prophylactic chlecystectomy elucidated on the basis of long-term follow-up on 526 non-operated cases. *Ann Surg* 1960; 151:153–162.

Gallstones: Statistical Considerations

Greg Freiherr

Gallstone disease is among the most common and least appreciated ailments in the world. On the basis of accumulated clinical data, an estimated 20 million Americans now have gallstones and another million will develop the disease each year. Although the prevalence is believed to hover around 10 percent, at least in Western industrialized nations, many more individuals are likely to have so-called silent stones. These cases are now being discovered with greater frequency as ultrasonography and CT scanning are being applied to large populations. Gallstones do not cause clinical symptoms unless they migrate and obstruct the cystic duct or common bile ducts, producing such problems as biliary colic or cholecystitis. Because many stones do not cause symptoms, assessing the true magnitude of gallstone disease has been difficult. Also complicating the assessment is the apparent geographic variance of gallstone incidence.

The average incidence of gallstones in European countries, for example, is believed to be about 25 percent.[1] In one study, performed in a German industrial town, the prevalence of gallstones was examined in 11,800 consecutive autopsies done from 1940 to 1975. The overall prevalence was 20.7 percent; 13.1 percent for men and 33.7 percent for women.[2] However, population study using ultrasonography to determine gallstone disease in the town of Sirmione, Italy, found an overall prevalence of just 11 percent; 6.7 percent in men and 14.6 percent in women ranging in age from 18 to 65.[3]

Some countries have extraordinarily high rates. In 14,768 autopsy records obtained from three university hospitals in Chile, 45 percent of women and 20 percent of men older than 20 years of age had gallstone disease.[4]

Although gallstone disease is believed to be rare in Africa, a recent study indicates that the clinical conditions resulting from the disease may themselves be underreported. A review of 100 cases of cholecystectomy performed at Baragwanath Hospital in South Africa from 1983 to 1985 found that the correct diagnosis of cholecystitis, obstructive jaundice, pancreatitis, or biliary colic was made on admission in only 41 percent of the cases. An average of 5 days passed before patients were correctly diagnosed. The researchers concluded that greater awareness of acute cholecystitis may be necessary in the black patient.[5] One may also wonder if the political climate and lack of extensive health care systems for certain segments of the population in some countries might result in underreporting.

Conversely, the incidence of symptomatic gallstones in Sweden appears to be actually declining as indicated by decreasing numbers of cholecystectomies and positive oral cholecystograms. Over a 10-year period, the cholecystectomy rate was reduced to 57 percent of the rate at the beginning of the study period, and the proportion of pathological cholecystograms was reduced to 35 percent of the beginning rate.[6]

In the United States, a nation of more than 237 million, an estimated 750,000 persons are discharged each year from short-term stays in nonfederal hospitals, with a diagnosis of cholelithiosis, according to the National Center for Health Statistics (NCHS). Of these cases, which are estimates based on the recently published National Health Survey, about 90 percent involve calculi of the gallbladder and 10 percent involve calculi of the bile duct. Approximately 16.4 percent of cholelithiasis cases are estimated to be complicated by acute cholecystitis.

Geography plays an important statistical role in the evaluation of cholelithiasis, even within nations. According to the NCHS, the southern United States has the largest number of cholelithiasis cases, followed by the north central, northeastern, and then western states. Accounting for regional population differences, however, the highest incidence is found in the north central states, followed by the northeastern, southern, and western states.

The majority of Americans—about 80 percent—form "cholesterol" stones, so named because they are composed of about 70 percent cholesterol, with lesser amounts of calcium salts, bile acids, bile pigments, fatty acids, proteins, and phospholipids. The remaining 20 percent form pigment gallstones that are composed primarily of calcium bilirubinate.

Based on data from the National Health Survey, the NCHS also concludes that gallstone incidence increases with patient age from virtually zero for those aged 15 or younger to 11.29 per 1000 persons over age 65. The next highest incidence—4.88 per 1000—appeared among persons aged 45 to 64.

Sex may also be a predictive factor, as the incidence appears to be higher in women than in men, although recent data has raised some doubts about the absolute legitimacy of this conclusion for all age groups. The NCHS data show that cholelithiasis is more prevalent in females than males, with women accounting for 68 percent of all cases. The largest difference, however, appears in the 15- to 44-year-old age group, in which female cases outnumber male cases five to one. Virtually no difference is apparent in the incidence of cholelithiasis among males and females aged 65 or older.

The connection between a higher occurrence of gallstones and advancing age is perhaps the single most important factor driving the development of alternatives to surgical intervention, particularly the noninvasive techniques of ESL and oral bile acid therapy. Whereas the overall mortality rate is just 1 percent from cholecystectomy—the therapy of choice for most patients with acute cholecystitis, porcelain gallbladder, or occlusion of the cystic duct—clinical reports indicate that the mortality rate jumps to about 10 percent in patients over the age of 70.

The increased surgical risk is reflected in the caution already being exercised with patients aged 65 and over. Whereas NCHS data indicate that 0.81 cholecystectomies are performed per diagnosed case of cholelithiasis for patients in the 15 to 44 age bracket, the ratio of surgical procedures per case decreases to 0.47 per diagnosed case in the age 65 plus category—even though this group experiences the highest incidence of cholelithiasis.

REFERENCES

1. Wechsler JG, Wenzel H, Swobodnik W, Splitt S, Janowitz P, Ditschuneit H: Dietary modification of bile lipids. *Leber Magen Darm* 1988; 18(1):46–54.
2. Balzer K, Goebell H, Breuer N, Ruping KW, Leder LD: Epidemiology of gallstones in a German industrial town (Essen) from 1940–1975. *Digestion* 1986; 33(4):189–197.
3. Barbara L, Sama C, Morselli Labate AM, Taroni F, Rusticali AG, Festi D, Sapio C, Roda E, Banterle C, Puci A, et al: A population study on the prevalence of gallstone disease: The Sirmione Study. *Hepatology* 1987; 7(5):913–917.
4. Nervi F, Duarte I, Gomez G, Rodriguez G, Del Pino G, Ferrerio O, Covarrubias C, Valdivieso V, Torres MI, Urzua A: Frequency of gallbladder cancer in Chile, a high-risk area. *Int J Cancer* 1988; 41(5):657–660.
5. Parekh D, Lawson HH, Kuyl JM: Gallstone disease among black South Africans. A review of the Baragwanath Hospital experience. *S Afr Med J* 1987; 72(1):23–26.
6. Norrby S, Fagerberg G, Sjodahl R: Decreasing incidence of gallstone disease in a defined Swedish population. *Scand J Gastroenterol* 1986; 21(2):158–162.

Overview of Bile Acid Adjuvant Therapy with Gallstone Lithotripsy

Mumtaz Ahmed

The era of extracorporeal shock wave lithotripsy (ESL) began in 1980 with fragmentation and elimination of renal calculi without surgical incision.[1,2] It is now the treatment of choice for most kidney stones less than 20 mm in diameter. Extracorporeal shock wave lithotripsy for small kidney stones is cost-effective, and the morbidity is less than that of open renal surgical procedures. A natural outcome of successful renal lithotripsy is to extend this technology to the management of gallstone disease. Cholelithiasis is much more prevalent than renal lithiasis, affecting approximately 20 million individuals in the United States. The course of the disease is highly unpredictable and may progress to biliary tract obstruction, jaundice, sepsis, hepatic injury, and even carcinoma of the gallbladder. If gallstone lithotripsy is found to be efficacious, safe, and cost effective, it will undoubtedly play a major role in the management of cholelithiasis, cholecystitis, and choledocholithiasis.

NEED FOR ADJUVANT THERAPY

For obvious anatomic reasons, it is unlikely that lithotripsy alone will be sufficient for removing all gallstone fragments from the pear-shaped gallbladder. In contrast, mechanical fragmentation of the kidney calculi by lithotripsy more or less guarantees a spontaneous passage of shattered stones through the ureter along with urine flow. Although invasive interventions to remove fragmented stones have been reported, they are uncommon following kidney lithotripsy. Gallbladder contractility is of paramount importance in the expulsion of gallstones. However, contractility is often impaired in inflammatory or chronic fibrosing gallstone disease and the trauma from shock waves might further affect it adversely. In addition, the cystic duct through which stone fragments must pass is narrow and tortuous because of mucosal duplications forming the spiral fold of Heister; and the common bile duct, unlike the ureter, lacks peristaltic activity. In an inflamed gallbladder, the pocket-like invaginations of the neck mucous glands may extend as pseudodiverticula and trap fragmented stones and other debris. Furthermore, sharp-edged fragments resulting from lithotripsy can act as irritants and cause abrasion or erosion of mucosa if not physically removed or dissolved promptly. Some of these fragments can also serve as nucleating agents in a cholesterol supersaturated bile—a likelihood in the majority of patients receiving lithotripsy.

Without litholytic adjuvant therapy, the stone fragments must be reduced by lithotripsy to a size that can easily pass through the tortuous cystic duct, the common bile duct, and the narrow ampulla of Vater. Obstruction to bile flow may lead to complications such as biliary colic, cholecystitis and cholangitis. Stone impaction at the orifice into the duodenum would induce reflux of bile up the main pancreatic duct, causing pancreatitis. In order to pulverize a gallstone(s) to sand-size particles to minimize complications, an excessive number of shock waves and/or more than one lithotripsy session may have to be employed. One of the common problems noted with lithotripsy of multiple calculi is that fragmentation of the first stone creates a fragment cloud that can hide other unfocused stones. As a result, focusing and fragmentation of the remaining stones are difficult and likely to provide residual fragments larger than those generated initially.[3]

Although there are no placebo-controlled clinical trials to evaluate the benefits of adjuvant bile acid therapy, the experience of Sackman and colleagues[3] should be noted. They reported that of the two patients who did not comply with the adjuvant bile acid therapy, only one showed disappearance of stones after lithotripsy. The other patient underwent two sessions of lithotripsy and still had gallstone fragments 11 months postlithotripsy. Another patient became pregnant 1 month after shock wave therapy, and the adjuvant bile acid treatment was discontinued. A follow-up examination 6 months later showed that small stones measuring less than 4 mm in diameter had aggregated into a 15-mm stone. Neubrand and associates[4] showed that dissolution of human cholesterol gallstones by glycoursodeoxycholic acid-lecithin solution was enormously enhanced in vitro if the stones were first fragmented with shock waves produced by a lithotriptor. They suggested that this enhancement was due to improved surface-area-to-volume relationship and changes in the surface structure of the stones.

For the reasons outlined above, fragmented stones following lithotripsy should be either removed mechanically or treated with an appropriate dissolving agent. A great majority (80 to 85 percent) of gallstones are primarily composed of cholesterol and are amenable to contact dissolution by chemical solvents such as monooctanoin and methyl tert-butyl ether (MTBE) or by administration of chenodeoxycholic acid or ursodeoxycholic acid to induce the formation of unsaturated bile. Both mono-octanoin and MTBE are potent dissolving agents and are able to solubilize cholesterol stones within hours or days. Unfortunately, they are toxic and require direct instillation into the gallbladder using invasive procedures. Bile acids, on the other hand, can be administered orally. They have been successfully used for more than a decade for dissolving cholesterol gallstones in symptomatic and asymptomatic patients.[5–18] Complete dissolution can be anticipated after 2 years of bile acid therapy in 30 to 40 percent of unselected patients with stones less than 20 mm in maximal diameter.[11,19–22] The dissolution rate with ursodeoxycholic acid increases to 50 percent if stones are floating and to 81 percent if the stones are less than 5 mm in diameter.[23] Thus, bile acid therapy is more effective in patients with small cholesterol calculi. This fact was further confirmed in the first 175 patients who underwent cholesterol gallstone lithotripsy and received adjuvant dissolution therapy with oral chenodeoxycholic acid and ursodeoxycholic acid. In patients with solitary stones of 20 mm or less in diameter, 45 percent completely disappeared within 2 months and 95 percent within 12 to 18 months after lithotripsy.[3] This experience has now been extended to more than 300 patients.[24]

PRETREATMENT WITH BILE ACIDS

Several United States and European lithotripsy protocols require 1 or 2 weeks of bile acid therapy prior to the lithotripsy procedure. The rationale behind pretreatment is to create cholesterol desaturation and increase the litholycity of bile before attempting stone fragmentation. Although this may be desirable, it may not be absolutely necessary for maximal efficacy of lithotripsy. In fact, if the stone is small, pretreatment may change its tensile strength sufficiently enough to make its disintegration more difficult. Moreover, bile acids after oral administration are readily absorbed from the small bowel and the bile acid pool recycles an average of 9 times per day.[25] Since the half-life of exogenous ursodeoxycholic acid appears to be 2 or 3 days,[26] significant bile acid concentrations can be attained within a few days after daily administration.

POST-LITHOTRIPSY TREATMENT

The time period required for complete dissolution of stone fragments with bile acid therapy following lithotripsy will be directly proportional to the size of resulting fragments and total stone volume, and inversely proportional to the cholesterol content. Gallbladder ultrasonograms should be performed a day after lithotripsy and then at least every 3 months during the bile acid adjuvant therapy to determine if additional lithotripsy or some other management of gallstones is needed. The dissolution therapy should be continued for 2 to 3 months after ultrasound examination of gallbladder is negative for gallstones, because stones less than 2 mm in size may not be visualized with ultrasound.

STONE RECURRENCE

The stone recurrence rate following successful lithotripsy is expected to be the same as observed with bile acid dissolution therapy alone, which is about 10 percent per year.[27,28] This is understandable because extracorporeal shock waves do not correct the metabolic defect that allows the synthesis of lithogenic bile. Sackmann and associates[3] evaluated 25 patients for 3 to 12 months after stone disappearance following lithotripsy and adjuvant bile acid therapy. In one patient, small stones recurred after 4 months, which were dissolved easily with 3 months of bile acid therapy. A follow-up schedule needs to be developed for patients who become free of gallstones after lithotripsy and bile acid therapy. Gallbladder ultrasound every 1 or 2 years should be able to identify recurrent stones soon after they are formed. Oral medical dissolution therapy alone should be sufficient in treating most of such recurrent stones.

BILE ACID SELECTION

Orally administered bile acids are rapidly absorbed from the bowel and efficiently cleared from the portal blood by the liver where they are conjugated with glycine or taurine before secretion into the bile. Only small quantities of unconjugated bile acids escape liver uptake and circulate in the peripheral blood. Gallbladder contraction stimulated by food consumption forces the concentrated bile into the common bile duct and then to the duodenum. Bile acids are primarily eliminated via the feces, and urinary elimination is negligible. The two bile acids that have been most commonly employed as litholytic agents are chenodeoxycholic acid and its 7-β-epimer, ursodeoxycholic acid. Although both bile acids are equally effective, many studies have established that ursodeoxycholic acid has a superior safety profile. Dissolution therapy with chenodeoxycholic acid has been associated with liver function test abnormalities.[6–8,18,29–33] Diarrhea is also common in patients receiving chenodeoxycholic acid.[5–9,18,31–35] These side effects are extremely rare with ursodeoxycholic acid.[11–16,19] Tint and co-workers[19] treated 53 patients with radiolucent gallstones with ursodeoxycholic acid in doses ranging from 250 to 1000 mg/day for 6 to 38 months. Overall, 42 of 53 patients (79 percent) achieved partial or complete dissolution. No patient developed diarrhea or abnormal liver chemistries during the treatment. Bachrach and Hofmann[36] reviewed data on 850 patients who received ursodeoxycholic acid for gallstone dissolution and found no evidence of drug-induced liver injury. Poupon and colleagues[37] recently treated 15 patients who had histologically confirmed primary biliary cirrhosis with ursodeoxycholic acid for 2 years. As a result, levels of alkaline phosphatase, alanine aminotransferase, gamma-glutamyltranspeptidase, and bilirubin fell significantly. Discontinuation of ursodeoxycholic acid therapy in three patients for 3 months resulted in deterioration of liver function tests that improved when the ursodeoxycholic acid therapy was resumed. In vitro experimental data also indicate that ursodeoxycholic acid is superior to other naturally occurring bile acids. When incubated with isolated hepatocytes, chenodeoxycholic and deoxycholic acids caused release of enzymes and plasma membrane damage. No such changes were seen after incubation with ursodeoxycholic acid even when hepatocytes were exposed to 3 times higher concentration than those used for chenodeoxycholic and deoxycholic acids. Lithocholic acid was the most toxic bile acid, causing cellular damage at concentrations one tenth of those of other bile acids.[38] All these data support that ursodeoxycholic acid can serve as a suitable adjuvant therapy with lithotripsy.

ACKNOWLEDGEMENT

The author thanks Dr. Alan Hofmann for helpful suggestions and review of the manuscript.

REFERENCES

1. Chaussy C, Brendel W, Schmiedt E: Extracorporeally induced destruction of kidney stones by shock waves. *Lancet* 1980; 2:1265–1268.
2. Chaussy C, Schmiedt E, Jocham D, et al: First clinical experience with extracorporeally induced destruction of kidney stones by shock waves. *J Urol* 1982; 127:417–420.
3. Sackmann M, Delius M, Sauerbruch T, et al: Shock-wave lithotripsy of gallbladder stones, *N Engl J Med* 1972; 318:393–397.
4. Neubrand M, Sauerbruch T, Stellaard F, et al: In vitro cholesterol gallstone dissolution after fragmentation with shock waves. *Digestion* 1986; 34:51–59.
5. Danzinger RG, Hofmann AF, Schoenfield LJ, et al: Dissolution of cholesterol gallstones by chenodeoxycholic acid. *N Engl J Med* 1972; 286:1–8.
6. Bell GD, Whitney B, Dowling RH: Gallstone dissolution in man using chenodeoxycholic acid. *Lancet* 1972; 286:1213–1216.
7. Thistle JL, Hofmann AF: Efficacy and specificity of chenodeoxycholic acid therapy for dissolving gallstones. *N Engl J Med* 1973; 289:655–659.
8. Isher JH, Dowling RH, Mok HYI, et al: Chenodeoxycholic acid treatment of gallstones: A follow-up report and analysis of factors influencing response to therapy. *N Engl J Med* 1975; 293:378–383.
9. Barbara L, Roda E, Roda A, et al: The medical treatment of cholesterol gallstones: Experience with chenodeoxycholic acid. *Digestion* 1976; 14:209-219.
10. Okumura M, Tanikawa K, Chuman Y: Clinical studies on dissolution of gallstones using ursodeoxycholic acid. *Gastroenterol Jpn* 1977; 12:469–475.
11. Maton PN, Murphy GM, Dowling RH: Ursodeoxycholic acid treatment of gallstones: Dose response study and possible mechanism of action. *Lancet* 1977; 2:1297–1301.
12. Nakagawa S, Makino I, Ishizaki T, et al: Dissolution of cholesterol gallstones by ursodeoxycholic acid. *Lancet* 1977; 2:367–369.
13. Salvioli G, Salati R, Fratalocchi Lugli R: Ursodeoxycholic acid therapy for radiolucent gallstone dissolution. *Curr Ther Res* 1979; 26:995–1004.
14. Tokyo Cooperative Gallstone Study Group: Efficacy and indications of ursodeoxycholic acid treatment for dissolving gallstones: A multicenter double-blind trial. *Gastroenterology* 1980; 78:542–548.
15. Salen G, Colalillo A, Verga D, et al: Effect of high and low doses of ursodeoxycholic acid on gallstone dissolution in humans. *Gastroenterology* 1980; 78:1412–1418.
16. Allessandrini A, Ripoli F, Boscaini M, et al: A multicentre clinical trial on ursodeoxycholic acid: Effect of different dosages upon cholesterol gallstone dissolution. *Ital J Gastroenterol* 1980; 12:85–88.
17. Bateson MC, Hill A, Bouchier AD: Analysis of response to ursodeoxycholic acid for gallstone dissolution. *Digestion* 1980; 20:358–364.
18. Schoenfield LJ, Lachin JM, The Steering Committee, The National Cooperative Gallstone Study Group: Chenodiol (chenodeoxycholic acid) for dissolution of gallstones: The National Cooperative Gallstone Study: A controlled study of efficacy and safety. *Ann Inter Med* 1981; 95:257–282.
19. Tint GS, Salen G, Colalillo A, et al: Ursodeoxycholic acid: A safe and effective agent for dissolving cholesterol gallstones. *Ann Intern Med* 1982; 97:351–356.
20. Meredith TJ, Williams GV, Maton PN, et al: Retrospective comparison of 'cheno' and 'urso' in the medical treatment of gallstones. *Gut* 1982; 23:382–289.
21. Roda E, Bazzoli F, Morselli AM, et al: Ursodeoxycholic acid vs. chenodeoxycholic acid as cholesterol gallstone-dissolving agents: A comparative randomized study. *Hepatology* 1982; 2:804–810.
22. Podda M, Zuin M, Dioguardi ML, et al: Gallstone dissolution after 6 months of ursodeoxycholic acid (UDCA): Effectiveness of different doses. *J Int Med Res* 1982; 10:59–63.
23. Actigall (ursodiol) Package Insert, 1988.
24. Paumgartner G, Sackmann M, Holl J, et al: Extracorporeal shock wave lithotripsy of gallstones.

Int Mtg Pathochem Pathophysio Pathomech Biliary Sys Bologna, Italy, 1988; 110.

25. Mok HYI, von Bergmann K, Grundy SM: Regulation of pool size of bile acids in man. *Gastroenterology* 1977; 73:684.
26. Actigall (ursodiol) Summary Basis of Approval, 1988.
27. Ruppin DC, Dowling RH: Is recurrence inevitable after gallstone dissolution by bile acid treatment? *Lancet* 1982; 1:181–185,
28. Lanzini A, Jazrawi RP, Kupfer RM, et al: Gallstone recurrence after medical dissolution: An overestimated threat *J Hepatology* 1986; 3:241–246.
29. Stiehl A, Ast E, Czygan P: Elevated serum transaminase following treatment of patients with cholesterol gallstones with chenodeoxycholic acid. *Inn Med* 1976; 3:75–80.
30. Stiehl A, Czygan P, Kommerell B, et al: Ursodeoxycholic acid versus chenodeoxycholic acid: Comparison of their effects on bile acid and bile lipid composition in patients with cholesterol gallstones. *Gastroenterology* 1978; 75:1016–1020.
31. Stiehl A, Raedsch R, Czygan P, et al: Effects of biliary bile acid composition of biliary cholesterol saturation in gallstone patients treated with chenodeoxycholic acid and/or ursodeoxycholic acid. *Gastroenterology* 1980; 79:1192–1198.
32. Nakayama F: Oral cholelitholysis—cheno versus urso: Japanese experience. *Dig Dis Sci* 1980; 25:129–134.
33. Iwamura K: Clinical studies on cheno- and ursodeoxycholic acid treatment for gallstone dissolution. *Hepatogastroenterology* 1980; 27:26–34.
34. Mok HYI, Bell GD, Dowling RH: Effect of different doses of chenodeoxycholic acid on bile-lipid composition and on frequency of side-effects in patients with gallstones. *Lancet* 1974; 2:253–257.
35. Capron JP, Dupas, JL, Capron-Chivrac D, et al: Unconjugated hyperbilirubinemia during treatment with chenodeoxycholic acid. *Gastroenterology* 1979; 77:121–122.
36. Bachrach WH, Hoffmann AF: Ursodeoxycholic acid in the treatment of cholesterol cholelithiasis: Part II. *Dig Dis Sci* 1982; 27:833–856.
37. Poupon R, Poupon, RE, Calmus Y, et al: Is ursodeoxycholic acid an effective treatment for primary biliary cirrhosis? *Lancet* 1987; 1:834–836.
38. Scholmerich J, Becher MS, Schmidt K, et al: Influence of hydroxylation and conjugation of bile salt on their membrane-damaging properties: Studies on isolated hepatocytes and lipid membrane vesicles. *Hepatology* 1984; 4:661–666.

Perspectives on the Treatment of Gallstones with Ursodeoxycholic Acid

Gerald Salen

Ursodeoxycholic acid ($3\alpha,7\beta$-dihydroxycholanoic acid) (Fig 1) is a naturally occurring bile acid that constitutes about 1 to 2 percent of the bile acids in human bile. First identified in polar bear bile in 1903, this 7β-hydroxy bile acid is also the major bile acid in the nutria (M. Coypus). [1] Although well known for more than 20 years as a treatment of biliary distress and dyspepsia in Japan, ursodeoxycholic acid was not tested as a gallstone-dissolving agent until 1977. Successful dissolution occurs in 30 to 80 percent of subjects with cholesterol gallstones, depending on their size and number (Fig 2).[2–8] Calcified or pigment stones do not respond to this treatment.

Ursodeoxycholic acid is a second-generation bile acid, having replaced chenodeoxycholic acid, its 7α-hydroxy epimer as the preferred nonsurgical litholytic treatment for gallstones. The major reasons for ursodeoxycholic acid's effectiveness are:

1. Biliary cholesterol secretion diminishes markedly during therapy.[9,10]
2. Hepatic bile acid synthesis is not inhibited by ursodeoxycholic acid.[11,12]
3. The 7β-hydroxy group of ursodeoxycholic acid resists bacterial dehydroxylation.[13–16]
4. Ursodeoxycholic acid is virtually free of side effects and toxicity.[1,5]

To better understand these mechanisms, it is important to consider several features in the pathogenesis of gallstones. It is now amply authenticated in gallstone subjects that lithogenic bile that is supersaturated with cholesterol is secreted by the liver and not produced in the gallbladder. Thus, although stones form in the gallbladder, defective liver cholesterol and bile acid metabolism are responsible for the lithogenic bile.[17,18] Two factors contribute (Table 1): (1) The liver accumulates cholesterol because HMG CoA reductase, the rate-controlling enzyme in cholesterol biosynthesis, is overactive; and (2) bile acid synthesis is reduced (50 percent lower activity of cholesterol 7α-hydroxylase, the rate-determining enzyme for bile acid synthesis), which limits bile acid pool size and micellar cholesterol solubilization. As a result, hepatic cholesterol rises and biliary cholesterol secretion increases. When the micellar solubility limit in bile is exceeded, cholesterol monomers (molecules) precipitate as microcrystals, beginning the stone-forming process.

Treatment (15 mg/kg/day) results in a 50 percent enrichment of the bile with ursodeoxycholic acid, the remaining 50 percent being composed of the primary bile acids, cholic acid and chenodeoxycholic acid and their bacterial derivatives (Table 2). Hepatic cholesterol secretion declines markedly (lithogenic index falls; Table 2) because synthesis is inhibited by ursodeoxycholic acid, as evidenced by the reduction in hepatic HMG CoA reductase activity.[2,4] Interestingly, despite reduced hepatic synthesis, plasma

COOH

HO OH

3α, 7β-dihydroxycholanoic Acid
Ursodeoxycholic Acid

FIG 1.
Structure of ursodeoxycholic acid.

cholesterol and triglyceride levels are unchanged by ursodeoxycholic acid.[6]

When ursodeoxycholic acid enters the intestine, certain anaerobic bacteria attack and remove the hydroxy group at C-7.[13–15] When this happens, lithocholic acid, a monohydroxy bile acid that causes cholestasis and liver damage, is formed. However, studies with human intestinal bacteria have demonstrated that the 7β-hydroxy group of ursodeoxycholic acid is more resistent to 7-dehydroxylation than is the 7α-hydroxy group of chenodeoxycholic acid. Thus, not only is less lithocholic acid produced, but more ursodeoxycholic acid is available to be reabsorbed from the intestine. Consequently, the effective litholytic dose of ursodeoxycholic acid is about 30 percent lower than with chenodeoxycholic acid. It is also important to remember that a portion of the ursodeoxycholic acid that enters the intestine is epimerized to chenodeoxycholic acid by bacteria.[13]

With regard to side effects, about 5 percent of ursodeoxycholic acid–treated subjects experience transient diarrhea. However, it is mild and of short duration; treatment does not have to be discontinued. Moreover, liver function tests that include serum levels of bilirubin, aminotransferases (SGOT-SGPT), and alkaline phosphatase remain normal during ursodeoxycholic acid treatment and, as noted before, serum cholesterol concentrations do not increase.[1,11,19]

After gallstone dissolution, it is important to periodically evaluate subjects, since gallstones may recur in 50 percent of subjects. Preliminary studies suggest that recurrence can be prevented by continued therapy with ursodeoxycholic acid. However, since long-term administration may be required, maintenance therapy has not been recommended. Moreover, even if stones recur, treatment with ursodeoxycholic acid should be as effective the second time. Also, no further

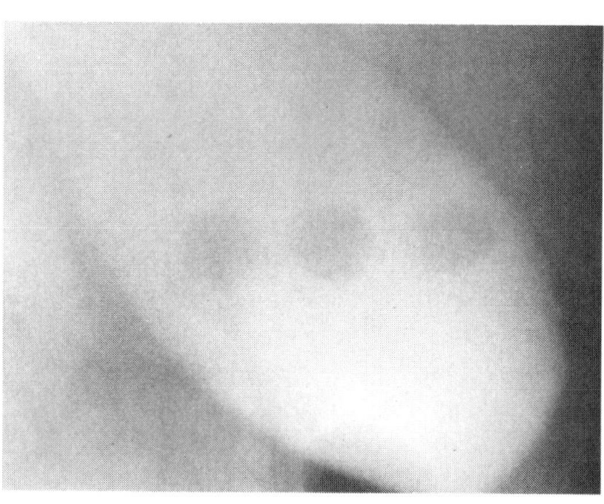

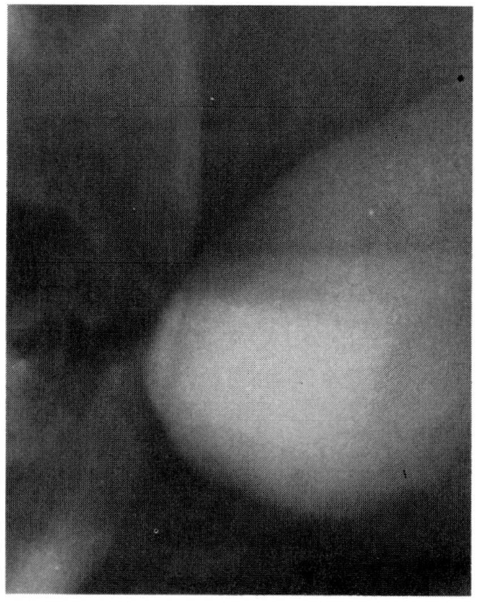

FIG 2.
Oral cholecystogram *(left)* (upright) showing three radiolucent gallstones. After 6 months of ursodeoxycholic acid (15 mg/kg/day), gallstones have dissolved *(right)*.

TABLE 1.

Activities of Hepatic Cholesterol and Bile Acid Regulating Enzymes*

	CONTROL N = B		GALLSTONE N = 9
HMG CoA reductase (pmoles/mg protein/min)	61±7.4		77.3±10.6
		p<0.001†	
Cholesterol 7α-hydroxylase (pmoles/mg protein/min)	18.2±3.7		9.6±4.4
		p<0.001†	
Liver cholesterol (mg/g)	3.4±0.5		5.3±2.2
		p<0.06	

*HMG CoA reductase and cholesterol 7α-hydroxylase activities were measured in liver microsomes according to the method of Salen et al.[18]
†Student t-test.

TABLE 2.

Effect of Ursodeoxycholic Acid (1000 mg/day) in Biliary Bile Acid Composition and Lithogenic Index

	PERCENTAGE OF BILE ACIDS		
	PRETREATMENT N = 9	POST-TREATMENT, N = 9	P*VALUES
Cholic acid	32±14	15±7	<0.05
Deoxycholic acid	27±17	15±12	<0.02
Chenodeoxycholic acid	37±14	22±5	<0.05
Lithocholic acid	2.3±1.7	0.6±0.8	<0.05
Ursodeoxycholic acid	1.7±2.4	48±11	<0.0001
Lithogenic index[6]	1.6±0.4	1.0±0.4	<0.05

*Student t-test.

therapy may be necessary in the 50 percent of subjects who do not reform gallstones.

In summary, ursodeoxycholic acid has proved to be a safe and effective therapy for cholesterol gallstones. It works by correcting the hepatic cholesterol and bile acid metabolic abnormalities. Side effects are minor, but stones may reform when ursodeoxycholic acid is discontinued.

REFERENCES

1. Ward A, Brogden RN, Heel RC, et al: Ursodeoxycholic acid: A review of its pharmacological properties and therapeutic efficacy. *Drugs* 1984; 27:95–131.
2. Maton PN, Murphy GM, Dowling RH: Ursodeoxycholic acid treatment of gallstones, dose response study and possible mechanism of action. *Lancet* 1977; 2:1297–1301.
3. Kutz K, Schulte A: EFfectiveness of ursodeoxycholic acid in gallstones therapy (abstract) *Gastroenterology* 1977; 73:632.
4. Salen G, Colalillo A, Verga D, et al: The effect of high and low doses of ursodeoxycholic acid on gallstone dissolution in humans. *Gastroenterology* 1980; 78:1412–1418.
5. Tokyo Cooperative Gallstone Study Group: EFficacy and indications of ursodeoxycholic acid treatment for dissolving gallstones: A multicenter double-blind trial. *Gastroenterology* 1980; 78:548–548.
6. Tint GS, Salen G, Colalillo A, et al: Ursodeoxycholic acid: A safe and effective agent for dis-

solving cholesterol gallstones. *Ann Intern Med* 1982; 97:351–356.

7. Nakagawa S, Makino I, Liskzohic I, et al: Dissolution of cholesterol gallstones by ursodeoxycholic acid. *Lancet* 1977; 2:367–369.
8. Fromm H, Roat JW, Gonzalez V, et al: Comparative efficacy and side effects of ursodeoxycholic and chenodeoxycholic acids in dissolving gallstones: A double-blind study. *Gastroenterology* 1983; 85:1257–1264.
9. Von Bergmann K, Gutsfeld M, Schulze-Hagen K, et al: Effects of ursodeoxycholic acid on biliary lipid secretion in patients with radiolucent gallstones, in Paumgartner G, Stiehl A, Gerok W (eds): *Biologic Effects on Bile Acids*. Lancaster, England, MTP Press, 1979, pp 61–66.
10. Schersten T, Lindblad L: Biliary cholesterol during ursodeoxycholic acid secretion in man, in Paumgartner G, Stiehl A, Gerok W (eds): *Biologic Effects of Bile Acids*. Lancaster, England, MTP Press, 1979, pp 53–60.
11. Tint GS, Salen G, Shefer S, et al: Oral ursodeoxycholic acid (UDCA) does not inhibit primary bile acid synthesis, but is a quantitatively important precursor for chenodeoxycholic acid (CDCA) (abstract). *Gastroenterology,* 1986; 90: 1776.
12. Hardison WGM, Grundy SM: Effect of ursodeoxycholate and its taurine conjugate on bile acid synthesis and cholesterol absorption. *Gastroenterology* 1984; 87:130–135.
13. Fedorowski T, Salen G, Tint GS, et al: Transformation of chenodeoxycholic and ursodeoxycholic acid by human intestinal bacteria. *Gastroenterology* 1979; 77:1068–1073.
14. Albini E, Marca G, Mellerio G: Further observations on the in vitro metabolism of chenodeoxycholic acid and ursodeoxycholic acid. *Arzneimittelforschung* 1982; 32:1554–1557.
15. White BA, Fricke RJ, Hylemon PB: 7β-Dehydroxylation of ursodeoxycholic acid by whole cells and cell extracts of the intestinal anaerobic bacterium, Eubacterium species VPI 12708. *J Lipid Res* 1982; 23:145–153.
16. Bazzoli G, Fromm H, Sarva RP, et al: Comparative formation of lithocholic acid from chenodeoxycholic and ursodeoxycholic acids in the colon. *Gastroenterology* 1982; 83:753–760.
17. Vlahcevic ZR, Bell CC, Buhac I, et al: Diminished bile acid pool size in patients with gallstones. *Gastroenterology* 1970; 59:165–173.
18. Salen G, Nicolau G, Shefer S, et al: Hepatic cholesterol metabolism in patients with gallstones. *Gastroenterology* 1975; 69:676–684.
19. Bachrach WH, Hofmann AF: Ursodeoxycholic acid in the treatment of cholesterol lithiasis. *Dig Dis Sci* 1982; 27:833–356.

Rationale of Bile Acid Therapy After Biliary Lithotripsy

Alan F. Hofmann

For the past century, symptomatic gallbladder disease caused by the presence of gallbladder stones has been treated by cholecystectomy and has been viewed as a surgical disease.[1] The discovery that gallstones could be dissolved slowly by oral therapy with chenodiol[2] and/or ursodiol[3] offered an alternative to those patients with cholesterol stones in visualizing gallbladders who were at increased risk for surgery. An overview of the current status of cholesterol dissolution by oral administration of ursodiol is summarized in the previous two contributions by G. Salen and M. Ahmed.

In the past 3 years, two new nonsurgical approaches have been introduced. The first is biliary lithotripsy with adjuvant bile acid therapy;[4] the second is percutaneous gallbladder catheterization with contact dissolution using cholesterol solvents.[5] The safety and efficacy of these two procedures are now being explored in multicenter studies.

The purpose of this brief review is to summarize the rationale for adjuvant oral bile acid therapy after the biliary lithotripsy procedure. It will be proposed that there are two groups of patients: those for whom adjuvant bile acid therapy is essential and those for whom it is not. It will be argued that these two groups of patients cannot be distinguished in advance at present and are unlikely to be distinguishable in the future. If this reasoning is correct, it is appropriate to initiate adjuvant bile acid therapy in all patients receiving biliary lithotripsy.

BACKGROUND

The formation of cholesterol gallstones requires supersaturated bile in the gallbladder.[6] The liver secretes supersaturated bile, and a gallbladder must be present. In most patients with cholesterol gallstones, there is more rapid nucleation of cholesterol crystals from filtered bile ex vivo[7,8] because of the presence of pronucleating factors.[9,10] There is likely to be abnormal retention of cholesterol crystals because of defective gallbladder contraction in gallstone patients.[11–13] In addition, gallbladder pH is higher in gallstone patients,[14] which results in gallbladder bile remaining supersaturated in calcium carbonate.[15]

The oral administration of chenodiol or ursodiol causes hepatic bile to change from being supersaturated in cholesterol to being unsaturated in cholesterol. Bile acid feeding experiments were initiated with the view that exogenous bile acids should correct the diminished bile acid pool known to be present in cholesterol gallstone patients.[16] However, subsequent experiments indicated that the mechanism of action of these natural 3,7-dihydroxy bile acids was to decrease cholesterol secretion rather than increase bile acid secretion.[17–20] Biliary cholesterol secretion is considered to involve bile acid-stimulated secretion of cholesterol/phospholipid vesicles from the hepatocyte.[21] During bile acid therapy, these vesicles should have a lower cholesterol/phospholipid ratio.

Further studies indicated that the mechanism of action of these two natural bile acids was not identical. Chenodiol, a hydrophobic dihydroxy bile acid, probably does not influence cholesterol absorption,[22–24] but down-regulates cholesterol biosynthesis since hepatic HMG CoA reductase activity falls[20,25–27]; this enzyme is known to be a rate-limiting enzyme for cholesterol biosynthesis.[28] At the same time, it also causes decreased bile acid biosynthesis,[20,27,29,30] presumably because of decreased hepatic cholesterol 7-hydroxylase activity[20]; this enzyme is known to be a rate-limiting enzyme for bile acid biosynthesis.[31] Biliary cholesterol secretion, which ultimately derives mostly from endogenous cholesterol biosynthesis, falls.[17–20,29] Hepatocyte LDL receptors are down-regulated, and the plasma cholesterol level increases.[32]

Ursodiol, on the other hand, appears to diminish cholesterol absorption.[24,33–35] There is little effect on hepatic HMG CoA reductase activity,[26,27,36] and bile acid biosynthesis remains unchanged[29,37] or somewhat lower,[38] indicating that the regulatory effects of ursodiol are much weaker than those of chenodiol. Cholesterol secretion into bile falls for two reasons: first, the vesicles induced by ursodiol contain a lower cholesterol/phospholipid ratio than those induced by other bile acids[39–41]; and second, the intestinal absorption of exogenous and endogenous cholesterol is less, as noted. Hepatocyte LDL receptor activity is unchanged, and ursodiol does not affect plasma cholesterol levels.[42]

It is of interest to contrast the effect of ursodiol with β-sitosterol. This plant sterol, when given in large quantities, decreases cholesterol absorption.[22] However, in contrast to ursodiol, it is likely that HMG CoA reductase levels increase[43]; and β-sitosterol administration does not decrease cholesterol secretion in cholesterol gallstone patients.[22]

Biliary lithotripsy fragments stones. It is unlikely to influence hepatic enzymes, biliary lipid secretion, cholesterol nucleation, gallbladder motility, or gallbladder pH. All the metabolic, secretory, and motility defects that were present before lithotripsy are likely to persist.

Cholecystectomy, just as lithotripsy, does not influence these pathogenetic factors. However, cholecystectomy removes the gallbladder, and the presence of a gallbladder by definition is essential for the formation of gallbladder stones. The gallbladder offers a reservoir for crystal and stone retention. Gravity can promote sedimentation of crystals or stones away from the gallbladder neck, decreasing their chance of evacuation during gallbladder contraction; crystal retention is essential for the formation of gallstones. When the gallbladder is removed, the small intestine becomes the site of storage of biliary lipids. Residence time here is a matter of hours so that crystals, even if they were to be formed, would not be retained.

ADJUVANT BILE ACID THERAPY

After successful biliary lithotripsy, gallstone fragments are present in supersaturated bile. In such bile, nucleation of cholesterol and deposition onto the fragment surface should occur more rapidly; expulsion of fragments should be defective in the majority of gallstone patients because of the known gallbladder motility defect present in such patients.[11–13]

These considerations led the Munich group of Sauerbruch, Sackmann, Paumgartner, Delius, Hepp, Brendel, and colleagues to give a mixture of chenodiol and ursodiol in conjunction with biliary lithotripsy.[44] Bile acid therapy was commenced several weeks before shock wave therapy, because it takes several weeks to replace circulating endogenous bile acids by orally administered exogenous bile acids.[45] A mixture of chenodiol and ursodiol was chosen for several reasons. First, at the time of study, the mixture was the most prescribed form of bile acid therapy in Germany. Second, at least one study had suggested that the mixture dissolves desaturated bile more effectively[46] and gallstones more rapidly than ursodiol alone.[47] Third, the mixture is less costly than ursodiol alone, because ursodiol is produced by a chemical modification of chenodiol.

The results of the Munich study indicate that elimination of all imagable fragments requires up to 1 year.[4,44] During that time, either fragments pass spontaneously through the cystic duct, down the common duct, and into the intestine or they dissolve. The frequent bouts of biliary pain in the treated patients suggest that stone fragments are passing and causing momentary obstruction in the cystic duct. Bile is unsaturated in such patients, and because gallstones dissolve in unsaturated bile, there must be continued dissolution of gallstone fragments. The density of these fragments can be considered to be that of cholesterol gallstones—1.040 to 1.060.[48] Bile has a density close to that of saline—1.009. Thus, fragments will sediment in bile according to Stokes' law. Sedimentation can be toward the neck of the gallbladder or toward the fundus. Senior and colleagues,[49] extending earlier data of Wolpers,[50] have presented evidence that during bile acid therapy gallstones dissolve at a rate *averaging* 1 mm (diameter) per month. Accordingly, if fragments vary from 1 to 6 mm in diameter, they will require 1 to 6 months to dissolve, on the average.

The second consideration regarding passage versus dissolution of fragments is the size of the fragment in relation to the functional diameter of the cystic duct. It is attractive to speculate that the cystic duct "valves" act to prevent sedimentation and adherence of particulate material during transit.

There is little information on the size-density relationships of particles that can be expelled from the human gallbladder, although studies in dogs indicate that particles less than 2 mm in diameter may be expelled by gallbladder contraction.[51] Sludge, which is composed of small particles containing a mixture of calcium bilirubinate crystals, cholesterol crystals, and mucoprotein,[52] is expelled spontaneously in most individuals.[8,52,53] The cephalosporin ceftriaxone may form insoluble calcium salts in the gallbladder; these usually pass spontaneously.[54]

DESIRABILITY OF ADJUVANT BILE ACID THERAPY

These considerations indicate that the natural history of cholesterol fragments formed by a lithotripsy procedure should either be expelled spontaneously or, if retained, grow in size by the accretion of cholesterol crystals. Growth should occur on all crystals, irrespective of their chemical composition. Despite the presence of growing gallstones, the patient's symptoms should improve if episodes of cystic duct obstruction have no longer occurred. Expulsion of calculi requires that crystals are brought to the gallbladder neck by either gravity or gallbladder contraction and that they be sufficiently small to be swept through the cystic duct during gallbladder emptying.

When bile acid therapy is initiated, bile will gradually become unsaturated in cholesterol. The dose must be sufficient and the patient must be compliant. Fragments will dissolve or when they become small enough will be evacuated from the gallbladder during gallbladder contraction (Fig 1).

A major question is whether the elimination of all particulate material should diminish stone recurrence. Perhaps noncholesterol particles, which are frequently present in the center of cholesterol gallstones, will be retained in all gallstone patients whether or not bile acid therapy is initiated.

UNCERTAINTIES

In the patient who has undergone lithotripsy-induced gallstone fragmentation, there are multiple unknowns. First, the exact size distribution of the fragments produced by lithotripsy cannot be quantified. These may sediment to the gallbladder neck or the fundus, depending on the patient's living pattern and abdominal anatomy. Gallbladder contractility varies, as does the functional size of the cystic duct.

All these considerations suggest that the safest course is to eliminate all fragments by dissolution in unsaturated bile. Dissolution will be unnecessary in that fraction of patients in whom all fragments pass spontaneously. What is the size of that fraction? It may well vary from center to center, depending on the completeness of the fragmentation by lithotripsy and will also be influenced by patient selection. In principle, it should be possible to define that fraction by observing patients after lithotripsy and omitting bile acid therapy. Some patients will pass their

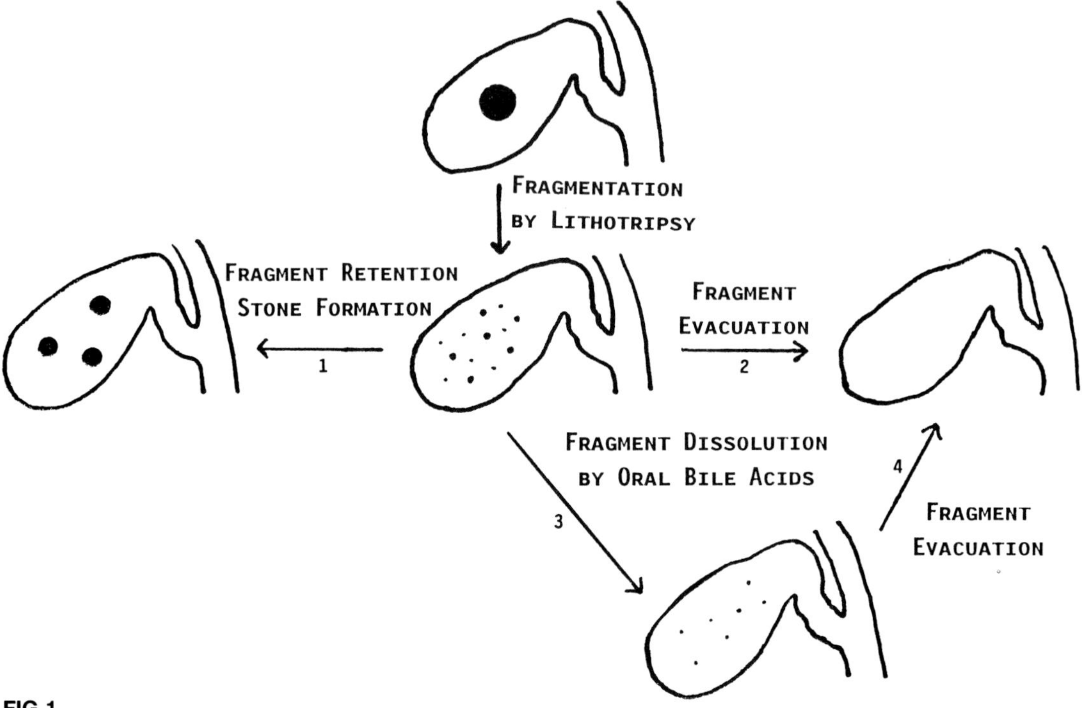

FIG 1.
Fate of solitary cholesterol gallstone treated by lithotripsy with or without adjuvant bile acid therapy. If the fragments are retained, they may grow in which case treatment is a failure *(arrow 1).* The fragments, if sufficiently small, may be evacuated by gallbladder contraction alone *(arrow 2).* If bile acid therapy is initiated, the fragments will become smaller *(arrow 3);* some may be expelled and others may dissolve *(arrows 3 and 4).* The end result is gallstone elimination. Institution of bile acid therapy eliminates the possibility of fragment retention and growth.

fragments; in others, fragments should become larger. The latter can then be treated with bile acid therapy, but time will have been lost; and it is not known whether such stones will respond. For example, if the presence of stone fragments caused a low-grade inflammation of the mucosa, resulting in acquired calcification, such stones would not respond to "delayed" bile acid therapy.

The questions raised here can be answered by the scientific method. Burhenne and colleagues (personal communication) are treating patients with lithotripsy and no adjuvant bile acid therapy. The Dornier Medical Systems trial in the United States will assign patients to receive either bile acid therapy or placebo therapy.

CONCLUSION

Lithotripsy will become an important treatment for symptomatic gallbladder disease only if it results in complete stone elimination in a short time without a high risk of recurrence. Its convenience and cost must outweigh its being nondefinitive therapy. Dissolution by adjuvant bile acid therapy should enhance spontaneous expulsion and is likely to become a standard component of biliary lithotripsy therapy. It has been recognized for many years that the most ideal patients for medical therapy were those with multiple small stones. In a sense, lithotripsy is best for converting the least ideal patient for bile acid therapy (one with a large solitary gallstone) to the most ideal patient (one with multiple small gallstones).

The most rapid dissolution of fragments is achieved by contact dissolution with organic solvents, such as methyl tert-butyl ether (MTBE). At present, this is placed in the gallbladder most commonly by percutaneous catheter.[5,55–57] although instillation by retrograde cholangiography has been reported.[58] A promising line of study might be the instillation of MTBE or other potent, safe solvents by cholangiography or other techniques before lithotripsy so that gallstone fragments could be dissolved in a matter of hours. In this way, a procedure would be available that offered complete gallstone elimination without a surgical procedure. The costs and benefits of surgical care would have to be weighted against the costs of possible future recurrence.

The merging of two unrelated techniques—gallstone fragmentation by lithotripsy and bile desaturation by metabolic therapy—is an exciting event. It will mean that biophysicists and biochemists will work together to develop improved therapies for this ancient malady. From this turbulent interface, progress is sure to come.

REFERENCES

1. Way W, and Sleisenger MH: Acute cholecystitis, in Sleisenger MH, Fordtran JS (eds): *Gastrointestinal Disease*. Philadelphia, WB Saunders, Co, 1983.
2. Danzinger RG, Hofmann AF, Schoenfield LJ, et al: Dissolution of cholesterol gallstones by chenodeoxycholic acid. *N Engl J Med* 1972; 286:1–8.
3. Makino I, Shinozaki K, Yoshino K, et al; Dissolution of cholesterol gallstones by ursodeoxycholic acid. Jap. J. Gastroenterol. 1975; 72:690–702.
4. Sackmann M, Delius M, Sauerbruch T, et al: Shock-wave lithotripsy of gallbladder stones: The first 175 patients. *N Engl J Med* 1988; 318:393–397.
5. Allen MJ, Borody TJ, Bugliosi TF, et al: Rapid dissolution of gallstones in humans using methyl tert-butyl ether. *N Engl J Med* 1985; 312:217–220.
6. Grundy SM: Mechanisms of cholesterol gallstone formation. *Semin Liver Dis* 1983; 3:97–111.
7. Holan KR, Holzbach T, Hermann RE, et al: Nucleation time: A key factor in the pathogenesis of cholesterol gallstone disease. *Gastroenterology* 1979; 77:611–617.
8. Gollish SH, Burnstein MJ, Ilson RG, et al: Nucleation of cholesterol monohydrate crystals from hepatic and gall-bladder bile of patients with cholesterol gallstones, *Gut* 1983; 24:836–844.
9. Gallinger S, Harvey PRC, Petrunka CN, et al: Biliary proteins and the nucleation defect in cholesterol cholelithiasis, *Gastroenterology* 1987; 92:867–875.
10. Drapers JAG, Groen AK, Stout JPJ, et al: Quantification of cholesterol nucleation promoting activity in human gallbladder bile. *Clin Clim Acta* 1987; 165:295–302.
11. Forgacs IC, Maisey MN, Murphy GM, et al: Influence of gallstones and ursodeoxycholic acid therapy on gallbladder emptying. *Gastroenterology* 1984; 87:299–307.
12. Kishk SMA, Darweesh RMA, Dodds WJ, et al: Sonographic evaluation of resting gallbladder volume and postprandial emptying in patients with gallstones. *Am J Roentgenol* 1987; 148:875–879.
13. Thompson JC, Fried GM, Ogden WD, et al: Correlation between release of cholecystokinin and contraction of the gallbladder in patients with gallstones. *Ann Surg* 1982; 195:670–676.
14. Shiffman ML, Moore EW: Defective acidification leads to $CaCO_3$ supersaturation of gallbladder bile in patients with all types of gallstones (abstract). *Gastroenterology* 1988; 94:A591.
15. Rege RV, Moore EW: Pathogenesis of calcium-containing gallstones: Canine ductular bile, but not gallbladder bile, is supersaturated with calcium carbonate. *J Clin Invest* 1986; 77:21–26.
16. Thistle JL, Schoenfield LJ: Induced alterations in composition of bile of persons having cholelithiasis. *Gastroenterology* 1971; 61:488–496.
17. Northfield TC, LaRusso NF, Hofmann AF, et al: Biliary lipid output during three meals and an overnight fast. II. Effect of chenodeoxycholic acid treatment in gallstone subjects. *Gut* 1975; 16:12–17.
18. Einarsson K, Grundy S: Effects of feeding cholic acid and chenodeoxycholic acid on cholesterol absorption and hepatic secretion of biliary lipids in man. *J Lipid Res* 1980; 21:23–34.
19. von Bergmann K, Epple-Gustfeld M, Leiss O: Differences in the effects of chenodeoxycholic and ursodeoxycholic acid on biliary lipid secretion and bile acid synthesis in patients with gallstones. *Gastroenterology* 1984; 87:136–143.
20. Key PH, Bonorris GG, Marks JW, et al: Biliary lipid synthesis and secretion in gallstone patients before and during treatment with chenodeoxy-

cholic acid. *J Lab Clin Med* 1980; 95:816–826.

21. Coleman R: Biochemistry of bile secretion. *Biochem J* 1987; 244:249–261.
22. Tangedahl TN, Thistle JL, Hofmann AF, et al: Effect of beta-sitosterol alone or in combination with chenic acid on cholesterol saturation of bile and cholesterol absorption in gallstone patients. *Gastroenterology* 1979; 76:1341–1346.
23. Ponz de Leon M, Carulli N, Loria P, et al: The effect of chenodeoxycholic acid (CDCA) on cholesterol absorption. *Gastroenterology* 1979; 77:223–230.
24. Leiss O, von Bergmann K, Streicher U, et al: Effect of three different dihydroxy bile acids on intestinal cholesterol absorption in normal volunteers. *Gastroenterology* 1984; 87:144–149.
25. Ahlberg J, Angelin B, Einarsson K: Hepatic 3-hydroxy-3-methylglutaryl coenzyme A reductase activity and biliary lipid composition in man: Relation to cholesterol gallstone disease and effects on cholic acid and chenodeoxycholic acid treatment. *J Lipid Res* 1981; 22:410–422.
26. Maton PN, Ellis JH, Higgins MJP, et al: HMG-CoA reductase in cholelithiasis: Effects of ursodeoxycholic and chenodeoxycholic acids. *Eur J Clin Invest* 1980; 10:325–332.
27. Carulli N, Ponz de Leon M, Zironi F, et al: Hepatic cholesterol and bile acid metabolism in subjects with gallstones: Comparative effects of short-term feeding of chenodeoxycholic acid and ursodeoxycholic acid. *J Lipid Res* 1980; 21:35–43.
28. Myant NB: *The Biology of Cholesterol and Related Steroids*. London, William Heinemann Medical Books, Ltd, 1981, pp 360–364.
29. Nilsell K, Angelin B, Leijd B, et al: Comparative effects of ursodeoxycholic acid and chenodeoxycholic acid on bile acid kinetics and biliary lipid secretion in humans: Evidence for different modes of action on bile acid synthesis. *Gastroenterology* 1983; 85:1248–1256.
30. Danzinger RG, Hofmann AF, Thistle JL, et al: Effect of oral chenodeoxycholic acid on bile acid kinetics and biliary lipid composition in women with cholelithiasis. *J Clin Invest* 1973; 52:2809–2821.
31. Bjorkhem I: Mechanism of bile acid biosynthesis in mamalian liver, in Danielsson H, Sjovall J (eds): *Sterols and Bile Acids*. Amsterdam, Elsevier Science Publishers, BV, 1985, pp 231–278.
32. Albers JJ, Grundy SM, Cleary PA, et al and the National Cooperative Gallstone Study Group: National Cooperative Gallstone Study: The effects of chenodeoxycholic acid on lipoproteins and apolipoproteins. *Gastroenterology* 1982; 82:638–646.
33. Ponz de Leon M, Carulli N, Loria P, et al: Cholesterol absorption during bile acid feeding: Effect of ursodeoxycholic acid (UDCA) administration. *Gastroenterology* 1980; 78:214–219.
34. Salvioli G, Lugli R, Pradelli JM: Cholesterol absorption and sterol balance in normal subjects receiving dietary fiber or ursodeoxycholic acid. *Dig Dis Sci* 1985; 30:301–307.
35. Hardison WGM, Grundy SM: Effect of ursodeoxycholate and its taurine conjugate on bile acid synthesis and cholesterol absorption. *Gastroenterology* 1984; 87:130–135.
36. Angelin B, Ewerth S, Einarsson K: Ursodeoxycholic acid treatment in cholesterol gallstone disease: Effects on hepatic 3-hydroxy-3-methylglutaryl coenzyme A reductase activity, biliary lipid composition, and plasma lipid levels. *J Lipid Res* 1983; 24:461–468.
37. Bertolotti M, Carulli N, Menozzi D, et al: In vivo evaluation of cholesterol 7-alpha-hydroxylation in humans: Effect of disease and drug treatment. *J Lipid Res* 1986; 27:1278–1286.
38. Frenkiel PG, Lee DWT, Cohen H, et al: The effect of diet on bile acid kinetics and biliary lipid secretion in gallstone patients treated with ursodeoxycholic acid. *Am J Clin Nutr* 1986; 43:239–250.
39. Sama C, LaRusso NF, Lopez del Pino V, et al: Effects of acute bile acid administration on biliary lipid secretion in healthy volunteers. *Gastroenterology* 1982; 82:515–525.
40. Carulli N, Loria P, Bertolloti M et al: Effects of acute changes of bile acid pool composition on biliary lipid secretion. *J Clin Invest* 1984; 74:614–624.
41. Gilmore IT, Stokes K, Hofmann AF, et al: Differing acute effects of chenodeoxycholyl conjugates and ursodeoxycholyl conjugates on biliary phospholipid and cholesterol secretion in gallstone patients (abstract). *Gastroenterology* 1980; 79:1020.
42. Bachrach WH, Hofmann AF: Ursodeoxycholic acid in the treatment of cholesterol cholelithiasis: A review. *Dig Dis Sci* 1982; 27:737–761, 833–856.
43. Shefer S, Hauser S, Lapar V, et al: Regulatory effects of sterols and bile acids on hepatic 3-hydroxy-3-methylglutaryl CoA reductase and cholesterol 7α-hydroxylase in the rat. *J Lipid Res* 1973; 14:573–580.
44. Sackmann M, Delius M, Sauerbruch T, et al: Extracorporeal shock wave lithotripsy of gallbladder stones: Results in 101 treatments (abstract). *Gastroenterology* 1987; 92:1608.
45. Iser JH, Murphy GM, Dowling RH: Speed of change in biliary lipids and bile acids with chenodeoxycholic acid: Is intermittent therapy feasible? *Gut* 1977; 18:7–15.
46. Podda M, Zuin M, Dioguardi ML, et al: A com-

bination of chenodeoxycholic acid and ursodeoxycholic acid is more effective than either alone in reducing biliary cholesterol saturation. *Hepatology* 1982; 2:334–339.

47. Podda M, Zuin M, de Fazio C, et al: Comparison of the efficacy and safety of ursodeoxycholic acid alone and in combination with chenodeoxycholic acid in patients with radiolucent gallstones: A randomized controlled trial, in Paumgartner G, Stiehl A, Gerok W (eds): *Bile Acids and the Liver,* Lancaster, England, MTP Press Limited, 1987, pp 347–352.

48. Akerlund A: Die Verfeinerung der roemtgemologischen Gallensteindiagnostik durch Untersuchung der Sedimentierungs- und Schichtungsverhaeltnisse in der Gallenblase. *Acta Radiol* 1938; 19:23–43.

49. Senior JR, Johnson MF, DeTurck DM, et al: Kinetics of cholesterol gallstone dissolution during bile acid therapy with chenodiol or ursodiol (in preparation).

50. Wolpers C: Cholelitholyse die gallensteinlosung ihre praktischen ergebnisse. *Der Kassenarzt* 1982; 22:3763-3770.

51. Delius M, Enders G, Brendel W: Passage of stone fragments from the gallbladders of dogs. *Surg Gynecol Obstet* 1988; 166:241–244.

52. Lee SP, Nicholls JF: Nature and composition of biliary sludge, *Gastroenterology* 1986; 90:677–686.

53. Messing B, Bories C, Kunstlinger F, et al: Does total parenteral nutrition induce gallbladder sludge formation and lithiasis? *Gastroenterology* 1983; 84:1012–1019.

54. Schaad UB, Tschappeler H, Lentze MJ: Transient formation of precipitations in the gallbladder associated with ceftriaxone therapy, *Pediatr Infect Dis* 1986; 5:708–710.

55. Zakko SF, Hofmann AF, Schteingart C, et al: Percutaneous gallbladder stone dissolution using a microprocessor assisted solvent transfer (MAST) system (abstract). *Gastroenterology* 1987; 92:1793.

56. vanSonnenberg E, Hofmann AF, Neoptolemos J, et al: Gallstone dissolution with methyl-tert-butyl ether via percutaneous cholecystostomy: Success and caveats. *Am J Roentgenol* 1986; 146:856–867.

57. Hellstern A, Leuschner M, Fischer H, et al: Perkutan-transhepatische Lyse von Gallenblasensteinen mit Methyl-tert-butyl-ather. *Dtsch Med Wschr* 1988; 113:506–510.

58. Sauerbruch T, Holl J, Kruis W, et al: Dissolution of gallstones by methyl tert-butyl ether. (letter to editor). *N Engl J Med* 1985; 313:385–386.

Percutaneous Access for Gallbladder Interventions: Catheter Cholecystostomy

Peter R. Mueller, M.D.
E. vanSonnenberg, M.D.

Recent experience in several centers has demonstrated the feasibility, clinical efficacy, and low complication rate of percutaneous gallbladder interventions.[1–6] Because of its superficial location, the gallbladder is easily localized by real-time ultrasonography for subsequent fluorosopic or ultrasound-guided catheter puncture and drainage.

Surgical cholecystostomy has long been accepted as a compromise procedure in the elderly and/or high-risk patients with acute cholecystitis.[7] However, the high perioperative mortality rate of 6 to 20 percent and high morbidity rate have been major factors in limiting the role of surgical cholecystostomy.[8, 9] In the last 5 years, percutaneous cholecystostomy (PC) has proved to be a viable substitute for surgery. More than 250 cases have now been reported in the literature, with an overall significant complication rate of less than 3 percent.[1–6] Like surgical cholecystostomy, percutaneous cholecystostomy (PC) had been found useful in "temporizing" prior to cholecystostomy in elderly and very ill patients.[1, 10–12] PC has also been definitive in the treatment of acalculous cholecystitis.[13] In addition, PC has utility in diagnostic cholangiography and decompression of the obstructed biliary tree in place of or as a backup to percutaneous transhepatic cholangiography and drainage.[1, 14, 16]

INDICATION

Table I outlines the principal indications for percutaneous access to the gallbladder. They include acute calculous or acalculous cholecystitis, empyema, or pericholecystic abscess in patients considered medically unsuitable for surgical cholecystostomy. Cholecystostomy drainage has also been employed for decompression of obstructive jaundice as an alternative approach when conventional percutaneous transhepatic drainage has either failed or appears technically unsuitable because of nondilated intrahepatic bile ducts. More recently, percutaneous cholecystostomy has been utilized as an access route to perform dissolution of gallstones with solvent methyl-tert-butyl-ether (MTBE).

TABLE 1.
Percutaneous Catheter Cholecystostomy: Indications

Decompression of acute gallbladder sepsis—calculous or acalculous cholecystitis hydrops, empyema, pericholecystic abscess
Palliative drainage of obstructive jaundice (failed or nonfeasible endoscopic or transhepatic approach)
Catheter access for contact gallstone dissolution (MTBE)

ACCESS ROUTE

Cross-sectional imaging is critical to the success of percutaneous cholecystostomy. The radiologist's ability to image the gallbladder and select a safe percutaneous access route with the use of real-time ultrasound has enabled interventional radiologists to insert needles and catheters directly into the gallbladder (Figs 1, 2). Initial imaging is usually performed with real-time ultrasound and then combined with fluoroscopic observation. In cases of difficulty with the access route, computed tomography may be used to direct the approach, particularly if intervening bowel is felt to be in the way.

To avoid bile leakage, an anterior or anterior lateral transhepatic approach to the gallbladder has been used by most investigators. Puncture into the upper third of the gallbladder near its attachment to the liver has a theoretical advantage of reducing the risk of bile leakage into the peritoneal cavity. The added protection of overlying liver also would theoretically enable a small leak to be tamponaded by hepatic parenchyma. Several investigators have used both the transhepatic and free-wall routes with no significant complications reported. In a review of 100 consecutive CT scans, however, Warren and associates[17] stressed that in 13 percent of patients, bowel was interposed between the gallbladder fundus and the skin entry site. They stated that the shortest and safest route in most patients was via the transhepatic approach (Fig 3). Suggestions for a removable "anchoring device" to fasten the gallbladder to the anterior abdominal wall and allow subhepatic fundal puncture of the gallbladder without bile leakage have also been reported.[18] The direct fundal approach eliminates hepatic trauma associated with the large sheaths sometimes required for percutaneous gallstone removal.

TECHNIQUE

The preferred method of entry into the gallbladder—whether by single puncture "one-stick technique" or a tandem technique and whether by Seldinger or trocar method—still remains unsettled. Trocar insertion of a needle-catheter system is preferred by some, since it has the advantage of placement by single puncture and avoids the potential bile leak and catheter positioning problems encountered with guide wire exchange. Others have found the trocar method difficult, requiring repeated punctures, because of inability to place the catheter within the gallbladder. Many investigators prefer the Seldinger technique or a modification thereof. The Seldinger technique can be performed with a simple needle, guide wire, dilator, and catheter system. Modifications of the Seldinger technique include a removable hub needle with coaxial placement of a large needle system[5] (Fig 4). Hawkins has developed a preloaded catheter system that allows for a single "stick" technique.[11, 19] Theoretically these systems reduce complications due to bile leak or inadvertent puncture of other organs from multiple needle punctures.

Regardless of the actual needle or catheter assembly required, the puncture technique should be done with a short downward thrust to effectively pierce the anterior gallbladder wall. Because of the gallbladder's mobility and potential to collapse as it is punctured, a slow, gradual entry may simply displace the gallbladder away from the needle tip without penetrating.

Several catheter systems may be used for drainage of the gallbladder or instillation of stone-dissolving agents. Simple pigtail catheters with a limited number of side holes, Cope loop catheters, accordion catheters, or even specially designed catheters have been used.[10–14, 20] The main differences among the variety of catheters are the size and whether they may be inserted by trocar or Seldinger technique. Most catheters usually vary between 5 and 8 French in size and have the similar characteristic of a limited number of side holes such that side holes are only within the gallbladder itself. Catheter fixation is done in the routine fashion.

RESULTS

More than 250 successful percutaneous cholecystostomies have been reported in the literature.[16] In patients who have presented with gallbladder empyema, relief of pain and defer-

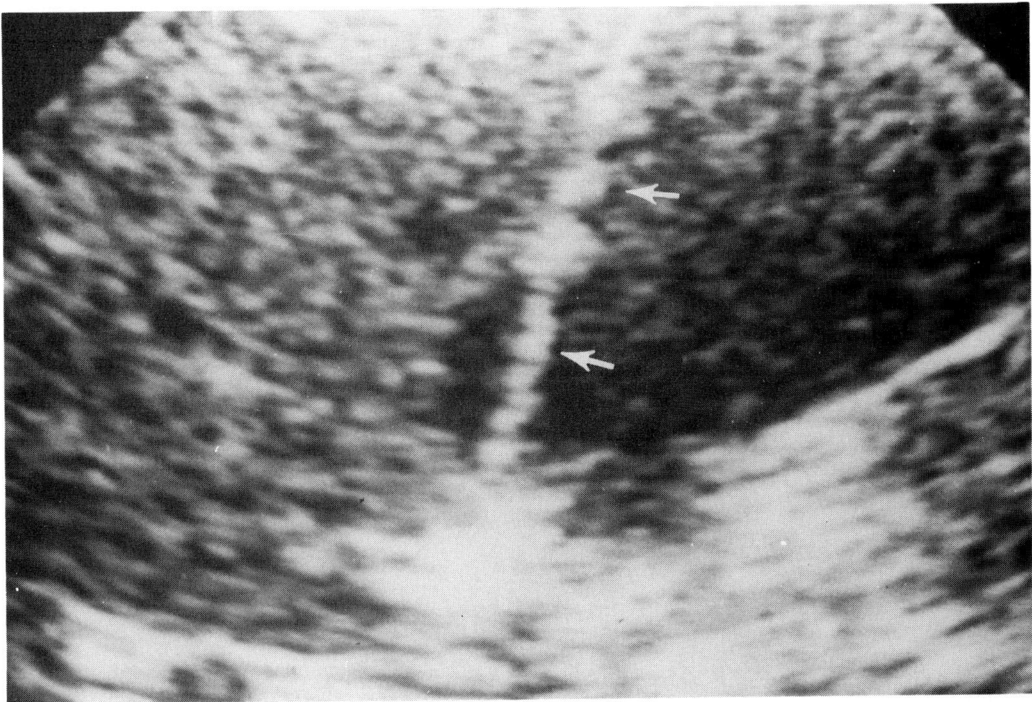

FIG 1.
Ultrasound-guided transhepatic approach for percutaneous cholecystostomy: Sagittal ultrasound demonstrates a 7 French catheter *(arrows)* placed transhepatically into the gallbladder via the trochar technique.

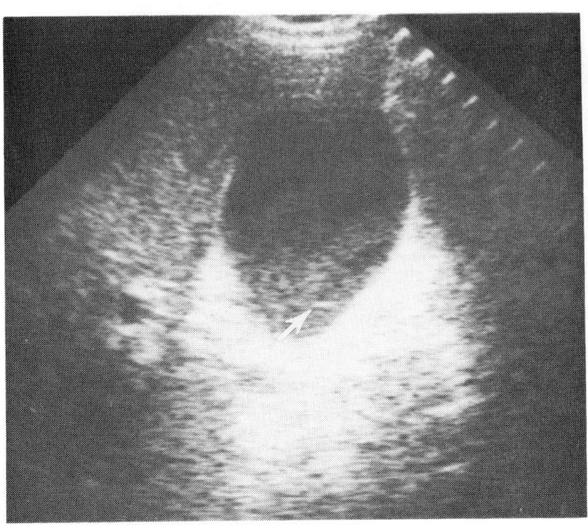

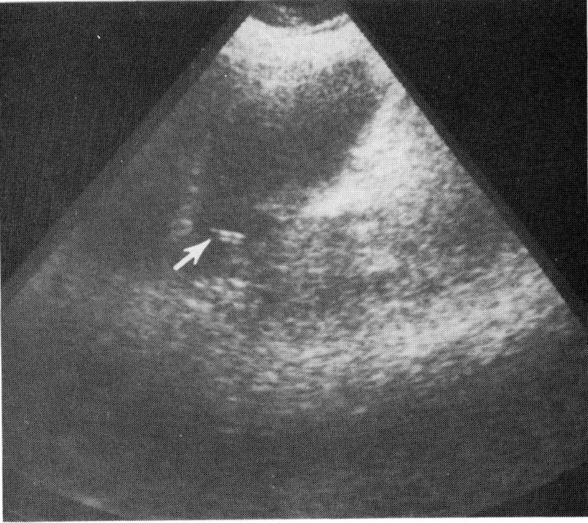

FIG 2.
Ultrasound-guided percutaneous cholecystostomy performed at the patient's bedside; 72-year-old patient status postrepair of a left hip fracture with increasing liver function test, distended gallbladder, and fever. **A.** Transverse ultrasound demonstrates large, distended gallbladder that is sludge filled. A 20-gauge needle placed transhepatically for aspiration *(arrow)* is seen in the most dependent portion of the gallbladder as an echogenic focus. A 7 French catheter was placed for drainage. **B.** Longitudinal sonogram obtained immediately after aspiration of 120 cc of bile demonstrates decrease in the volume size of the gallbladder. A portion of the catheter *(arrow)* is visualized in the dependent portion of the gallbladder.

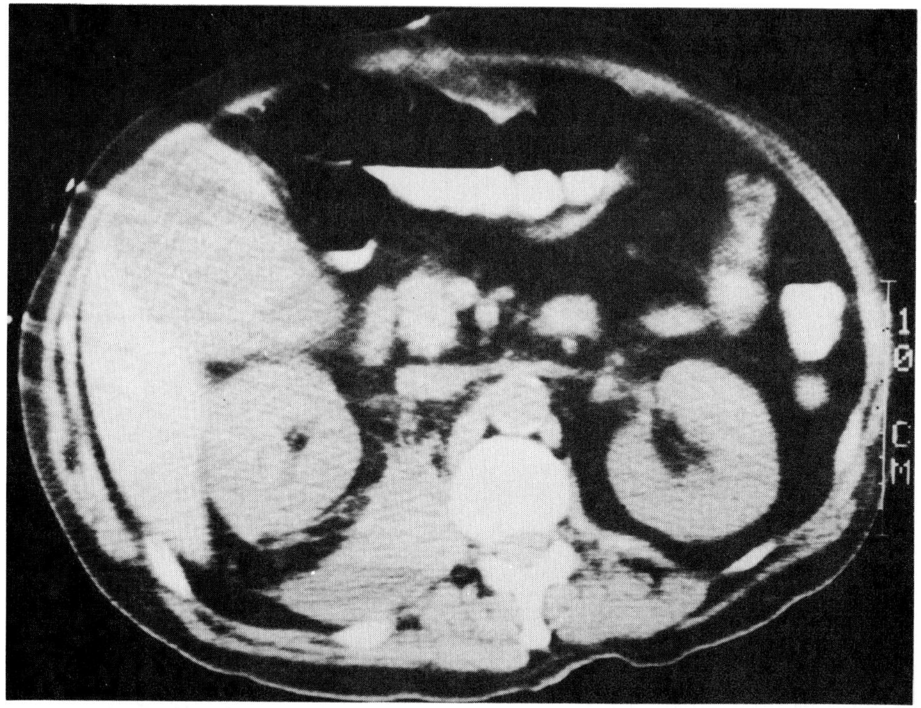

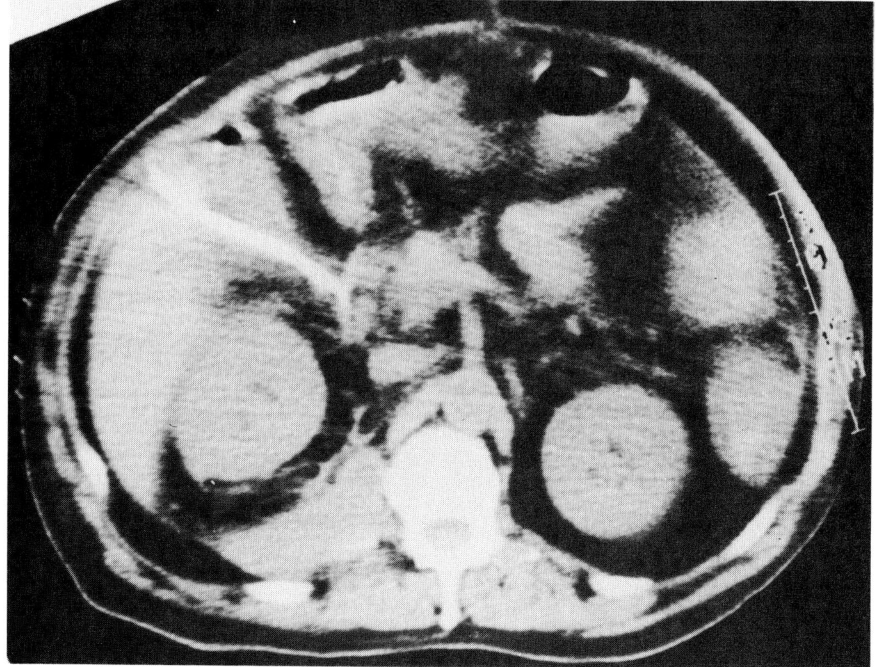

FIG 3.
CT scan for access route planning. **A.** CT performed after initial diagnostic needle puncture confirms absence of interposed bowel. **B.** CT postcatheter insertion shows successful decompression with no transgression of bowel.

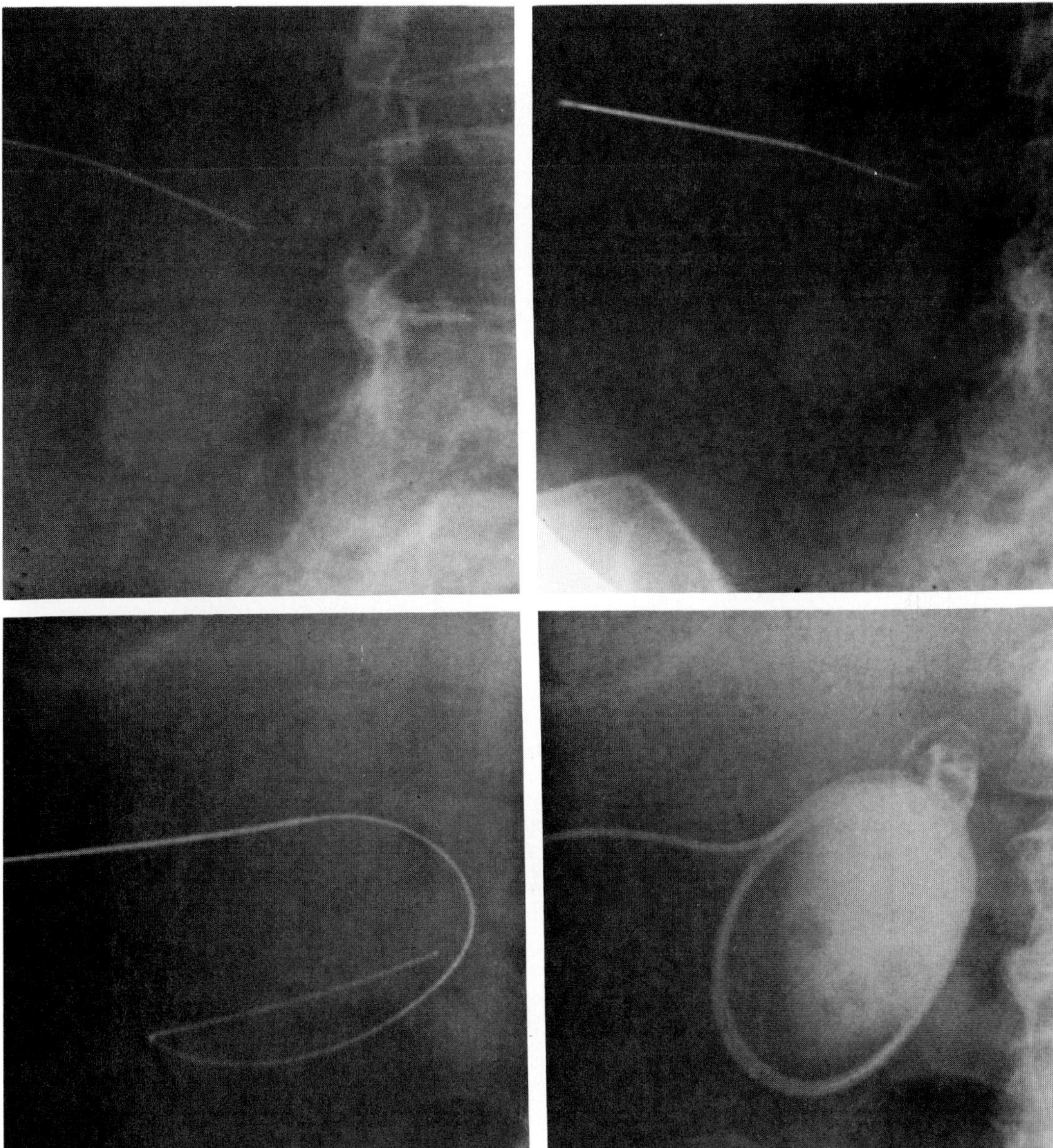

FIG 4.
Use of ultrasound and fluoroscopy with "one-stick" Seldinger method for placement of catheter in the gallbladder. The initial ultrasound was performed at the fluoroscopy table, and the gallbladder was marked on the skin. **A.** A 22-gauge removable hub needle was placed using ultrasound guidance. **B.** The hub was removed from the inner 22-gauge needle and an 18-gauge needle was passed over the 22 gauge. A slight amount of opacification of the gallbladder is seen from injection of the 22-gauge needle. **C.** An 0.038 guide wire was inserted through the 18-gauge needle directly into the gallbladder. **D.** A 6 French catheter is seen coiled into the gallbladder. Injection of the gallbladder demonstrates several small stones.

vescence can usually be promptly observed following placement of the catheter for drainage. If calculi are demonstrated in the gallbladder, they may be managed by methyl-tert-butyl-ether injection or, after a delayed period to develop a tract, by percutaneous extraction via stone basket or other mechanical means. Cholecystocholangiography can be performed via the PC catheter and may document the presence of gallstones, patency of cystic duct, or coincidentally associated common duct pathology in patients.

COMPLICATIONS

The most commonly reported complication from PC has been bile leakage. By a combination of phone and literature, we recently surveyed over 250 cases; eight cases of bile leakage had occurred. In general, the amount of leakage has been small and caused only transient right upper quadrant irritation. Only two cases have required surgical intervention.

Several investigators have emphasized adequate decompression of an obstructed biliary system to avoid bile leak.[1-6] Even in decompressed systems, however, too early removal of a PC catheter can lead to leakage of bile from the gallbladder. Most authors suggest waiting several days for a tract to develop prior to removing the catheter (Fig 5). One report notes adherence of the gallbladder to the abdominal wall only 1 week after placement of percutaneous cholecystostomy catheter.[16] The most common time period for removal is 10 days to 2 weeks.

Postprocedure sepsis has not been a common complication. In fact, sepsis has been an indication for performance of percutaneous cholecystostomy in patients with gallbladder empyema. Extensive experience with percutaneous transhepatic cholangiography over the years has shown the risk of septicemia can be reduced by avoiding undue distention of the biliary tree with contrast medium and by using preprocedure antibiotics. Only small-volume contrast injections should be made during the initial procedure; wait 24 to 48 hours after decompression to perform a definitive diagnostic study.

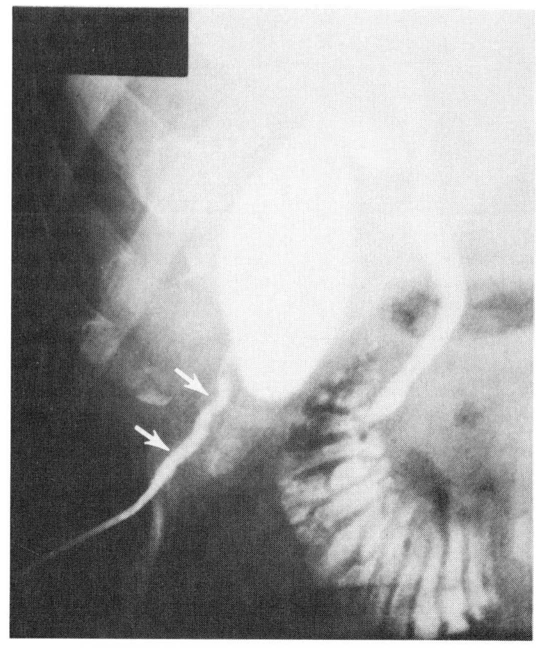

FIG 5.
Fluoroscopic spot film demonstrating a well-developed tract between the gallbladder and the skin *(arrows)*. The percutaneous cholecystostomy catheter was originally placed for decompression of the biliary system and removal of gallstones. After the procedure, the catheter remained in place for 14 days and then was removed under fluoroscopic guidance.

Four cases of severe vagal reactions have been associated with PC, one of which led to a nonfatal cardiac arrest.[21] The proposed etiology of this reaction is uncertain, but it is felt to be due to manipulation of a severely distended hydropic gallbladder. In addition, each of the patients in whom this reaction occurred had underlying cardiac disease or recent myocardial infarction. Although not a large number of these types of cases has been reported, suggestions for minimizing the risk of vagal reaction include limitation of gallbladder manipulation, removal of bile and injection of contrast in small aliquots, and use of atropine. In all cases, continuous blood pressure and ECG monitoring are strongly advised during PC.

Other potential but uncommon complications of PC include inadvertent puncture of nontarget organs, hemorrhage, and pneumothorax.

REFERENCES

1. Hawkins IF: Percutaneous cholecystostomy. *Sem In Rad* 1985; 2(1):97–103.
2. McGahan JP: A new catheter design for percutaneous cholecystostomy. *Radiology* 1988; 166:49–52.
3. McGahan JP, Lindfors KK: Acute cholecystitis: Diagnostic accuracy of percutaneous aspiration of the gallbladder. *Radiology* 1988; 167:669–671.
4. Pearse DM, Hawkins IF, Shaver R, Vogel S: Percutaneous cholecystostomy in acute cholecystitis and common duct obstruction. *Radiology* 1984; 152:365–367.
5. vanSonnenberg E, Wittich GR, Casola G, et al: Diagnostic and therapeutic percutaneous gallbladder procedures. *Radiology* 1986; 160:23–26.
6. Vogelzang RL, Nemcek AA. Percutaneous cholecystostomy: Diagnostic and therapeutic efficacy. *Radiology* 1988; 168:29–34.
7. Moore EE, Kelly GL, Driver T. Eiseman B: Reassessment of simple cholecystostomy. *Arch Surg* 1979; 114:515–518.
8. Skillings JC, Kumar C, Hinshaw JR: Cholecystostomy: A place in modern biliary surgery? *Am J Surg* 139:865–9, 1980.
9. Welch JP, Malt RA: Outcome of cholecystostomy. *Surg Gynecol Obstet* 1972; 135:7171–20.
10. Elyaderani M, Gabriele OF: Percutaneous cholecystostomy and cholangiography in patients with obstructive jaundice. *Radiology* 1979; 130:601–602.
11. Shaver RW, Hawkins IF, Soong J: Percutaneous cholecystostomy. *AJR* 1982; 138:1133–1136.
12. Teplick SK, Wolferth CC, Hayes MF, Amrom G: Percutaneous cholecystostomy in obstructive jaundice. *Gastroint Radiol* 1982; 7:259–261.
13. Eggermont AM, Lameiras JS, Jeekel J: Ultrasound guided percutaneous transhepatic cholecystostomy for acute acalculous cholecystitis. *Arch Surg* 1985; 120:1354–1358.
14. Bean WJ, Calonje MA, Aprill CN, Geshner J: Percutaneous catheterization of the gallbladder with ultrasonic guidance. *South Med J* 1979; 72(5):612–614.
15. Fromm H: Gallstone dissolution therapy: Current status and future prospects. *Gastroenterology* 1986; 91:1560–1567.
16. vanSonnenberg E, Hofmann AF, Neoptolemus J, Wittich GR, Princethal RA, Wilson SW: Gallstone dissolution with MTBE via percutaneous cholecystostomy: Success and caveats. *AJR* 1986; 146:865–867.
17. Warren LP, Kadir S, Dunnick NR: Percutaneous cholecystostomy: Anatomic considerations. *Radiology* 1988; 168:615–616.
18. Cope C: Percutaneous subhepatic cholecystostomy with removable anchor. Abstract presented at American Roentgen Ray Society Meeting, May, 1988.
19. Hawkins IF: New fine needle for cholangiography with optional sheath for decompression. *Radiology* 1979; 131:252–253.
20. Caridi JG, Hawkins IF: Single-step placement of a self-retaining "accordion" catheter. *AJR* 1984; 143:337–340.
21. vanSonnenberg E, Wing VW, Pollard JW, Casola G: Life-threatening vagal reactions associated with percutaneous cholecystostomy. *Radiology* 1984; 151:377–380.

Dissolution of Cholesterol Gallbladder Stones With Methyl Tert-Butyl Ether

J. L. Thistle, B. T. Petersen, C. E. Bender and H. J. Williams

More than 10 percent of the population in the United States have or have had gallstones, and 80 percent of these stones are composed predominantly of cholesterol. Efforts to dissolve gallstones with cholesterol solvents are predicated on the premise that removal of the cholesterol will allow the remaining stone components, primarily calcium bilirubinate and calcium carbonate, to be aspirated from the gallbladder or passed spontaneously. Very effective cholesterol solvents have been utilized in the laboratory for decades but have been too toxic or impractical for clinical use. Diethyl ether, for example, rapidly dissolves cholesterol but has a boiling point of 35°C and expands 225-fold when introduced into the body.

IN VITRO STUDIES

Methyl tert-butyl ether (MTBE) is an aliphatic ether that is liquid at body temperature and has a high capacity for dissolving cholesterol[1,2] (Table 1). Acute toxicity studies of MTBE when administered topically or parenterally to several animal species have demonstrated tolerance similar to that of diethyl (anesthetic) ether. In sufficient dosage, both ethers can induce general anesthesia and have the potential for inducing intravascular hemolysis. Both ethers are flammable and potentially explosive above 1.5 volume percent in air. MTBE is more stable and less volatile than diethyl ether, however.

HUMAN STUDIES OF MTBE

The use of MTBE in the United States is investigational, and human studies require FDA permission. Delivery of MTBE by percutaneous transhepatic catheter has been easily and safely accomplished, utilizing a CT scan to assess the hepatic-gallbladder interface and plan the optimal gallbladdder entry route. Placement of a 5F (1.7 mm) catheter (Cook Inc., Indianapolis, IN) under fluoroscopic guidance has been uniformly accomplished using local and intravenous anal-

TABLE 1.

Methyl Tert-Butyl Ether

Structure: $CH_3 - 0 - C(CH_3)_2 - CH_3$

$$\begin{array}{c} CH_3 \\ | \\ CH_3 - 0 - C - CH_3 \\ | \\ CH_3 \end{array}$$

Boiling point: 55°C

Cholesterol solubilizing capacity: 14 g/dL

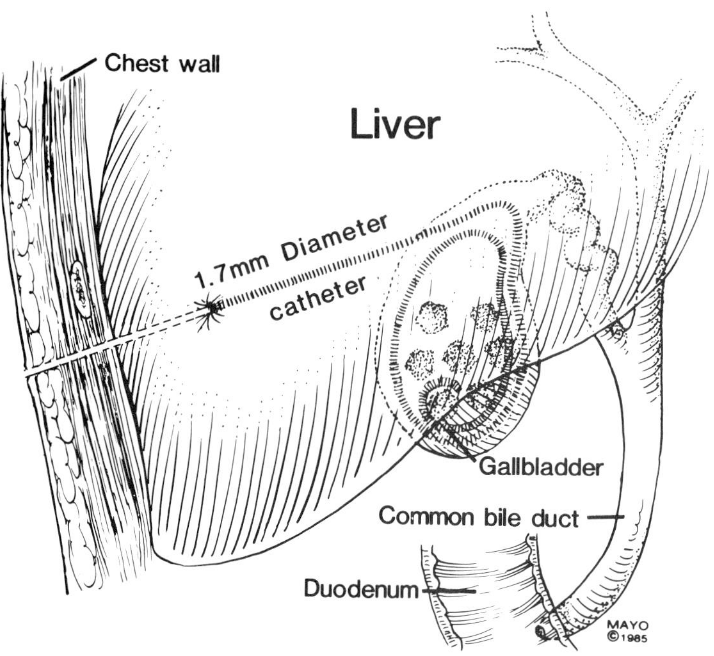

FIG 1.
Placement of percutaneous transhepatic catheter through the gallbladder-hepatic interface with 1.5 loops of catheter in the gallbladder and pigtail located in the fundus.

gesia (Fig 1). Patients with cirrhosis or coagulopathies have not been treated.[3,4]

TREATMENT CRITERIA

Patients studied have had biliary symptoms, a patent cystic duct, and a high probability of soluble cholesterol stones. Soluble cholesterol stones obstructing the gallbladder neck or cystic duct could be dissolved, but these cannot be clearly differentiated from a fibrotic occlusion secondary to chronic cholecystitis, which would leave the patient with a hydrops. Safe, effective methods for completely ablating both the cystic duct and the secretory gallbladder mucosa have not been established. We have not used MTBE in patients with acute cholecystitis or pancreatitis, and no animal data relevant to MTBE use under these circumstances are available. MTBE is available as a high-performance liquid chromatography (HPLC) laboratory solvent. For investigational use, we redistill it, gas chromatograph it to confirm purity, and millipore filter it (0.22 μ) under sterile conditions.

METHODOLOGY

Dissolution treatment can be initiated immediately after catheter placement, provided extravasation of radiopaque contrast media at the catheter entry site is not apparent using anticipated treatment volumes. This treatment volume of MTBE is determined fluoroscopically by infusing contrast medium sufficient to envelop the stones and then adding contrast until it begins to enter the cystic duct (the overflow volume). Usually 3 to 5 mL is an effective treatment volume and 10 to 20 mL or more is required to exceed the gallbladder capacity. Overflow does not grossly appear to correlate with infusion pressure because it occurs well before complete gallbladder filling or physiologic fasting gallbladder volume is achieved.

After complete aspiration of bile, continuous

cycling of the treatment volume of MTBE can be initiated, starting with 1 to 2 mL and increasing as tolerated to the prescribed treatment volume. Patients often notice discomfort when MTBE is first introduced. Although usually transient and tolerable, patient discomfort is minimized by administering an analgesic such as butorphanol 0.5 to 1 mg intravenously. Sedation is minimized so that development of any anesthetic effect from MTBE will not be masked. Nausea and emesis are infrequent and have responded to prochlorperazine suppositories.

Once a comfortable exchange volume and rate of infusion and aspiration of MTBE are established, this regimen is continued, using glass syringes and materials stable in MTBE. This procedure may be easily performed by a well-trained and supervised clinical assistant. Complete evacuation of bile and MTBE from the gallbladder after each aspiration stroke and avoidance of reinfusion of bile, stone debris, or infusion of air will optimize efficacy and provide complete control over the intragallbladder volume and thus risk of overflow. Acute or persistent overflow or extravasation of MTBE from the gallbladder could induce intravascular hemolysis, general anesthesia, and possibly duodenitis. This is easily avoided but must not be neglected. Fail-safe pump systems to administer and stir carefully controlled volumes of MTBE are under development.

To assure optimal stone and catheter positioning, fluoroscopic assessment should be performed every 2 to 4 hours. Dissolution of stones encircled by the catheter pigtail is much more rapid than at the opposite end of the gallbladder (Fig 2). Stones can usually be corralled or floated into the newly emptied fundus, but occasionally the pigtail must be repositioned to accomodate the location of the residual stones. If the pigtail is positioned in the fundus rather than the proximal end of the gallbladder, a large treatment volume can be instilled without overflow. This also avoids infusing MTBE adjacent to the catheter entry site, usually in the upper third of the gallbladder.

Once stone dissolution is complete, the catheter can be removed with a guide wire and fluoroscopy. This may be accomplished the same day the catheter was placed if dissolution has been completed. We have continued dissolution treatment for 1 to 2 hours when no further stone material can be detected fluoroscopically. Leakage of bile after catheter removal has been infrequent, and only one patient has required replacement of the catheter for this purpose. We have had no symptoms or signs of leakage since initiating placement of Gelfoam in the transhepatic tract at the time of catheter removal.

The morning following catheter removal, a gallbladder ultrasound will determine most accurately whether radiologically inapparent debris remains. Patients can then resume a normal diet and activity as tolerated, usually returning home that day and to work the following day or week.

FOLLOW-UP AND STONE RECURRENCE

Residual stone debris, when present, has consisted of particles 1 to 3 mm in diameter, detectable only by ultrasound, and has remained asymptomatic. We are monitoring patients by ultrasound after 6 to 12 months and then annually to define the incidence of stone recurrence and to assess postdissolution natural history.

SEQUENTIAL EXTRACORPOREAL SHOCK WAVE LITHOTRIPSY AND MTBE FRAGMENT DISSOLUTION

Because passage of stone fragments following ESL often results in pain and occasionally in duct obstruction or pancreatitis, rapid fragment dissolution immediately following lithotripsy is appealing. In addition, intact cholesterol stones with one or more layers of noncholesterol material may be difficult to dissolve with MTBE. Lithotripsy should allow the ether access to the cholesterol and fragment and residual material to fine debris, which may be aspirated or passed spontaneously. Our preliminary experience combining these two techniques in dogs and then in humans with partially calcified cholesterol

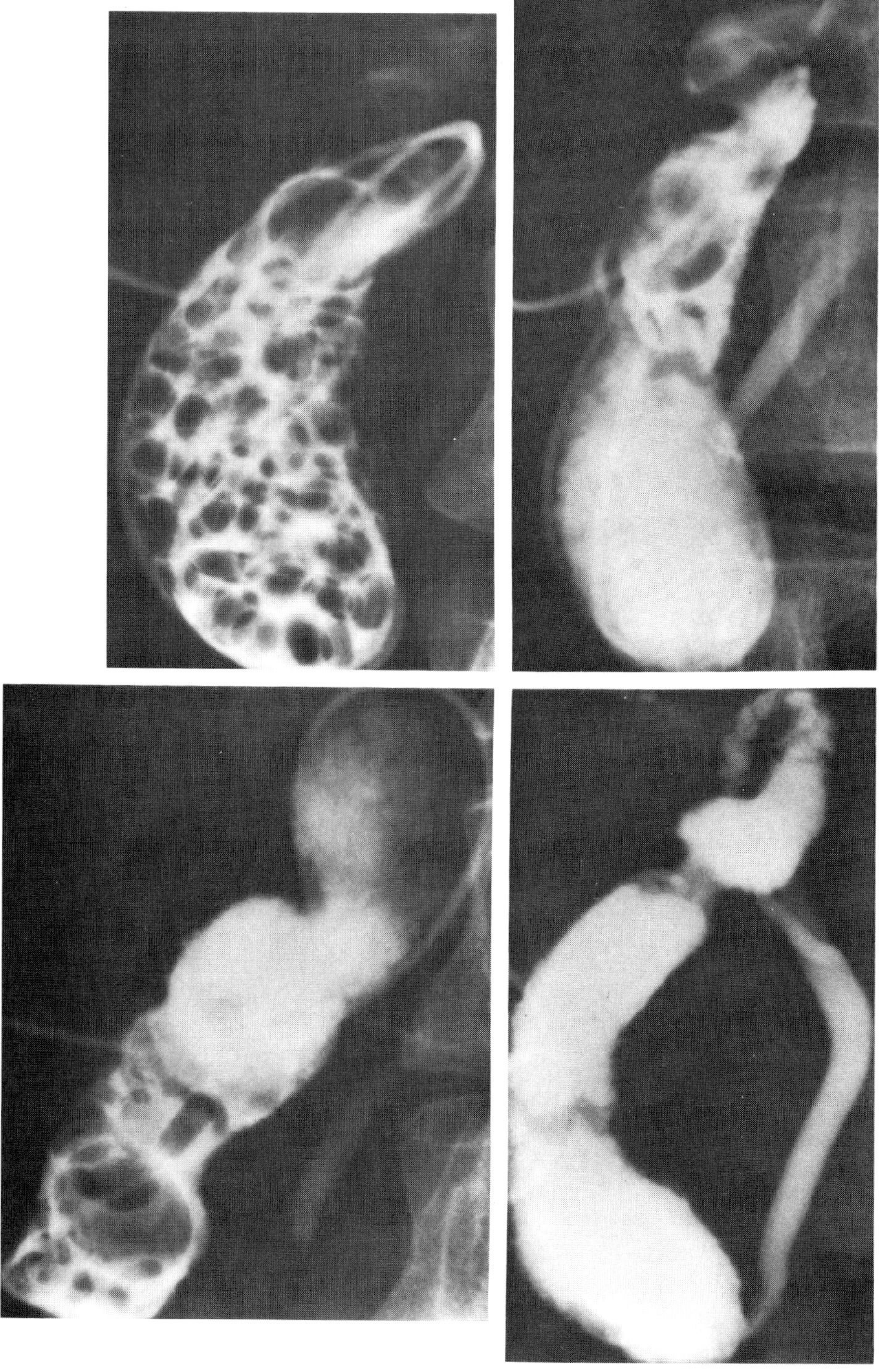

FIG 2.
See legend on facing page.

stones suggests that this approach is feasible and potentially safe and effective.[5,6]

REFERENCES

1. Allen MJ, Borody TJ, Bugliosi TF, et al: Cholelitholysis using methyl tertiary butyl ether. *Gastroenterology* 1985; 88:122–125.
2. Allen MJ, Borody TJ, Thistle JL: In vitro dissolution of cholesterol gallstones: A study of factors influencing rate and a comparison of solvents. *Gastroenterology* 1985; 89:1097–1103.
3. Allen MJ, Borody TJ, Bugliosi TF, et al: Rapid dissolution of gallstones by methyl tert-butyl ether. *N Engl J Med* 1985; 312:217–220.
4. Thistle JL: Direct contact dissolution of gallstones. *Seminars in Liver Disease* 1987; 7:311–316.
5. Peine CJ, May GR, Nagorney DM, et al: Same day sequential extracorporeal shock wave lithotripsy and methyl tert-butyl ether dissolution of gallstones in dogs: Effect on gallbladder mucosa and MTBE absorption. *Hepatology* 1986; 6:1206.
6. Peine CJ, Petersen BT, Williams HJ, et al: Fragmentation and dissolution of calcified cholesterol gallstones using extracorporeal shock wave lithotripsy and methyl tert-butyl ether in humans. *Hepatology* 1987; 7:113.

FIG 2.
A. Large and medium-sized radiolucent cholesterol gallstones filling the gallbladder as demonstrated by contrast infusion via 5F transhepatic percutaneous catheter placed as illustrated in Fig. 1. **B.** Dissolution of all stones in fundus after 3 hours of MTBE dissolution therapy. **C.** Residual stones in the upper half of the gallbladder have been manipulated with guide wire and/or floated into fundus for most rapid dissolution. **D.** Complete dissolution of stones after 3 additional hours of treatment. Gallbladder mucosal fold noted in midgallbladder. Biliary duct system normal and drains freely into duodenum. Ultrasound the following morning demonstrated no residual stones.

Radiologic Aspects of MTBE Therapy

Gerald R. May, M.D.

Initial experience with the contact solvent methyl tert butyl ether (MTBE) for the dissolution of cholesterol gallstones indicates that it is a safe and effective technique.[1-3] The radiologic aspects of the procedure are vital to the success of the technique. Increasing experience with the use of MTBE has led to modifications in the radiologic techniques that have increased the chances of success with the procedure. The following is a review of the radiologic aspects of the procedure based on experience with 75 cases.

There are three aspects of the MTBE dissolution procedure in which radiologic exams and/or techniques are used: (1) the preprocedure evaluation, in which a determination of gallbladder anatomy, cystic duct patency, and stone composition is necessary; (2) the placement, maintenance, and removal of the cholecystostomy catheter; and (3) follow-up exams of the gallbladder after MTBE gallstone dissolution to identify residual debris and detect stone recurrence. The following questions about these aspects of the procedure seem important and have been partially answered by early experience with the procedure: (1) Can gallstone composition be determined prior to the procedure? (2) Under what conditions is short-term percutaneous cholecystostomy for MTBE therapy safe? (3) What technical factors increase the speed of stone dissolution and minimize the side effects of MTBE? and (4) What is the best method to identify residual debris or recurrent stones in the gallbladder?

PREPROCEDURE EVALUATION

The initial diagnosis of gallstones is made in almost all cases by ultrasound exam.[4] Further radiologic examination is then directed toward evaluating the composition of the stones, the presence of a patent cystic duct, and the exclusion of any anatomic anomalies that would make percutaneous cholecystostomy difficult or unsafe. With few exceptions, gallstone composition and cystic duct patency cannot be determined by ultrasound. Ultrasound can detect anatomic anomalies of the gallbladder and evaluate the gallbladder-liver interface. Cystic duct stones are very difficult to dissolve or extract; converting a hydrops with stones to a hydrops without stones by MTBE therapy would not be particularly useful. Therefore, all patients are screened for cystic duct patency by oral cholecystography after a double dose of either iopanoic acid or sodium tyropanoate. Any opacification of the gallbladder by the contrast is taken as proof of cystic duct patency. In an otherwise healthy, ambulatory patient, nonopacification of the gallbladder is reliable evidence of cystic duct obstruction. If the stones float in the contrast, they can be assumed to be cholesterol stones (Fig 1). The size and shape of the gallstones

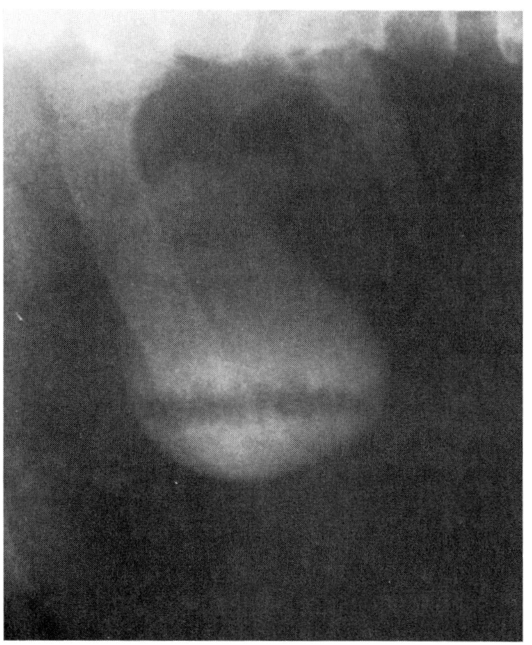

FIG 1.
Oral cholecystogram, decubitus view, demonstrates floating gallstones, an indicator of high cholesterol content.

seen on the oral cholecystogram provide a clue to the ease of stone dissolution with MTBE. Single round or oval stones and multiple faceted stones are usually easier to dissolve (have a higher cholesterol content) than multiple tiny stones with irregular surfaces or multiple stones of warying sizes and shapes (Fig 2). Radionuclide biliary scans (with HIDA derivatives) can also be used to evaluate cystic duct patency. In a few cases, however, radionuclide scans have indicated cystic duct patency in the presence of small, partially obstructing cystic duct stones that proved impossible to dissolve or extract (Fig 3).

Initial laboratory and clinical experience with MTBE indicate that most noncalcified stones will dissolve in MTBE; therefore, evaluation of stone composition is directed toward detection of calcium in the stones. A CT scan of the gallbladder is the most sensitive technique for the demonstration of calcification in gallstones.[5–7] The presence of any amount of calcification greater than a few tiny flecks makes successful stone dissolution with MTBE unlikely. A few stones, despite having no detectable calcification

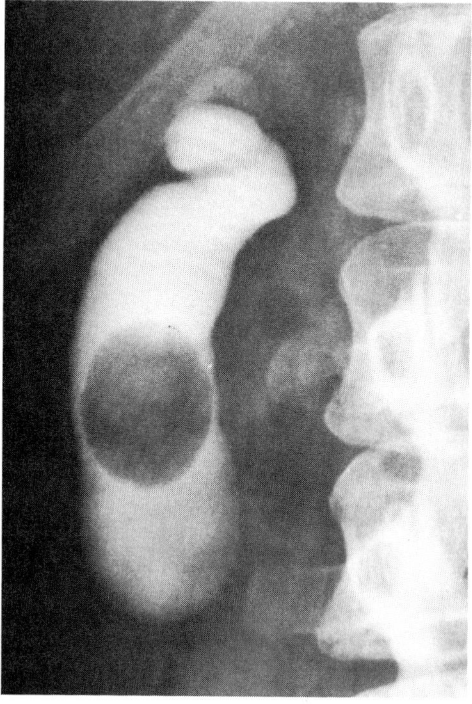

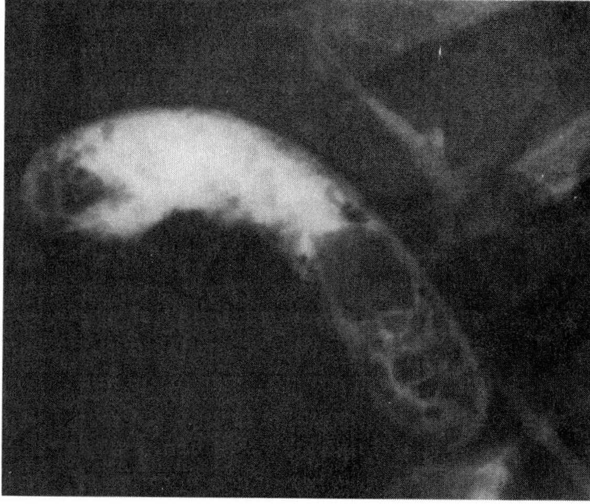

FIG 2.
A. A single oval gallstone, dissolved by MTBE in four hours. **B.** Multiple stones of varying sizes and shapes dissolved by MTBE in four days (about 30 hours of MTBE injections).

by CT, will still be very resistant to MTBE dissolution. Even in the same gallbladder, stones may have different compositions so that their resistance to MTBE disolution varies widely. The efficacy of obtaining a plain abdominal film to look for stone calcification prior to the CT scan is uncertain. The ideal CT technique for the detection of stone calcification has not been established. Our current protocol uses 5 mm contiguous slices through the gallbladder. To prevent partial volume effects that could simulate stone calcification, oral and intravenous contrast are not given. The ideal gallbladder for this procedure has a long area of close contact with the liver with no fat interposed between the gallbladder and liver (Fig 4). Initially, we excluded patients whose gallbladders were not closely applied to the liver; subsequent experience with a small number of patients indicates that the procedure can still be done in these patients, but that local extravasation of MTBE about the catheter entry site is more likely to occur, especially immediately after catheter placement (Fig 5). In addition, initial catheter placement in these patients is more difficult, as the gallbladder is quite mobile. If local extravasation occurs, it will usually resolve if the catheter is left in place for 24 to 28 hours before the MTBE injections resume. A few patients have had anatomic anomalies, usually bowel interposed between the gallbladder or liver and abdominal wall, which have made cholecystostomy impossible. One patient had a small hemangioma detected in the liver along the usual course of the cholecystostomy cathether.

CHOLECYSTOSTOMY CATHETER PLACEMENT, MAINTENANCE, AND REMOVAL

Important technical factors increasing the safety of short-term percutaneous cholecystostomy for MTBE gallstone dissolution are the use of small-diameter catheters, use of a transhepatic route for catheter placement through the site where the gallbladder and liver are in close contact, and secure placement of the catheter within the gallbladder with the distal end of the catheter as distant from the cystic duct as possible. Factors increasing the speed of dissolution of the gallstones are the proximity of the distal end of the catheter to the stones, design of the catheter and sideholes to increase solvent turbulence during injection, and MTBE injection technique.

The initial puncture of the gallbaldder is done via a right lateral transhepatic approach (either intercostal or subcostal) with a 22-gauge needle. Localization of the gallbladder can be done either by fluoroscopy (after ingestion of oral cholecystographic contrast) or by ultrasonography. In my own experience, gallbladder puncture has been more easily performed with fluoroscopic guidance, as selection of the gallbladder entry site is easier. The needle puncture is usually successful on the first or second pass, and puncture of the opposite wall of the gallbladder is more easily avoided. The procedure is performed with local anesthetic and small doses of intravenous analgesics and sedatives. A variety of needles, guide wires, and dilators have been used with success. Care should be taken to produce only a single puncture site in the proximal or middle third of the lateral border of the gallbladder. The number of guide wire and dilator exchanges should be minimized. In this regard, a long, 22-gauge puncture needle with a detachable hub with a 4 French or 5 French dilator preloaded on the shaft of the needle has been very useful. Dilation of the tract to a diameter greater than 5 French should be avoided, as this will increase the risk of extravasation of MTBE about the catheter entry site. Excessive guide wire manipulation and entry of the guide wire into the cystic duct should also be avoided. Distention of the gallbladder by coiling of the guide wire within the gallbladder is usually the most uncomfortable part of the procedure for the patient, and additional analgesic is frequently necessary at this time. Careful observation of the pulse and blood pressure should be done to detect any evidence of a vagal response to gallbladder distention,[8] particularly in those patients with a history of cardiac disease (Fig 6). The guide wire that in my experience is most frequently successful is the large-radius (15 mm) "J" configuration. A small-radius (1.5 or 3 mm)

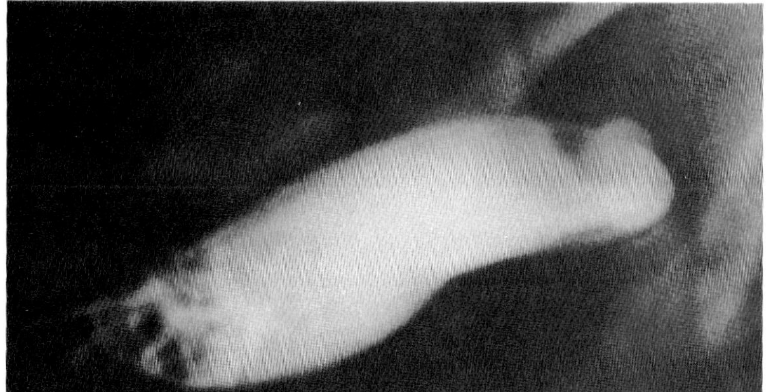

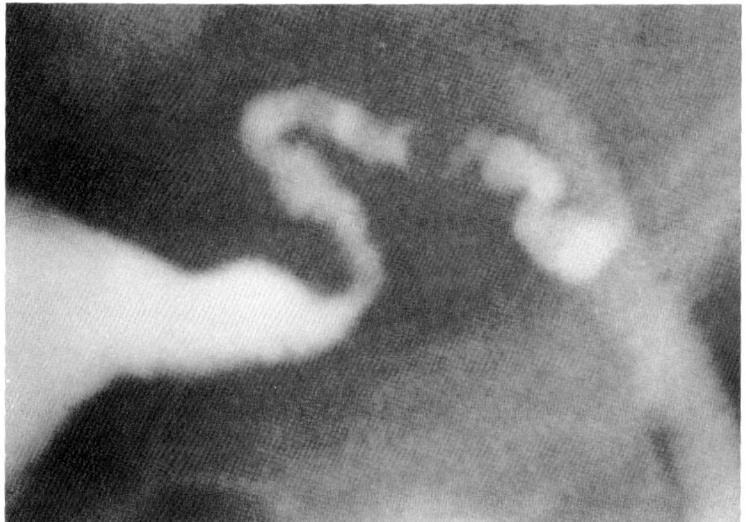

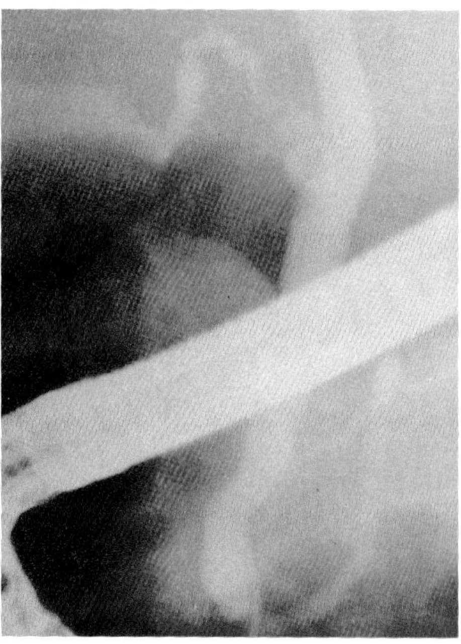

FIG 3.
A, B. There are multiple small stones in the gallbladder and a nonobstructing stone in the cystic duct; the radionuclide biliary scan was normal. The stones in the gallbladder were dissolved with MTBE, but the cystic duct stone could not be dissolved or extracted; therefore, the cholecystostomy catheter was removed. **C.** 6 months later, after an episode of biliary colic, and ERCP shows that the cystic duct stone has passed.

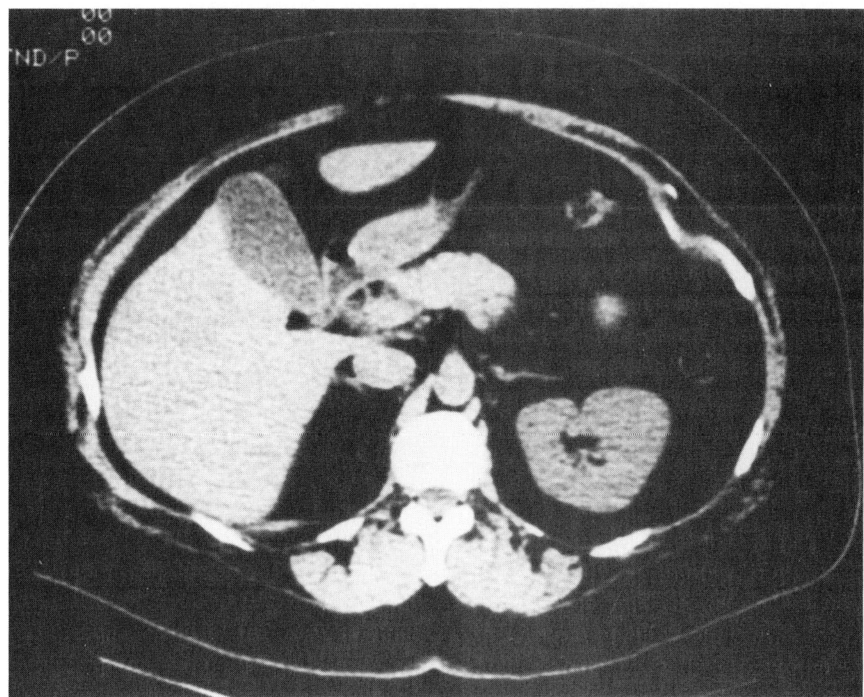

FIG 4.
CT scan of the gallbladder shows no evidence of gallstone calcification and demonstrates a long area of close contact between the gallbladder wall and liver.

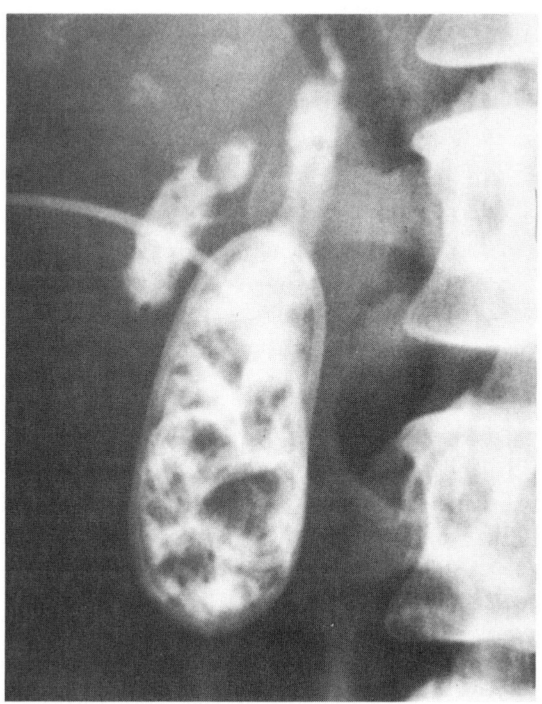

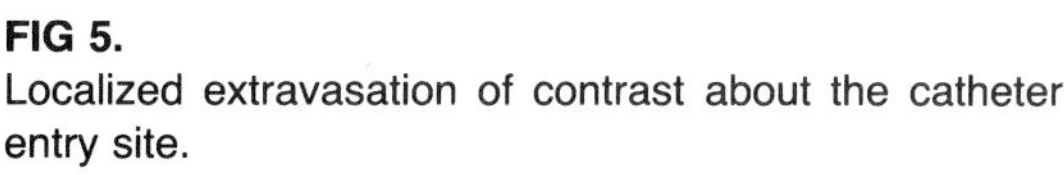

FIG 5.
Localized extravasation of contrast about the catheter entry site.

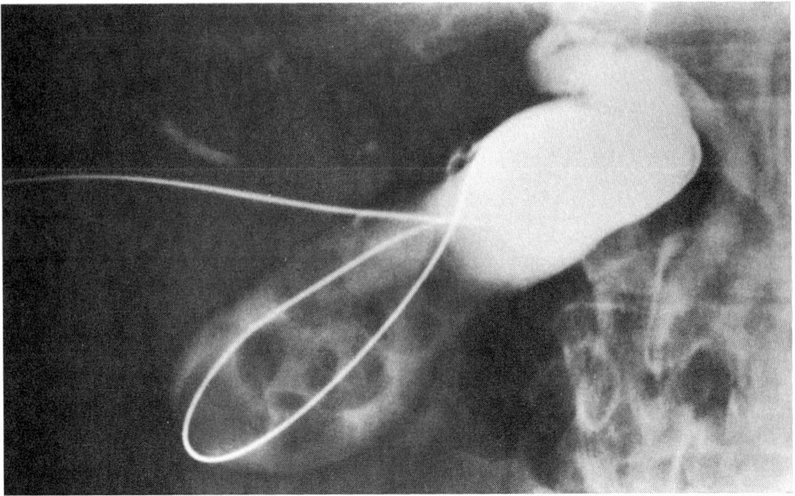

FIG 6.
Coiling of the guide wire within the gallbladder.

"J" and a malleable-tip torque control wire are also occasionally useful. Usually, a single dilation of the tract with a 4 or 5 French dilator is sufficient to allow catheter placement. The catheter used is a modified 5 French polyethylene pediatric nephrostomy catheter with a 2 cm diameter pigtail tip and multiple sideholes placed along the inner aspect of the pigtail. The pigtail tip of the catheter should be placed in the gallbladder fundus—placing an extra loop of the catheter in the gallbladder decreases the chances of catheter dislodgement. The gallstones are maneuvered into the region of the pigtail via gravity (most stones float in contrast and sink in bile or saline) or by pushing them with the guide wire or catheter (Fig 7).

After the catheter is placed, the gallbladder is completely aspirated and small amounts of contrast are slowly injected, while the volume of injected contrast needed to produce entry of contrast into the cystic duct and common bile duct is assessed. A volume of MTBE significantly less than this amount is then selected as the initial injection volume. Usually this will be in range of 3 to 5 cc of MTBE. The cholecystostomy catheter is then fixed to the skin by suture or tape, and the MTBE injections are begun by hand with a glass syringe. The MTBE is injected as rapidly as possible, allowed to remain in the gallbladder for a few minutes, and then aspirated. Any aspirated bile is separated from MTBE and discarded; the MTBE is then reinjected. At 20 to 30 minute intervals, the MTBE is discarded and fresh MTBE is used. Catheter position and stone dissolution is checked with fluoroscopy at 3 to 4 hour intervals or sooner if the patient's condition suggests a change in catheter position or the catheter becomes difficult to inject or aspirate. If the stones move away from the pigtail portion of the catheter, an attempt is made to reposition the stones into the fundus of the gallbladder adjacent to the pigtail (Fig 8). During times when MTBE is not being injected, the catheter is attached to an external collection bag and allowed to drain via gravity. After gallstones can no longer be identified by cholangiography, the MTBE injections are continued for another hour or two. The final cholangiogram should include opacification of the cystic duct and bile ducts to exclude stone fragments in these areas (Fig 9). At this point, the gallbladder is thoroughly irrigated with saline, and then the catheter is removed over a guide wire.

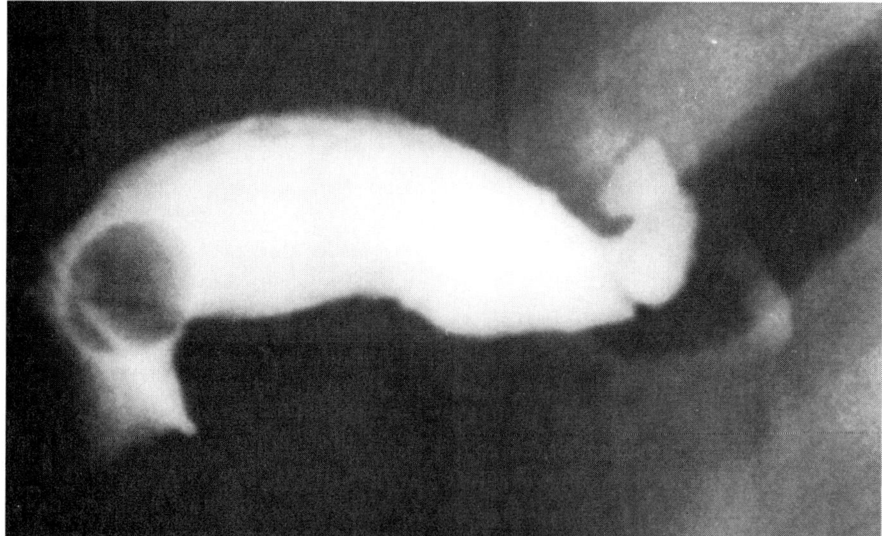

FIG 7.
The pigtail portion of the cholecystostomy catheter lies in the fundus of the gallbladder adjacent to the stone.

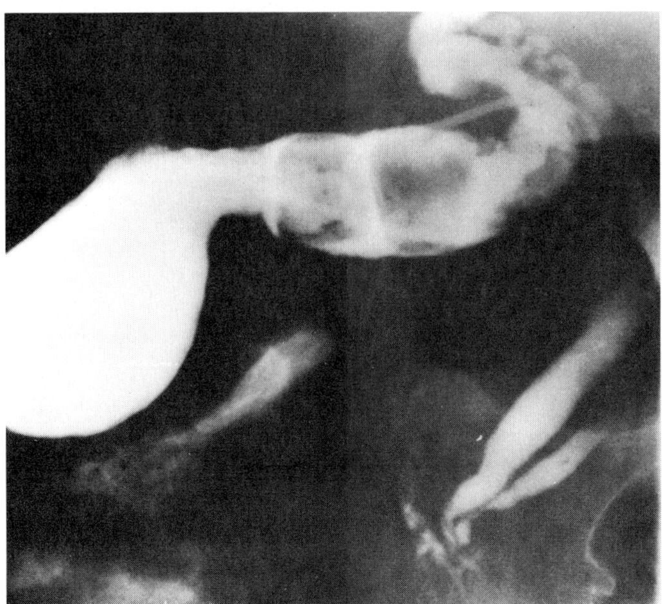

FIG 8.
Interval cholecystogram shows the stones have moved away from the pigtail portion of the catheter (in the fundus). The stones were repositioned by gravity into the fundus, and MTBE injections resumed.

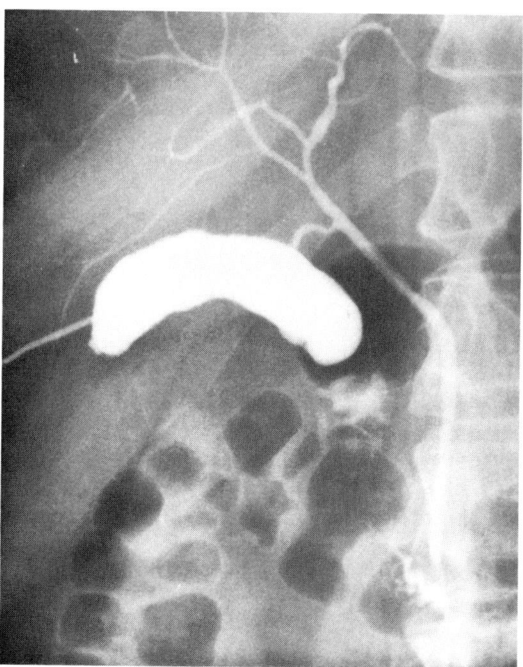

FIG 9.
Normal cholangiogram done just prior to catheter removal. Note patent cystic duct and normal bile ducts.

TECHNICAL PROBLEMS AND REFINEMENTS

Catheter-related complications are for the most part minor in nature. The commonest complication is partial catheter dislodgment from the gallbladder. Usually this occurs when the catheter remains in the gallbladder overnight. In most cases, the catheter is repositioned over a guide wire and the MTBE injections are then resumed (Fig 10). In some patients, partial catheter dislodgment is asymptomatic; in others, right upper quadrant pain develops. In no patient has catheter dislodgment resulted in a significant extravasation of bile or MTBE. Most patients have small amounts of bleeding into the gallbladder during catheter placement. This clears quickly and is of no clinical significance. One patient with friable gallbladder mucosa had a large amount of bleeding into the gallbladder after extensive catheter manipulation. This cleared after overnight observation without specific therapy. A few patients had transient asymptomatic episodes of cystic duct obstruction during MTBE injection, presumably related to small stone fragments entering the cystic duct. Many of these episodes resolved spontaneously. Those that did not were treated by gentle catheterization of the cystic duct with disimpaction of the stone fragment or extraction of the fragment with a stone basket (small stone baskets that can be passed through the lumen of a 6 French straight catheter are available). One patient had several common bile duct stones pulled back into the gallbladder with a stone basket and then dissolved with MTBE. A few patients with stone fragments resistant to MTBE had the fragments crushed with the stone basket. The fragments were then either dissolved with MTBE or irrigated out with saline. After catheterization of the cystic duct or basketing of stone fragments, it is necessary to maintain gallbladder catheterization with external drainage overnight to allow any edema or hemorrhage to clear. Major complications of the procedure include localized extravasation of MTBE around the catheter entry site and bile leak from the gallbladder after catheter removal. Localized extravasation of MTBE usually occurs during the initial MTBE injections immediately after catheter placement and causes intense localized pain. Injection of contrast will usually demonstrate the extravasation. Leaving the cholecystostomy catheter in place for 24 to 48 hours before resuming the MTBE injections allows a more secure tract to form. One patient developed right upper quadrant pain and low-grade fever after catheter removal that resolved 48 hours without specific therapy and presumably represented a mild case of bile peritonitis.

FOLLOW-UP EXAMS

Initial experience with ultrasound exams done prior to cholecystostomy catheter removal demonstrated the difficulty of detecting or excluding small stone fragments when the cholecystostomy catheter was still in place. The initial follow-up ultrasound exam is now done immediately after catheter removal. No significant perihepatic or pericholecystic fluid collections have been iden-

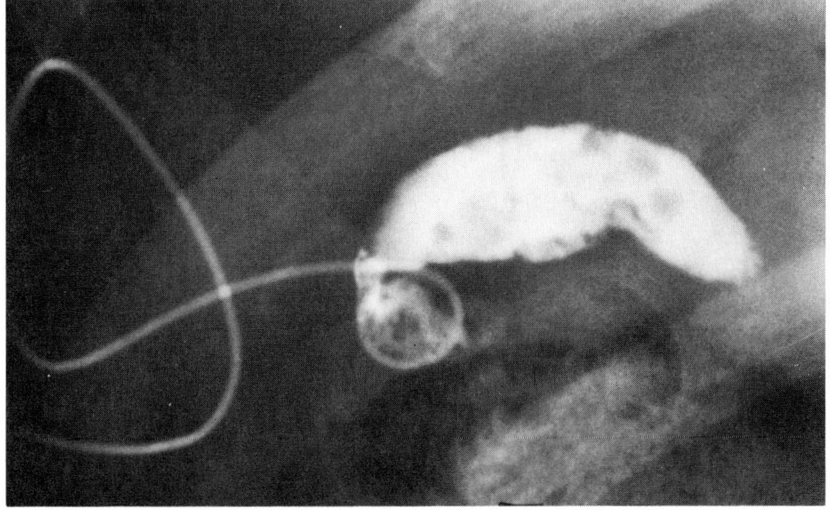

FIG 10.
Partial dislodgment of the catheter from the gallbladder. Note the loop of catheter lying between the surface of the liver and the abdominal wall.

tified. Approximately half of the patients have small echogenic foci within the gallbladder that do not have accompanying acoustical shadows and frequently are immobile (Fig 11). Presumably these foci represent small bits of insoluble debris. In at least some patients, follow-up exams have demonstrated that the echogenic foci are no longer present. Routine follow-up exams by ultrasound are the most sensitive technique for detecting recurrent stones and have detected small, asymptomatic gallstone recurrences in several patients.

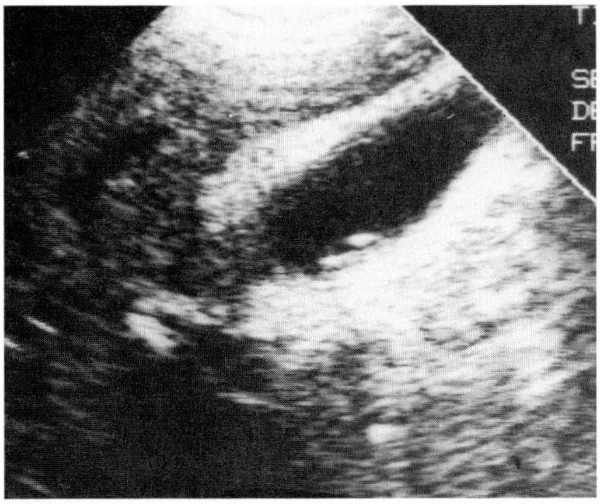

FIG 11.
Follow-up ultrasound exam after MTBE dissolution demonstrates debris in the gallbladder. A repeat exam done 1 year later was normal.

SUMMARY

Initial experience with radiologic aspects of MTBE gallstone dissolution indicates that pre-procedure radiologic evaluation can identify most, but not all, patients with gallstones insoluble in MTBE. Careful catheter placement and attention to technical details, such as catheter position, increase the safety and speed of the dissolution procedure. Short-term percutaneous cholecystostomy with a small-diameter catheter is a safe and well-tolerated technique for MTBE delivery. Further improvements in catheter design, for example, the use of multiple-lumen catheters for continuous infusion and aspiration of MTBE or the use of some sort of catheter or balloon to occlude the cystic duct during MTBE injections, may increase the safety and speed of the procedure. The development of transcatheter mechanical or laser devices to fragment stones prior to MTBE injection might also improve the success of the procedure. The discovery of a safe and effective agent or device to ablate the gallbladder lumen would improve the long-term results of the procedure.

REFERENCES

1. Allen MJ, Borody TJ, Bugliosi TF, et al: Rapid dissolution of gallstones by methyl tert-butyl ether. Preliminary observations. *N Engl J Med* 1985; 312:217–220.
2. Van Sonnenberg E, Wittich GR, Casola G, et al: Diagnostic and therapeutic percutaneous gallbladder procedures. *Radiology* 1986; 160:23–26.
3. Van Sonnenberg E, Hofmann AF, Neoptolemus J, et al: Gallstone dissolution with methyl-tert-butyl ether via percutaneous cholecystostomy: Success and caveats. *AJR* 1986; 146:865–868.
4. Cooperberg PL. Gibney RG: Imaging of the gallbladder, 1987. *Radiology* 1987; 163:605–613.
5. Moss AA, Filly RA, Way LA: In vitro investigation of gallstones with computed tomography. *JCAT* 1980; 4:827–831.
6. Havrilla TR, Reich NE, Haaga JR, Seidelmann FE, Cooperman AM, Alfidi RJ: Computed tomography of the gallbladder. *Am J Roentgenol* 1978; 130:1059–1067.
7. Barakos JA, Ralls PW, Lapin SA, et al: Cholelithiasis: Evaluation with CT. *Radiology* 1987; 162:415–418.
8. Van Sonnenberg E, Wing VW, Pollard JW, Casola G: Life-threatening vagal reactions associated with percutaneous cholecystostomy. *Radiology* 1984; 151:377–380.

Mechanical and Laser Techniques for Ablation of Common Duct Stones

Robert H. Schapiro, M.D.
Norman S. Nishioka, M.D.
Peter B. Kelsey, M.D.

The current techniques for shock wave lithotripsy of common duct stones ideally require direct endoscopic intervention in the common duct to make them effective. An endoscopic sphincterotomy is needed to allow passage of the stone fragments split off by lithotripsy. In addition, a route for introduction of contrast is needed to allow the current lithotripters to zero in on the stone or stones to be crushed. Usually this is done by means of an endoscopically placed nasobiliary drain. Alternatively, contrast may be introduced and fragments removed from the common duct by means of a surgically placed T-tube. Because these prerequisites for lithotripsy both presuppose a route for direct manipulation in the duct, it is reasonable to ask what else can be accomplished via the endoscope to rid the duct of stones too large to pass through a papillotomy or too difficult to extract through a T-tube tract. This chapter details techniques for immediate stone removal available at the time of initial endoscopic sphincterotomy, and then focuses upon a promising though still cumbersome approach that we have been specifically investigating here at the Massachusetts General Hospital, the fragmentation of stones by direct application of pulsed laser energy.

What makes a stone oversized? How well can we predict that a stone will not pass after endoscopic sphincterotomy? A stone diameter of 1.5 cm has been the traditional separation between extractable and oversized stones, but clearly the ability to remove a stone endoscopically is a function of the size of the papillotomy. A stone impacted at the ampulla for a protracted period of time causes marked enlargement of the ampulla and common duct and may permit a considerably more extensive papillotomy than is possible when a stone has been recently passed out of the gallbladder. Another factor, the surprising flexibility of tissues, may permit spontaneous passage of oversized stones after recent papillotomy. On two occasions in the last month, when patients were being prepared for laser fragmentation of common duct stones clearly larger in diameter than the available papillotomy, we found that all the stones had spontaneously passed. One should never proceed to surgery or to an expensive fragmentation technique until at least several days postpapillotomy to confirm that stones are still present.

Another problem in stone extraction relates to the available equipment. Fogarty balloons easily slip around stones when there is resistance in the duct. Stone-retrieval baskets can pull a stone forcefully through a papillotomy, but once committed disentangling a stone from the basket is difficult if the stone is truly too large. The spector of emergency surgery to extract an impacted stone basket can chill the aggressiveness of any endoscopist. Newer baskets have been designed to obviate this problem. A series of detachable parts allow the endoscope to be withdrawn with the basket still engaged around the stone. A flexible but noncompressible metal overtube is then fitted over the stone basket and the basket wire is inserted into a device that allows the wire to be slowly tightened while exerting a great deal of mechanical force. The process is monitored under fluoroscopy because the endoscope has been removed. Eventually either the stone is fragmented or the basket breaks.

Although the foregoing suggests almost every stone problem has a solution, in practice, stone baskets are exceedingly difficult to use. They come in various shapes, octagonal or spiral, 3 or 4 wire, stiff or soft wired. All varieties work well in vitro but often will not open completely when in a bile duct. Successful stone entrapment requires a bile duct wider than the stone and a stone basket whose wires are spaced widely enough to admit the stone, but narrow enough to open completely in the bile duct. In addition, there can be only a minimum of angulation in the duct. A great deal of endoscopic expertise and personal patience is needed to manipulate these devices, and the overall rate of success for endoscopic extraction of large stones is not high. Nevertheless, better stone basket design in the future is possible. In terms of costeffectiveness, it is by far the most attractive approach.

In view of these limitations and the success of laser devices in fragmenting renal stones, we have investigated the possibilities of using this same modality for fragmentation of common duct stones. With kidney stones, access requires a percutaneous nephrostomy or ureteroscopy; in the common duct a sphincterotomy is usually already available. Much of the background feasibility work on laser fragmentation of biliary stones has been carried out by investigators in the Wellman Research laboratories here at the Massachusetts General Hospital.[1-3] These studies have shown that biliary stones can be fragmented easily in vitro. The use of continuous laser energy would produce too much heat, so the energy is delivered in short repetitive pulses of brief duration operating at high peak power. The laser used in our work is a flashlamp pumped tunable dye laser provided by the Candela Corporation of Wayland, Massachusetts. This was coupled to a flexible quartz fiber 200 μm in diameter with the laser energy delivered by direct application of the fiber to the stone. The ablation threshold, a measure of the energy required for initial damage to the stone, was measured across the visible spectrum of light. Although the threshold was somewhat lower at the shorter wavelengths, the laser was effective at all the wavelengths studied. An arbitrary wavelength of 504 nm was chosen for further experiments. Of interest, pigment stones were consistently more easily disrupted than cholesterol stones, presumably because they absorbed visible light more readily. Other studies revealed that the greater the amount of laser energy applied, the more rapid the fragmentation, although the size of the fragments produced also increased from 2 mm to a maximum of 8 mm. Finally, the process of stone fragmentation proceeded much more efficiently in a liquid medium than in air, although the density of the liquid did not seem to matter.

The process of fragmentation seems to occur in two stages, an induction period followed by a period of rapid removal. The latter does not seem to correlate with the time of impingement of maximum laser energy. The initial event appears to be the formation of a plasma, a gaseous collection of ions asnd electrons initially produced by laser heating of the stone. This plasma becomes opaque, absorbs the laser energy, and expands, generating intense stress waves and crevassing within the stone. The process of stone fragmentation is usually accompanied by an audible snap and a flash of visible light. There is not much thermal effect on surrounding tissues. The total laser energy used in fragmenting a typical stone would raise 1 cc of water only 4°C, even if completely converted to heat.

The tunable dye laser is not the only laser capable of producing stone fragmentation. A flashlamp pulsed neodymium YAG laser has been used by Dr. Christian Ell in Erlangen, Germany.[4] This laser operates at a wavelength of 1064 nm.

In our laboratory the safety of the fragmentation process was tested in an animal model using the pig, whose bile duct closely resembles the human bile duct. Stones were inserted in the bile duct in a stone basket assembly through which a quartz fiber could be coaxially passed and placed in direct contact with the stone. The animals were sacrificed from 7 days to 3 months after the fragmentation had been accomplished. In brief, these studies[5] demonstrated that the stones could be fragmented in situ without significant short- or long-term damage to the bile duct. Nevertheless, a potential for laser-induced injury was present. In a worst case scenario, the fiber was pressed perpendicularly against the bile duct wall and laser pulses delivered at various energy levels. Above 60 mj it was possible to produce pinpoint perforation of the duct with relative ease. Accordingly, in our human studies laser energy is kept between 20 and 60 mj. The pulse duration currently used is 1.2 us.

In summary, then, with reasonable care, pulsed laser energy can efficiently and safely fragment common duct stones. The problems are not in the laser but in the delivery system. For the laser to be effective, it has to be applied directly against the stone. Even a gap of a millimeter or two will markedly reduce efficiency. Attempts to use a stone basket containing a central channel for the laser fiber to entrap and immobilize the stones encountered the same frustrations inherent in the use of crushing baskets. We would need a means for direct visualization of the stone in the duct, that is, a choledochoscope, through which the laser delivery fiber could be passed. Recently, the Olympus corporation has developed a prototype model of a "mother-daughter" endoscope that meets this need. Their sideviewing "mother" ERCP scope, though not effective for standard duct cannulation, contains a 5.5 mm channel through which an independently controlled "daughter" scope can be passed which contains an 1.7 mm instrumentation channel and has the capacity for two-way deflection of its tip. Introduction of the "daughter" scope requires a previous papillotomy and is facilitated by the use of a guidewire passed through the "daughter" scope. Figure 1 depicts the instruments in use, with the "daughter" scope being inserted well up into the

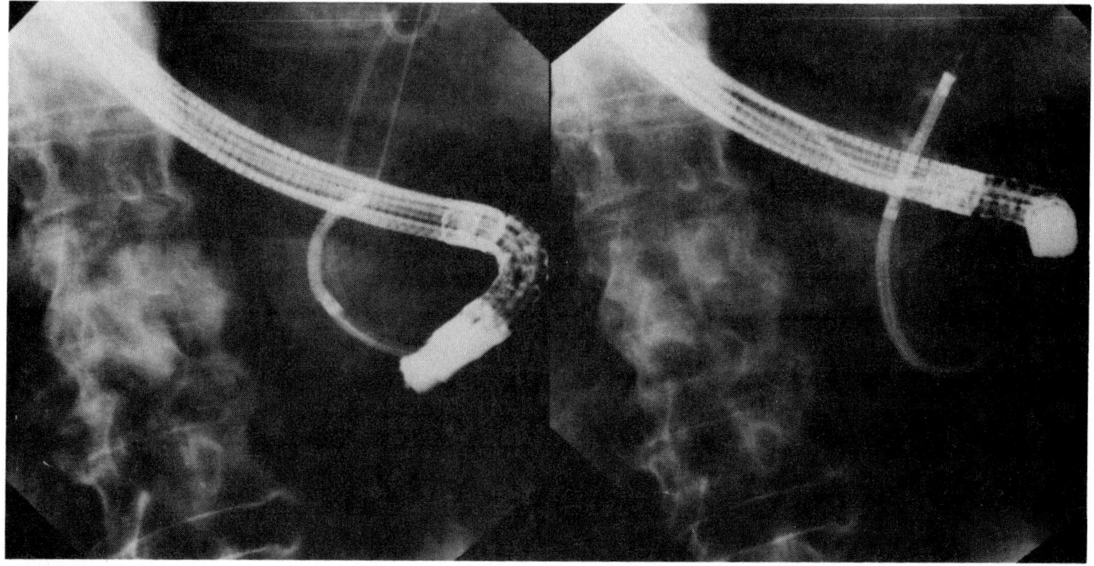

FIG 1.
A. Mother endoscope positioned opposite a previously sphincterotomized ampulla of Vater in a patient with a retained radiolucent common duct stone. A guide wire has been passed through the instrument channel of the daughter scope and anchored in the bile duct. A nasobiliary drain (*arrow*) is already present in the duct. **B.** The daughter scope has now been advanced over the guide wire and is positioned well into the common duct.

common duct. Alternatively, a conventional thin duodenoscope could be passed up a previously papillotomized duct or a fiberoptic bronchoscope passed through a T-tube tract or even through a previously created percutaneous, transhepatic tract.

Once the choledochoscope has been introduced into the bile duct, the quartz delivery fiber can be passed down the instrumentation channel and the tip visualized as it impacts against the stone. A radiopaque metal cladding on the tip allows it also to be visualized radiographically (Fig. 2).

A plastic sheath on the fiber reduces fragility. A nasobiliary drainage tube, previously inserted above the stone, is irrigated with saline to provide a fluid interface and to wash away the debris produced by fragmentation. In addition this prevents the stone from migrating proximally.

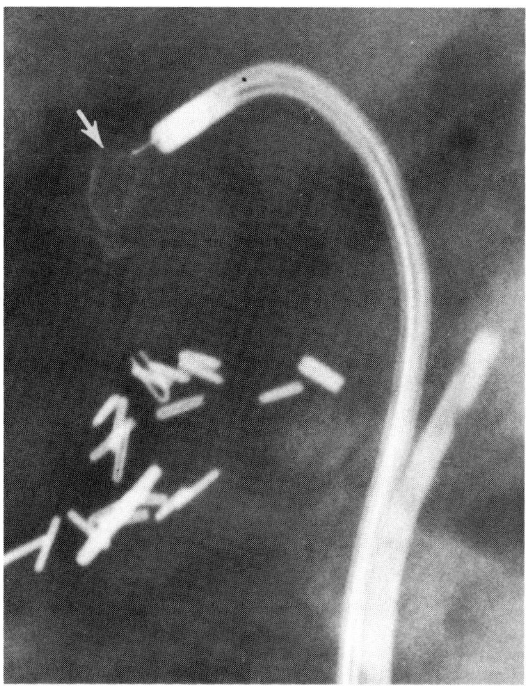

FIG 2.
A radiopaque stone impacted in the right hepatic duct is visualized using a choledochoscope passed through a T-tube tract. The metal-clad quartz delivery fiber protruding from the tip of the endoscope is positioned against the stone. A few smudgy appearing fragments are visible adjacent to the stone (*arrow*).

The experience with this technique in humans is still limited, although increasing almost weekly. At present we are aware of three groups that have performed laser lithotripsy of common duct stones in humans using the tunable dye laser: Dr. Peter Cotton's in Durham, North Carolina, Dr. Richard Kozarek's in Seattle, and ourselves. As best we can tally up the score, the procedure has been attempted in 16 patients, all with oversized stones refractory to all other nonsurgical techniques. In 12 patients at least partial fragmentation was accomplished, although in only 8 was the duct totally cleared of stone material. In addition, Dr. Ell in Erlangen reported 9 attempts with the Nd YAG laser.[4] In 8 at least partial fragmentation occurred, and in 6 the duct was cleared.

We are dealing with an emerging technology of demonstrated effectiveness, but one still flawed by the limitation of the delivery system. When that has reached the second and third generation of development, the problem of large common duct stones should be amenable to a reliable and less costly solution than shock wave lithotripsy.

REFERENCES

1. Nishioka NS, Levins PC, Murray, SC, Parrish JA, Anderson RR: Fragmentation of biliary calculi with tunable dye lasers. *Gastroenterology* 1987; 93:250–255.
2. Nishioka NS, Teng P, Deutsch TF, Anderson RR: Mechanism of laser-induced fragmentation of urinary and biliary calculi. *Lasers in the Life Sciences* 1987; 1:231–245.
3. Teng P, Nishioka NN, Farinelli WA, Anderson RR, Deutsch TF: Microsecond-long photography of laser-induced ablation of biliary and urinary calculi. *Lasers in Surgery and Medicine* 1987; 7:394–397.
4. Ell C, Hochberger J, Lux G, Demling L: Laser lithotripsy of gallstones by means of pulsed ND:YAG lasers: *Gastroenterology* 1988; 92:241.
5. Nishioka NN, Kelsey PB, Kibbi AG, Delmonico F, Parrish JA, Anderson RR: Laser lithotripsy: Animal studies of safety and efficacy. *Lasers in Surgery and Medicine* (in press).

Cystic Duct Occlusion and Gallbladder Sclerotherapy: An Experimental Approach To Prevent Gallstone Recurrence

Chrisoph D. Becker, MD
H. Joachim Burhenne, MD

Fragmentation of gallbladder calculi by extracorporeal shockwave lithotripsy[1,2] and recent advances in chemical dissolution therapy[3,4] have permitted nonsurgical treatment of cholecystolithiasis in selected patients. The indications for these new techniques have not been fully established yet, but the traditional therapeutic concepts for cholelithiasis will certainly change to some degree in the future. All of these nonsurgical substitutes for cholecystectomy, however, have one drawback in common: they cannot prevent recurrent gallstone formation, which has, for example, been observed in up to 50 percent of patients within a few years after successful dissolution therapy.[3,5] Repeat treatment or long-term oral chemoprophylaxis with ursodeoxycholic acid may therefore become necessary for many patients.

Definitive cure of cholecystolithiasis requires elimination of the functioning gallbladder, and cholecystectomy, therefore, remains the gold standard. Cholecystolithotomy has been abandoned because of an unacceptable rate of symptomatic gallstone recurrence on long-term follow-up,[6] and the role of cholecystostomy is generally limited to patients with acute cholecystitis who are too ill to undergo formal cholecystectomy.[7] At our institution, a relatively noninvasive combined surgical and radiologic "minicholecystostomy" approach has been used over several years in elderly and severely compromised patients with acute calculous gallbladder disease who were at a high anesthetic risk.[8,9] Following stone extractions through a wide surgical cholecystostomy tract under fluoroscopic control, the cholecystostomy catheter was removed and the gallbladder fistula left to close. The results of this treatment were excellent, and, in this patient group, recurrence was not necessarily a primary concern. Nevertheless, the potential for recurrent gallstone formation in the functioning gallbladder prompted us to search for a technique to defunctionalize the gallbladder by catheter via the cholecystostomy.[8]

We have developed a catheter technique that permits in situ ablation of the gallbladder in animals. This technique includes two steps: cystic duct occlusion[10] and chemical sclerotherapy of the gallbladder.[11]

CYSTIC DUCT OCCLUSION

Complete occlusion of the cystic duct must be considered an indispensable prerequisite for safe and successful gallbladder ablation because chemical sclerosants cannot be instilled safely into the gallbladder unless the common bile duct

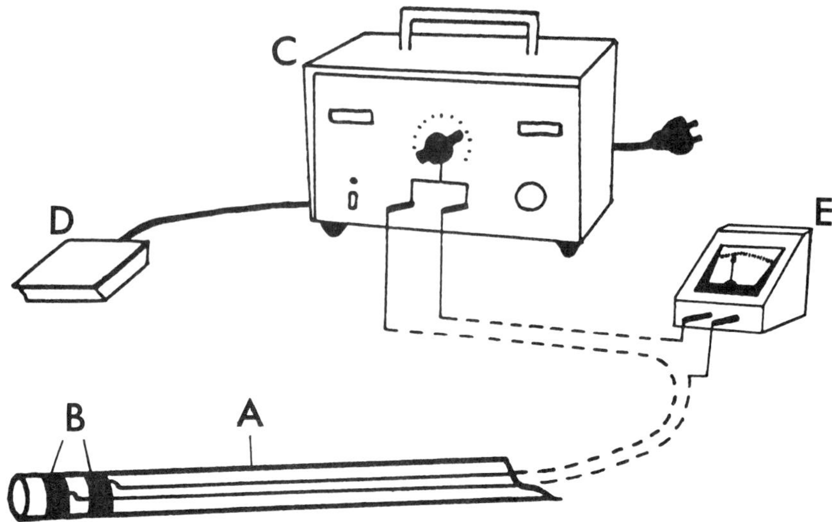

FIG 1.
Schematic of bipolar system for RF electrocoagulation of the cystic duct. A flexible polyethylene catheter (*A*) has an active tip consisting of two 1-mm stainless steel electrodes (*B*). The electrical circuit is completed by tissue contact between the two electrodes. Two insulated internal wires are connected with a bipolar electrosurgical RF generator (*C*), which is operated by a foot switch (*D*). An RF ammeter (*E*) permits monitoring of the current flow (in milliamperes) during electrocoagulation. (From Becker CD, Quenville NF, Burhenne HJ: Long-term occlusion of the porcine cystic duct by means of endoluminal radio-frequency electrocoagulation. *Radiology* 1988; 167:63–68. Used with permission.)

is protected by its functional disconnection from the gallbladder. The first experimental attempts at cystic duct occlusion by catheter in animals employed transcatheter embolization techniques (H. J. Burhenne and J. L. Stoller, unpublished data). Studies in dogs, rabbits,[12] and pigs (G. K. McLean, oral communication, 1987) demonstrated, however, that tissue adhesives and other embolization particles did not result in consistent and reproducible cystic duct occlusion. A tendency of the cystic duct to dilate around foreign bodies led to proximal or distal dislodgment of the embolization material. Reliable, consistent occlusion of the cystic duct would clearly require a localized, controlled destruction of the cystic duct mucosa.

Therefore, we developed a catheter technique to produce a circumferential endoluminal thermal lesion of the cystic duct epithelium.[10] A flexible, angiographic-type polyethylene catheter was modified for bipolar radiofrequency (RF) electrocoagulation (Fig 1). In a recent further modification, this catheter accommodates a guide wire[13] and can be introduced into the gallbladder and the cystic duct under fluoroscopic control either via a subhepatic cholecystostomy or via a percutaneous transphepatic approach through a 7 French Teflon sheath (Fig 2). Following placement of the active catheter tip under fluoroscopic control, repeat coagulations are performed for a few seconds. Dosage of the current is based on empirical data and monitored by means of an RF ammeter. Histologically, the RF technique causes circumscribed thermal necrosis

FIG 2.
Percutaneous insertion of coagulation catheter under sonographic and fluoroscopic guidance. **A.** Gallbladder puncture under ultrasonographic guidance. **B.** Opacification of gallbladder and bile ducts; negotiation of the cystic duct with guide wire under fluoroscopic control. **C.** Placement of the electrocoagulation catheter under fluoroscopic control. (Note radiopaque bipolar electrodes.)

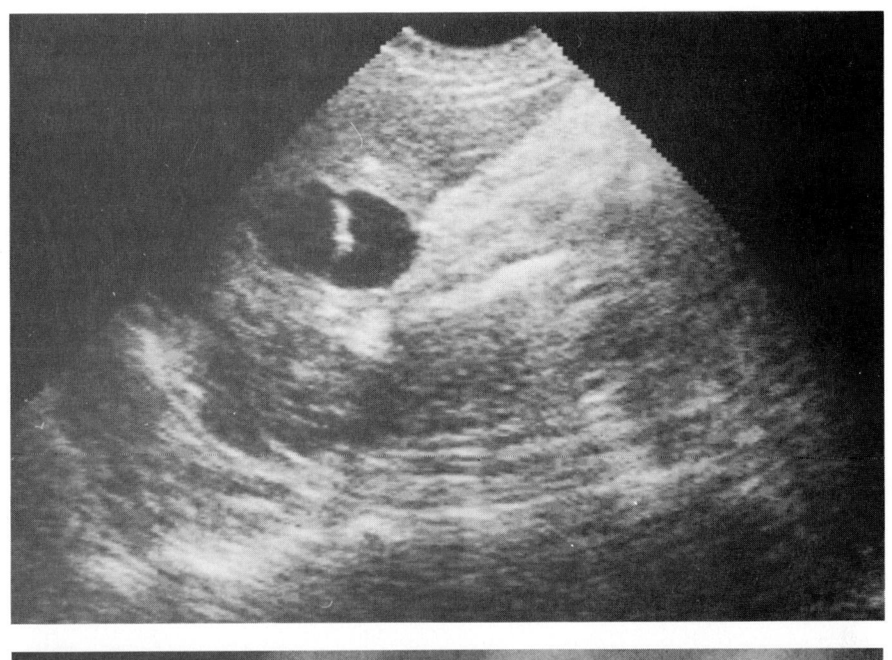

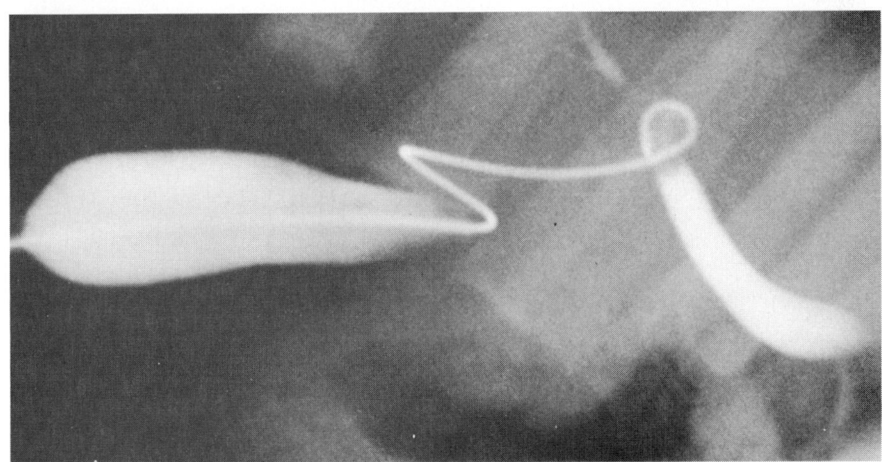

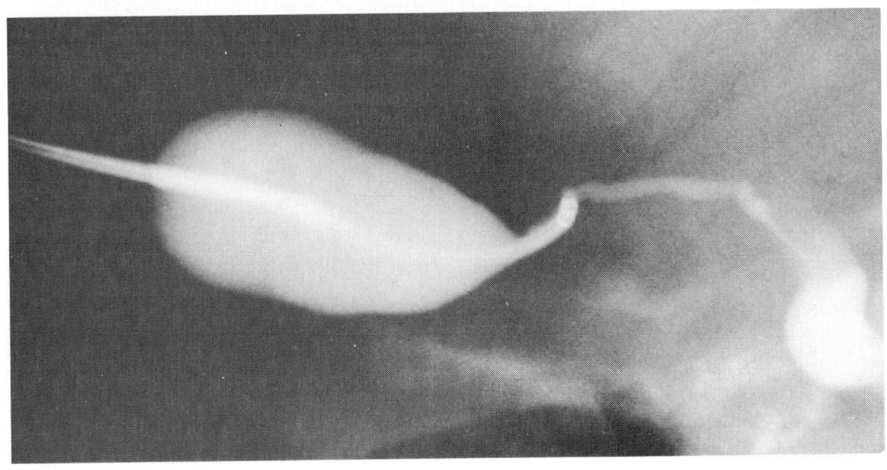

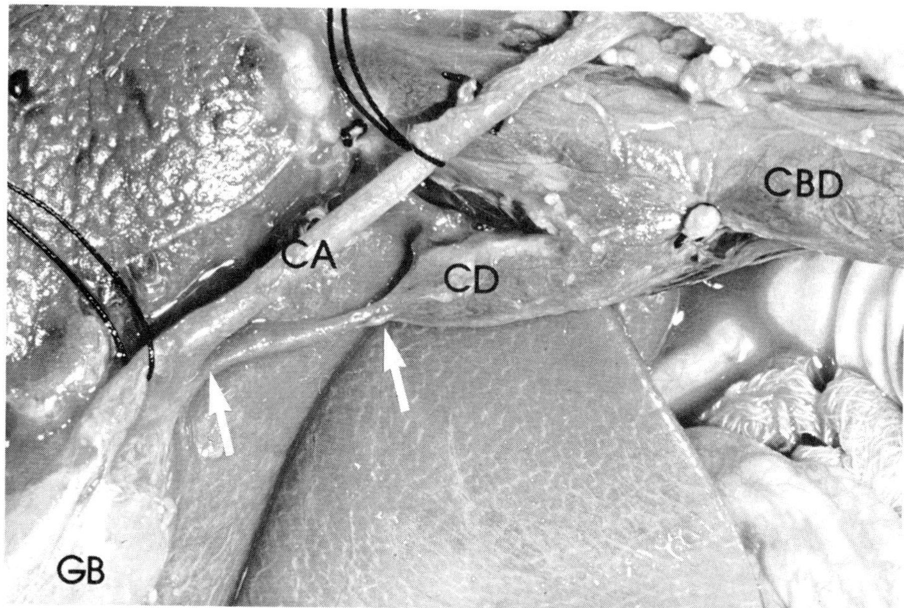

FIG 3.
The extrahepatic bile ducts and cystic artery have been dissected 4 months after cystic duct electrocoagulation. The coagulated portion of the cystic duct is obliterated and appears as a fibrotic string (*arrows*). The end of the normal cystic duct (*cd*) appears like a "remnant" similar to the findings following cholecystectomy. The patent cystic artery (*ca*) is seen as it crosses over the common hepatic duct to parellel the course of the cystic duct. *GB* = gallbladder, *CBD* = common bile duct. (From Becker CD, Quenville NF, Burhenne HJ: Long-term occlusion of the porcine cystic duct by means of endoluminal radio-frequency electrocoagulation. *Radiology* 1988; 167:63–68. Used by permission.)

of the cystic duct wall and induces an intense, chronic, inflammatory and fibroblastic reaction, which, in turn, obliterates the coagulated cystic duct segments within approximately 2 weeks. The circumferential coagulation effect is limited to a few millimeters in depth so that the adjacent structures, that is, the cystic artery, serosa, and liver, remain intact (Figs 3, 4). After successful results in our initial study,[10] we have used this technique successfully in over 40 animals. Long-term follow-up demonstrated no recanalization or re-epithelialization of the coagulated cystic duct segments (Figs 3, 4C). Occlusion of the porcine cystic duct by the RF technique can thus be considered reproducible and permanent.

CHEMICAL SCLEROTHERAPY OF THE GALLBLADDER

Gallbladder changes after cystic duct occlusion alone were studied in two groups of pigs. One group had subhepatic cholecystostomies and was followed over several weeks after the catheters were removed and the gallbladder fistulae left to close. Histology in these animals revealed mild to moderate chronic follicular cholecystitis; the gallbladder lumina were skrunken and contained white fluid or inspissated viscous material. The other group underwent cystic duct occlusion via a percutaneous transhepatic access; no drainage catheter was left behind. Ultrasound follow-up and postmortem studies demonstrated small collapsed gallbladders with inspissated materials in most of these animals; a small minority developed a gallbladder mucocele but not acute cholecystitis. Similar observations have been made by previous investigators after surgical cystic duct ligation in dogs.[14]

Cystic duct occlusion alone might thus be considered all that would be required in some instances to prevent formation of recurrent gallstones. However, the presence of an empty or mucous-filled, isolated gallbladder lumen is a

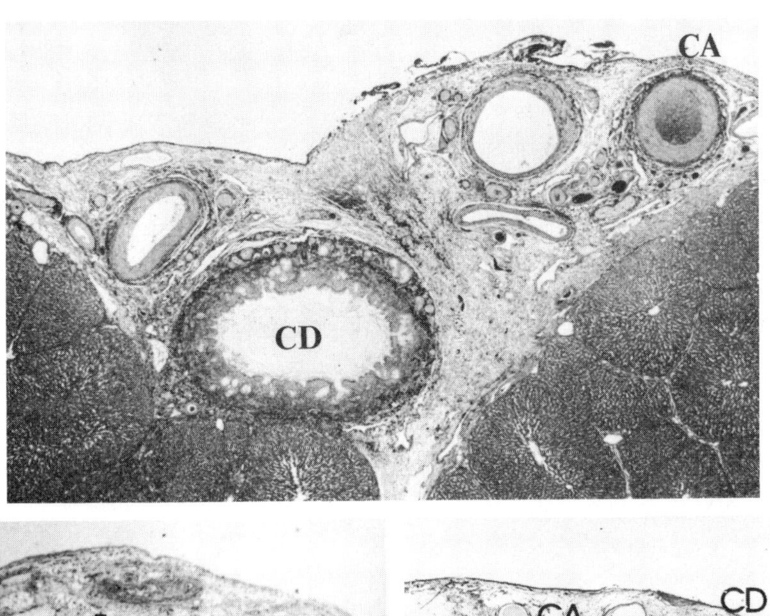

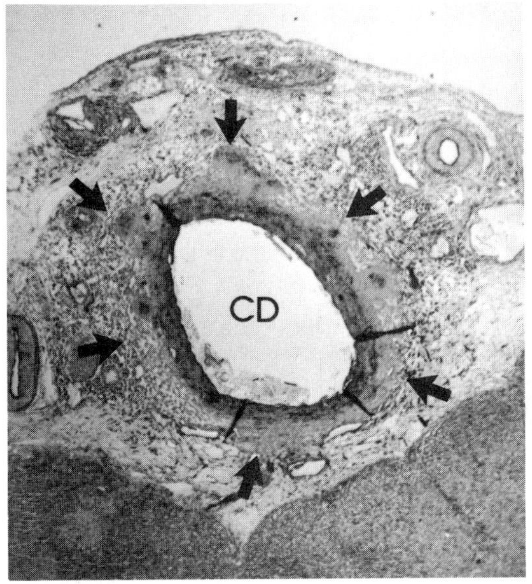

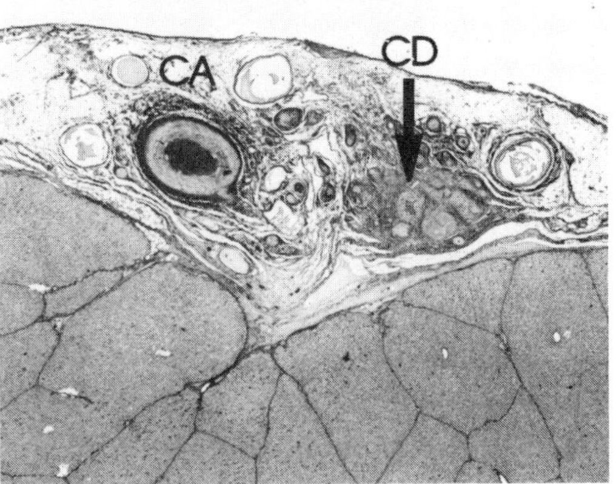

FIG 4.
Histologic effects of RF electrocoagulation. **A.** Normal porcine cystic duct (*CD*) lined by tall columnar epithelium. The duct wall contains mucin-secreting glands and is supported by loose connective tissue. *CA* = cystic artery. **B.** Immediate effect of electrocoagulation. The cystic duct (*CD*) mucosa has been destroyed. The area of acute tissue coagulation extends slightly beyond the cystic duct wall but does not involve the liver, the vessels, or the serosa (*arrows*). **C.** Four months after electrocoagulation, the cystic duct is obliterated by fibrous connective tissue. A pale, round structure consisting of dense fibrous connective tissue is seen. There is no residual cystic duct epithelium and no evidence of epithelial regeneration. The major vessels are well clear of the zone of fibrosis. *CA* = cystic artery. Note that the serosal surface and adjacent liver are intact. (Staining technique: Mallory trichrome).

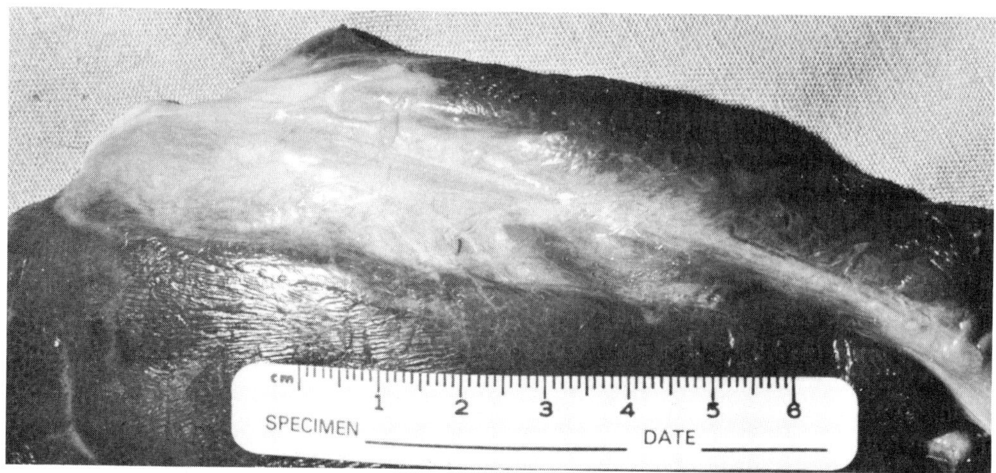

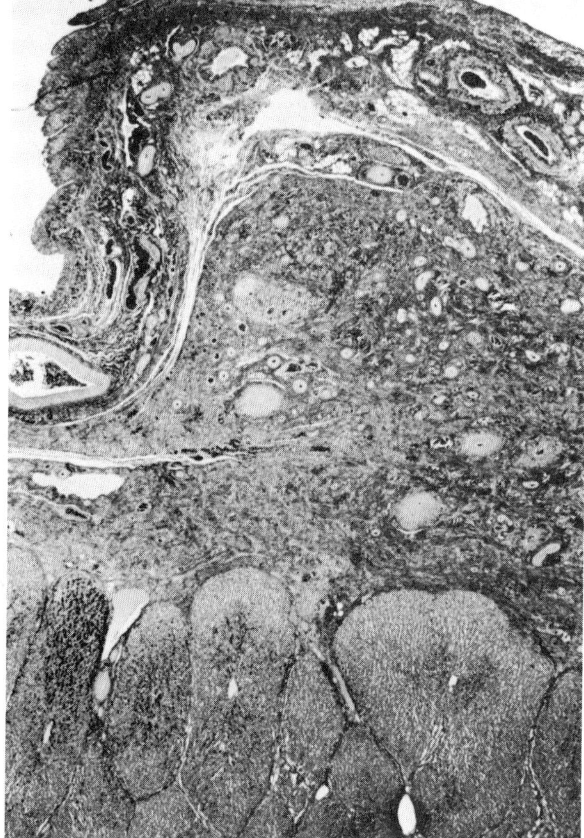

FIG 5.

A. Fibrosed porcine gallbladder 6 weeks after cystic duct occlusion and chemical sclerotherapy. No residual gallbladder lumen was present. **B.** Histologic section through the fibrosed gallbladder and adjacent liver demonstrates mature scar tissue without epithelial remnants. The vessels, however, are intact. (From Becker CD, Quenville NF, Burhenne HJ: Long-term occlusion of the porcine cystic duct by means of endoluminal radio-frequency electrocoagulation. *Radiology* 1988; 167:63–68. Used by permission.)

potential nidus for infectious complications. One might also argue that the potential risk of gallbladder adenocarcinoma—even though remote—cannot be ruled out. In another study, therefore, we attempted ablation of the gallbladder mucosa by means of chemical sclerotherapy after preliminary cystic duct occlusion. Our intentions were to obliterate the gallbladder lumen by fibrous scar tissue and to eradicate the entire gallbladder mucosa, which would ideally not only offer prevention of recurrent gallstone formation but also obviate the remote risk of adenocarcinoma of the gallbladder. At the same time, we evaluated whether this could be done safely, that is, without causing damage to the bile ducts and other adjacent structures.

The effect of a variety of sclerosing substances on the gallbladders of rabbits, with or without preliminary surgical ligation of the cystic duct, have been evaluated by several investigators with varying success.[12,15–17] In the second part of our study, we first occluded the cystic duct with the RF technique and then used a combination of two sclerosants that were already in clinical use for local and intravascular sclerotherapy: ethanol and sodium tetradecyl sulfate (Sotradecol).[11] These chemicals were instilled into the gallbladder in sequence to induce necrosis of the mucosa and promote subsequent fibrotic obliteration of the gallbladder lumen. Our histologic results in pigs indicate that a regimen consisting of 95 percent ethanol and 3 percent Sotradecol causes necrosis of the mucosa and the muscularis of the gallbladder within 2 weeks and induces fibrotic obliteration of the gallbladder lumen. Within 5 to 8 weeks, a mature, flat, subhepatic scar is all that remains of the gallbladder (Fig 5). In 9 of 10 animals, no residual intact gallbladder mucosa was found on serial histologic blocks after treatment with this regimen. At the same time, histology demonstrated that the bile ducts distal to the site of cystic duct occlusion remained unaffected by the chemicals and that there was no relevant damage to the liver and the other structures adjacent to the gallbladder.[11]

With further experience and refinement of our experimental technique, in situ ablation of the gallbladder may become clinically useful in patients who have been treated by a temporizing cholecystostomy and who would otherwise have to undergo elective cholecystectomy. Gallbladder ablation via the percutaneous approach may, eventually, enable definitive nonsurgical cure of cholecystolithiasis after successful gallstone fragmentation and dissolution therapy.[18]

REFERENCES

1. Sauerbruch T, Delius M, Paumgartner G, Holl J, et al: Fragmentation of gallstones by extracorporeal shock waves. *N Engl J Med* 1986; 314:818–822.
2. Sackmann M, Delius M, Sauerbruch T, et al: Shockwave lithotripsy of gallbladder stones: The first 175 patients. *N Engl J Med* 1988; 318:393–397.
3. Fromm H: Gallstone dissolution therapy. Current status and future prospects. *Gastroenterology* 1986; 91:1560–1567.
4. Allen MJ, Borody TJ, Bugliosi TF, May GR, LaRusso NF, Thistle JL: Rapid dissolution of gallstones by methyl tert-butyl ether: Preliminary observations. *N Engl J Med* 1985; 213:217–220.
5. Ruppin DC, Dowling RH: Is recurrence inevitable after gallstone dissolution by bile-acid treatment? *Lancet* 1982; 1:182–185.
6. Norrby S, Schönebeck J: Long-term results with cholecystolithotomy. *Acta Chir Scand* 1970; 136:711–713.
7. Skillings JC, Kumai PAC, Hinshaw JR: Cholecystostomy: A place in modern biliary surgery? *Am J Surg* 1980; 139:865–869.
8. Burhenne HJ, Stoller JL: Minicholecystostomy and radiologic stone extraction in high-risk cholelithiasis patients: Preliminary experience. *Am J Surg* 1985; 149:637–635.
9. Gibney RG, Fache JS, Becker CD, Nichols DM, Cooperberg PL, Stoller JL, Burhenne HJ: Combined surgical/radiological intervention for complicated cholelithiasis in high-risk patients. *Radiology* 1987; 165:715–719.
10. Becker CD, Quenville NF, Burhenne HJ: Long-term occlusion of the porcine cystic duct by means of endoluminal radio-frequency electrocoagulation. *Radiology* 1988; 167:63–68.
11. Becker CD, Quenville NF, Burhenne HJ: Gallbladder ablation by radiologic intervention: An experimental alternative to cholecystectomy. Submitted for publication.
12. Salomonowitz E, Frick MP, Simons RL, O'Leary JF, et al: Obliteration of the gallbladder without formal cholecystectomy: A feasibility study. *Arch Surg* 1984; 190:725–729.
13. Becker CD, Jameson M, Fache JS, Burhenne HJ: A bipolar catheter for endoluminal electrocoagu-

lation. *Radiology* (accepted for publication).

14. Morris CR, Hohf RP, Ivy AC: An experimental study of the role of stasis in the etiology of cholecystitis. *Surgery* 1952; 32:673–685.

15. Getrajdman GI, O'Toole K, Logerfo P, Laffey KJ, Martin EC: Transcatheter sclerosis of the gallbladder in rabbits: A preliminary study. *Invest Radiol* 1985; 20:393–398.

16. Remley KB, Cubberley DA, Watanabe AS, Nelson JA, Colby TV: Systemic absorption of gallbladder sclerosing agents in the rabbit. A preliminary study. *Invest Radiol* 1986; 21:396–399.

17. Getrajdman GI, O'Toole K, Laffey KD, Martin EC: Cystic duct occlusion and transcatheter sclerosis of the gallbladder in the rabbit. *Invest Radiol* 1986; 21:400–403.

18. Becker GJ, Kopecky K: Can the newer interventional procedures replace cholecystecotmy for cholelithiasis? The potential role of percutaneous cystic duct ablation. *Radiology* 1988; 167:275–279.

Prevention of Stone Recurrence After Lithotripsy: Oral Chemoprophylaxis

Enrico Roda, Franco Bazzoli, Davide Festi, Giuseppe Mazzella, Massimo Ronchi, Nicola Villanova, Roberto Frabboni

OVERVIEW

Chenodeoxycholic and ursodeoxycholic acids are effective in dissolving cholesterol gallstones;[1–5] however, the overall role of oral bile acid treatment in the management of gallstone disease is still debated. A major problem in the use of medical therapy is that, after dissolution and cessation of treatment, bile resaturates and gallstones may recur.[6] Similarly, the newer nonsurgical modes of treatment, such as solvent instillation into the gallbladder and the extracorporeal shockwave lithotripsy (ESL), are going to be evaluated in the light of the magnitude of the "postreatment recurrence" problem. In this chapter we will review some aspects of the pathochemistry and pathomechanics of gallstone recurrence, the data presently available regarding recurrence rates after nonsurgical treatment of cholesterol gallstones, and the possibility of preventing recurrence via postdissolution treatment with oral bile acids. Because of this final objective, the efficacy and safety of chenodeoxycholic and ursodeoxycholic acids administration will be also considered.

Presently, the management of gallbladder stones relies on three alternative approaches: (1) no treatment and expectant management with periodic clinical and ultrasound evaluation of the patient; (2) cholecystectomy; and (3) nonsurgical treatments, namely, oral bile acids, solvent (Methyl Tert Butyl Ether—MTBE) instillation into the gallbladder, and ESL.

If the patient is asymptomatic, expectant management can be adopted or dissolution by oral bile acids may be attempted. In the symptomatic patient, cholecystectomy still represents a safe and effective treatment, but, if stones are radiolucent and the cystic duct is patent, the nonsurgical treatments may be indicated. Dissolution by oral bile acids may be employed if stones are less than 15 mm in diameter, if biliary colic is infrequent, and if the patient prefers not to undergo surgery. A single stone equal or less than 3 cm in diameter or up to 3 stones of the same total volume may be fragmented by ESWL and further treated to promote fragment dissolution with adjuvant oral bile acids. MTBE instillation is indicated in symptomatic patients with radiolucent gallstones and a patent cystic duct, without any limitation regarding stone size and number.

GALLSTONE FORMATION AND RECURRENCE

All three of the approaches represent valid and rapidly evolving alternatives to surgical treatment. After dissolution (or fragmentation plus dissolution), however, in all thre situations, the metabolic, physical, and physicochemical abnormalities of gallstone disease appear to persist, and gallstone-free patients are at risk of developing recurrent gallstones. Recurrent gallstone formation, similar to primary lithogenesis, involves abnormalities of biliary cholesterol saturation, nucleation, and gallbladder motor function. In successfully treated patients, cholesterol saturation index, bile acid pool size, and biliary lipid secretion rates are similar, in one to four weeks after withdrawal of oral bile acid therapy, to those observed before treatment began.[7] One the basis of these results, Ruppin and Dowling named "gallstone disease without gallstones" or "postgallstone disease" the condition, prior to recurrent gallstone formation, in which the metabolic defect of cholesterol supersaturation has already recurred.

As for primary gallstone formation, cholesterol supersaturation is the prerequisite for cholesterol crystallization and stone growth. Alone, however it is not sufficient, and the presence of nucleating defects and gallbladder mucosal/motor dysfunction is also required. A nucleation defect was first demonstrated by Holan and associates in primary gallstone formation.[8] By measuring nucleation time, in fact, they were able to discriminate between normal and gallstone biles. Whether an excess of nucleating agents, a deficiency of crystallization inhibitors, or both is responsible for this nucleation defect is not known.[9, 10] However, this condition is likely to persist after dissolution (or fragmentation plus dissolution) and will further the progress of gallstones re-formation.

Gallbladder motor dysfunction has recently been shown to be present in subjects with gallstone disease. Slower and less complete gallbladder emptying and, consequently, stasis may favor crystal coalescence and stone growth.[11] In a recent study,[12] we have shown that gallbladder basal and residual volumes are significantly larger and that gallbladder emptying is significantly reduced in gallstone patients as compared to normal subjects. Also, in subjects who previously achieved gallstone dissolution with oral bile acids, we observed that basal and residual volumes, as well as percent gallbladder emptying, are similar to those observed in patients still having gallstones, indicating that gallbladder motor dysfunction persists after gallstone dissolution. Regarding the effect of ESL on gallbladder motor function, data are still very preliminary; however, the motility defect present in gallstone patients is not modified after ESL.[13] Supersaturated bile and nucleation defects will probably still be present after the newer nonsurgical means of therapy, and therefore gallstones are likely to recur with equal frequency as after oral bile acid therapy.

The only information now available regarding gallstone recurrence after ESL plus adjuvant oral bile acids is from the recent communication of Spengler and Paumgartner that about 10 percent of their patients exhibited stone recurrence after a mean follow-up period of 6 months after cessation of adjuvant litholytic therapy.[13] We must therefore refer to the literature concerning oral bile acid treatment in order to consider the frequency of gallstone recurrence after any of the nonsurgical managements and in order to individualize possible means of preventing it. Reported frequencies of gallstone recurrence vary from 28.5 to 64 percent; however, initial studies were conducted on relatively small numbers of patients and during short follow-up periods.[6, 14–18] For the same reasons, conflicting results have been reported as to the possibility of postdissolution treatment, particularly with long-term, low-dose oral bile acids, in preventing gallstone recurrence. Before we consider chemoprophylaxis of gallstone recurrence, a brief review of the current state of gallstone dissolution with oral bile acids appear to be timely.

ORAL BILE ACID CHEMOLYSIS

In the last few years, the knowledge pertaining to medical treatment of cholesterol cholelithiasis has been considerably enlarged by a number of studies from Europe, the United States, and Japan.[1–5] Presently, only two compounds have been proven to dissolve gallstones in humans: chenodeoxycholic acid and its 7-beta epimer, ursodeoxycholic acid. Both are bile acids that occur naturally in humans. The rationale for using oral bile acids to dissolve gallstones is, essentially, to reduce the ratio of cholesterol to bile acids plus phospholipids in bile. The bioavailability of both bile acids is excellent; after efficient intestinal absorption, they are transported, via the portal vein, to the liver where they are conjugated with taurine and glycine and resecreted into bile.[19] Therefore, the quantities of chenodeoxycholic and ursodeoxycholic acids in the systemic circulation are very small, but they reach high concentration in the enterohepatic circulation. This is crucial as their efficacy is related to biliary and not to serum concentrations. Both bile acids are effective in lowering the lithogenic index by reducing biliary cholesterol output, even though they achieve this differently.

Ursodeoxycholic acid, as suggested by acute bile acid pool replacement studies,[20] probably reduces cholesterol secretion because of its limited capacity for transporting cholesterol in micellar form through the canalicular membrane. Moreover, it seems to reduce the intestinal absorption of cholesterol and to induce a moderate enhancement of bile acid synthesis,[21] thus contributing to maintaining a normal or negative balance of cholesterol.

Chenodeoxycholic acid reduces cholesterol secretion only after chronic administration, possibly because of the inhibition of cholesterol synthesis,[22,23] and secretory coupling[20] and intestinal absorption[24] are not modified.

As for the clinical effects of chenodeoxycholic and ursodeoxycholic acids, because radiopaque pigment stones are insoluble even in unsaturated bile, only radiolucent, cholesterol-rich gallstones may be treated medically. Radiolucent gallstones, however, do not always mean cholesterol-rich gallstone; up to 20 percent of such stones are not cholesterol. Furthermore, oral bile acid therapy is not efficacious in dissolving stones with calcification either at the periphery or in the center. To dissolve gallstones in the gallbladder, bile, unsaturated in cholesterol by the administration of oral bile acids, must be able to easily enter the gallbladder lumen. A functioning gallbladder and gallstone radiolucency are fundamental prerequisites of oral bile acid therapy.

Stone size is another important factor to be considered for the prognosis of successful cholelitholytic treatment. Both bile acids are poorly and slowly effective on large stones (15 to 20 mm in diameter, or more). Because of the low surface-volume ratio and probably because of densely packed, laminated outer layers, large stones are more resistant to the effect of unsaturated bile.

In addition to stone type and size, dose is also an important factor influencing dissolution. In the National Cooperative Gallstone Study,[3] the doses of chenodeoxycholic acid were suboptimal (the highest dose was 750 mg/day) and the frequency of cholelitholysis was definitely lower than those obtained in other studies[4,5] in which a weight-related dosage of 15 mg/kg/day was adopted. Further evidence that a fixed dose of 750 mg/day chenodeoxycholic acid is inadequate is the observation that higher dissolution rates were obtained in those patients with less than ideal body weight and, consequently, receiving an higher dosage per kg/body weight. Presently, the accepted optimal dosage of chenodeoxycholic acid is 15 mg/kg/day. As far as ursodeoxycholic acid is concerned, the dosage should not be higher than 8 to 10 mg/kg/day; increasing the dose up to 15 mg/kg/day does not produce significant increases of dissolution rates.[4] However, the above dosage must be increased in obese gallstone patients up to 20 mg/kg/day chenodeoxycholic acid and, probably, to 15 mg/kg/day ursodeoxycholic acid. If the optimal dose is adopted and if patient selection is rigorous, a total dissolution rate of about 40 percent and even higher can be expected in those patients with "floating stones." This success rate is achieved with both bile acids; however, ursodeoxycholic acid–treated patients show an earlier response to treatment. In our comparative study, in fact, of the 42 total dissolutions obtained with ursodeoxycholic acid, 31 (73 percent) were achieved during the first 6-month period; of the 33 total dissolutions obtained with chenodeoxycholic acid, only 14 (42 percent) were achieved during the same period. In addition to the lower dose and the earlier response, ursodeoxycholic acid therapy has the advantage of not producing those side effects fequently observed in patients treated with chenodeoxycholic acid: diarrhea and hypertransaminasemia. Clinically important diarrhea has been reported in about 40 percent of the patients treated with chenodeoxycholic acid.[3-5] In several studies, some patients refused to continue the treatment because of this annoying side effect. Liver function test abnormality during chenodeoxycholic acid administration is related to a dose-dependent hypertransaminasemia that usually occurs in 15 percent of treated patients during the first 3 months of treatment and, in most cases, tends to normalization in 5 to 9 months.[3-5] Hypertransaminasemia has not been shown to be associated with significant, hystologically proven liver damage. However, patients on chenodeoxycholic acid should be carefully monitored with liver function test evaluation, at least during the first months of treatment. Because of its higher efficacy at a lower dosage and its absence of side effects, ursodeoxycholic acid is presently considered the bile acid of choice for cholesterol gallstone dissolution.

PROPHYLAXIS AFTER RECURRENCE

As before mentioned, available data regarding the prevention of gallstone recurrence by oral bile acid postdissolution treatment are conflicting. In the National Cooperative Gallstone Study, a continuous treatment with low-dose chenodeoxycholic acid (375 mg/day) did not significantly reduce the frequency of gallstone recurrence (23.9 percent), as compared with the frequency observed in the placebo-treated patients (28.5 percent), over a 3.5 year period.[15] The British/Belgian Study[25] did not demonstrate a significant difference between ursodeoxycholic acid (300 mg/day) and placebo-treated patients; however, the frequency of gallstone recurrence was reduced in the former group (treatment: 21 percent, placebo: 37 percent) In the same study, furthermore, a statistically significant prevention of gallstone recurrence by postdissolution treatment was observed on the basis of "high and low risk patients" (less or more than 9 months stone free before joining the trial). In a study from Sapin,[16] gallstone recurrence was observed in 60 percent of subjects without postdissolution treatment, while the prophylactic administration of low-dose chenodeoxycholic acid (250 mg/day) reduced the frequency to 25 percent. In the same study, chemoprophylaxis with ursodeoxycholic acid was fully successful, and none of the subjects in this group had recurrent gallstones.

Our experience on gallstone recurrence and chemoprophylaxis by long-term, low-dose ursodeoxycholic acid administration relates to a 12-year follow-up study.[26] The aims of this study were to determine the long-term recurrence rate after 96 occasions of successful oral bile acid treatment, to search for factors predictive of gallstone recurrence, and to observe the effect of continuous treatment with low-dose ursodeoxycholic acid. Gallstone recurrence was evaluated in 86 subjects, after 96 occasions of complete dissolution, as established by two consecutive oral cholecystograms and/or ultrasound examinations. In 36 cases, ursodeoxycholic acid was administered at the fixed dose of 300 mg/day, in the remaining 60 cases, treatment was withdrawn after dissolution was confirmed. Patients were controlled yearly by oral cholecystogram and/or ultrasound. The maximum length of follow-up was 12 years. Diagnosis of recurrence was established by the presence of gallstones on two consecutive examinations. Factors affecting gallstone recurrence were investigated by examining recurrence rates stratified by subgroups: postdissolution treatment, sex, age, degree of obesity, serum cholesterol and triglycerides, pretreatment gallstone size, and number and type of bile acids taken during previous therapy. The cumulative proportion of gallstone recurrence was calculated by the acturial life table method.

The cumulative proportion of gallstone recurrence was 12.5 percent in the first year, rising to 61 percent in the eleventh year. Stratifying subjects by whether or not they received postdissolution treatment, we observed that 300 mg/day of ursodeoxycholic acid significantly reduced the frequency of gallstone recurrence. The only predictive factor we have been able to identify was pretreatment gallstone number. Recurrence rates were significantly higher in those subjects who had pretreatment multiple stones than in those with pretreatment solitary stones. In considering age-related differences, some interesting observations may be made. Recurrence rates were higher in subjects older than 50. However, when subjects were further stratified by postdissolution treatment, recurrence was similar in both age groups of untreated patients, but a definite age-related difference was due to the effect of postdissolution treatment, which significantly reduced the recurrence rate in younger subjects but was ineffective in older ones. Therefore, successfully treated gallstone patients, and particularly those with multiple stones, are at risk of re-forming gallstones. The continous administration of ursodeoxycholic acid at the dose of 300 mg/day can prevent gallstone recurrence only in younger subjects.

Although very likely, whether these results are also applicable to post-ESL gallstone recurrence is not yet known. Only the broad diffusion of shockwave lithotripters and a large number of treated patients will allow the definition of post-ESL recurrence frequency in both untreated patients and those treated long-term with oral bile acid. Dose response studies are also needed to individualize the optimal dosage of ursodeoxycholic acid.

REFERENCES

1. Danzinger RG, Hofmann AF, Shoenfield LJ: Dissolution of cholesterol gallstones by chenodeoxycholic acid. *N Engl J Med* 1972; 286:1.
2. Makino I, Shginozaky K: Dissolution of cholesterol gallstones by ursodeoxycholic acid. *Jap J Gastroenterol* 1975; 72:690.
3. Schoenfield LJ, Lachin JM, The Steering Committee and the National Cooperative Gallstone Study Group: Chenodiol for dissolution of gallstones: The National Cooperative Gallstone Study. *Ann Intern Med* 1981; 95:257.
4. Roda E, Bazzoli F, Labate AMM, et al: Ursodeoxycholic acid vs Chenodeoxycholic acid as cholesterol dissolving agents: A comparative randomized study. *Hepatology* 1982; 2:804.
5. Fromm H, Roat JW, Gonzales V, et al: Comparative efficacy and side effects of ursodeoxycholic and chenodeoxycholic acids in dissolving gallstones. A double blind controlled study. *Gastroenterology* 1983; 85:1257.
6. Ruppin DC, Dowling RH: Is recurrence inevitable after gallstone dissolution by bile acid treatment? *Lancet* 1982; 1:181.
7. Ruppin DC, Murphy GM, Dowling RH, et al: Gall stone disease without gall stones—Bile acid and bile lipid metabolism after complete gallstone dissolution. *Gut* 1986; 27:559.
8. Holan KR, Holzbach RT, Hermann RE, et al: Nucleation time: A key factor in the pathogenesis of cholesterol gallstone disease. *Gastroenterology* 1979; 77:611.
9. Burnstein JM, Ilson RG, Petrunka CH, et al: Evidence for a potent nucleating factor in the gallbladder bile of patients with cholesterol gallstones. *Gastroenterology* 1983; 85:801.
10. Holżbach RT, Kibe A, Thiel E, et al: Biliary proteins: Unique inhibitors of cholesterol crystal nucleation in human gallbladder. *J Clin Invest* 1984; 73:35.
11. Pomeranz IS, Shaffer EA: Abnormal gallbladder emptying in a subgroup of patients with gallstones. *Gastroenterology* 1985; 88:787.
12. Frabboni R, Festi D, Bazzoli F, et al: Effect of bile acid treatment on gallbladder dynamics, in Paumgartner G, Stiehl A, Gerok W (eds.) *Trends in Bile Acid Research* (Falk Symposium N. 52) MTP Press Limited, Lancaster, 1988 (in press).
13. Spengler U, Sackmann M, Sauerbruch T, et al: Gallbladder motility before and after extracorporeal shock wave lithotripsy (ESWL). *Hepatology* 1987; 7:1113.
14. Sauerbruch T, Sackmann M, Holl J, et al: Extracorporeal shock wave lithotripsy of gallstones, in X International Bile Acid Meeting: *Trends in Bile Acid Research*. Freiburg, 1988; Abstract book, pp 59–60.
15. Marks JW, Lan SP, The Steering Committee and The National Cooperative Gallstone Study Group. Low dose chenodiol to prevent gallstone recurrence after dissolution therapy. *Ann Int Med* 1984; 100:376.
16. Perez Aguilar F, Breto M. Alfonso V, et al: Gallstone recurrence following cessation of dissolving treatment and during prophylactic administration of either low dose chenodeoxycholic acid (CDCA) or medium dose ursodeoxycholic acid (UDCA). *J Hepatol* 1985; 1:S305.
17. Tint GS, Salen G, Chazen D: Symptomatic gallstones are likely to reoccur after dissolution with ursodeoxycholic acid (UDCA) but this may be prevented by low dose UDCA. *Gastroenterology* 1987; 92:1787.
18. O'Donnell, Keaton KW: Success and failure in

the medical treatment of gallstones. *Gut* 1986; 27:A1234.

19. Van Berge Henegouwen GP, Hofmann AF: Pharmacology of chenodeoxycholic acid: II Absorbtion and Metabolism. *Gastroenterology* 1977; 73:300.

20. Sama C, La Russo NF, Lopez Del Pino V, et al: Effects of bile acid administration on biliary lipid secretion in healthy volunteers. *Gastroenterology* 1982; 82:515.

21. Hardison WGM, Grundy SM: Effect of ursodeoxycholic acid and its taurine conjugate on bile acid synthesis and cholesterol absorption. *Gastroenterology* 1984; 87:130.

22. Coyne MJ, Bonorris GG, Goldstein LI, et al: Effect of chenodeoxycholic acid and phenobarbital on the rate limiting enzymes of hepatic cholesterol and bile acid synthesis in patients with gallstones. *J Lab Clin Med* 1976; 87:281.

23. Ahlberg J, Angelin B, Einarsson K, et al: Hepatic 3-hydroxy-3-methylglutaril Coenzyme A reductase activity and biliary composition in man: Relation to cholesterol gallstone disease and effects of cholic and chenodeoxycholic acids treatment. *J Lipid Res* 1981; 22:410.

24. Einarsson K, Grundy SM: Effects of feeding cholic acid and chenodeoxycholic acid on cholesterol absorption and hepatic secretion of biliary lipid in man. *J Lipid Res* 1980; 21:23.

25. Hood K, Gleeson D, Ruppin DC, et al: The British/Belgian Gallstone Study Group's (BBGSG) postdissolution trial. *Gut* 1987; 28:A1359.

26. Villanova N, Bazzoli F, Frabboni R, et al: Gallstone recurrence after successful oral bile acid treatment: A follow-up study and evaluation of postdissolution treatment. *Gastroenterology* 1987; 92:1789.

Extracorporeal Shock Wave Lithotripsy of Bile Duct Stones

T. Sauerbruch

In 1985, the first patients with bile duct stones were treated by extracorporeal shock wave lithotripsy.[1] Since then the method has been readily applied all over the world.[2, 3, 4] However, when using predefined criteria for eligibility of patients with bile duct stones for extracorporeal shock wave lithotripsy (bile duct stones not amenable to routine endoscopic measures, sphincterotomy of the papilla of Vater performed, no coagulation disorders), less than 10 percent of patients referred for endoscopic extraction of their stones are candidates.[5]

Employing a kidney lithotripter (Fig. 1) with an x-ray location system and shock wave entry from the rear (the patients being in supine position), stone disintegration may be achieved in 90 percent of these patients (Figs. 2 through 5), and complete clearance of stones from the bile ducts can be obtained in about 80 percent of all patients.[5, 6] Intrahepatically located stones (Fig. 5) or stones in the upper part of the hepatic duct may also be treated by machines with an ultrasound location system originally constructed for the treatment of gallbladder stones.

Morbidity and mortality are relatively low compared with results of open surgery. In our own multicenter prospective clinical trial, the 30-day mortality rate was 0.9 percent and the in-hospital mortality rate was 1.8 percent in a high-risk group of patients (mean age 72 years, cholangitis rate about 25 percent).

Extracorporeal shock wave lithotripsy of bile duct stones, therefore, is considered to be a useful adjuvant method to endoscopic extraction of bile duct stones.

REFERENCES

1. Sauerbruch T, Delius M, Paumgartner G, et al: Fragmentation of gallstones by extracorporeal shock waves. *N Engl J Med* 1986; 314:818–822.
2. Staritz M, Floth A, Rambow A, et al: Shock wave lithotripsy of gallstones with second-generation device without conventional water bath (letter). *Lancet* 1987; 2:155.
3. Burhenne HJ, Fache JS, Gibney RG, et al: Biliary lithotripsy by extracorporeal shock waves: Integral part of nonsurgical intervention. *AJR* 1988; 150:1279–1283.
4. Ferruci JT: Biliary lithotripsy: What will the issues be? *AJR* 1987; 149:227–231.
5. Sauerbruch T, Stern M, and the Study Group for Shock Wave Lithotripsy of Bile Duct Stones: Fragmentation of bile duct stones by extracorporeal shock waves: A new approach to biliary calculi after failure of routine endoscopic measures. *Gastroenterology* 1988, in press.
6. Sauerbruch T, Holl J, Sackmann M, et al: Treatment of bile duct stones by extracorporeal shock waves. *Semin Ultrasound, CT, MR* 1987; 8:155–161.
7. Sauerbruch T: Behandlungen von Gallensteinen durch extrakorporale Stoßwellen. Erste Erfahrungen. *Akt Chir* 1988; 23:58–65.

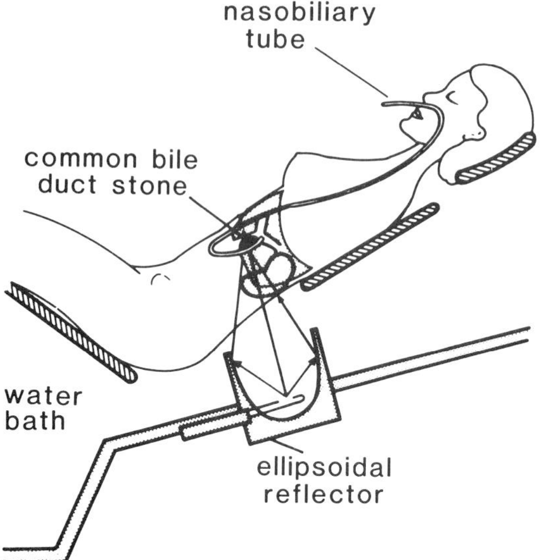

FIG 1.
Treatment of bile duct stones by extracorporeally induced shock waves. The patient is partly immersed in a water bath in supine position using a kidney lithotripter. Location of the stone into the shock wave focus is achieved by x-ray. The stones are visualized by giving dye through an endoscopically placed nasobiliary tube. (From Sauerbruch T, Holl J, Sackmann M, et al: Treatment of bile duct stones by extracorporeal shock waves. *Semin Ultrasound, CT, MR* 1987; 8:155. Used by permission.)

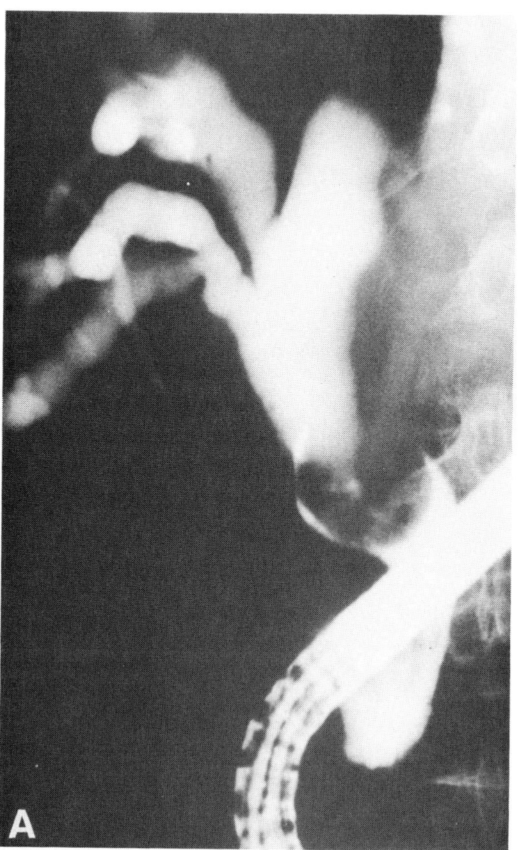

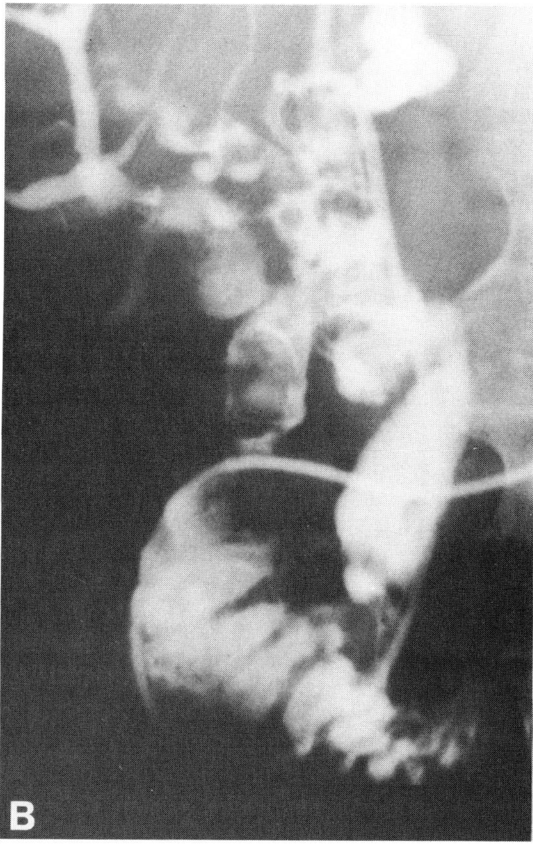

FIG 2.
Common bile duct stone before (**A,** endoscopic retrograde cholangiogram) and immediately after shock wave lithotripsy (**B,** retrograde cholangiogram via a nasobiliary tube). The stone was disintegrated, and most fragments moved into the upper part of the biliary tree.

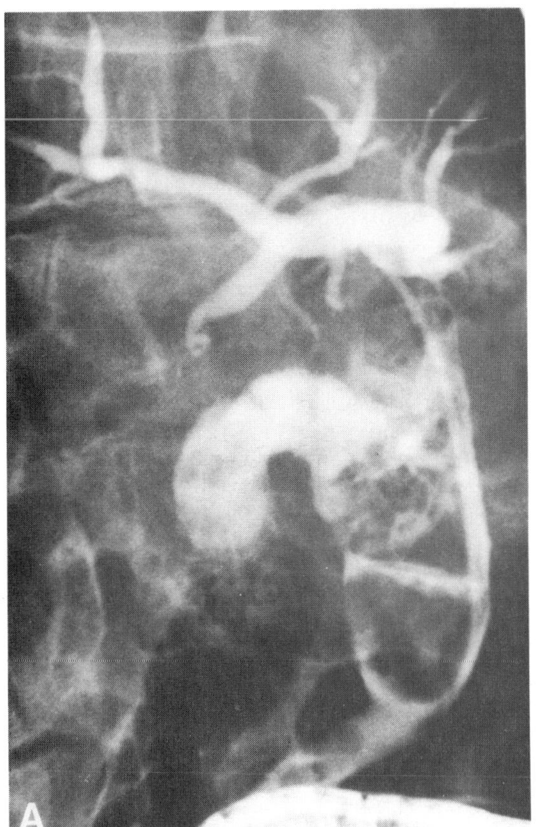

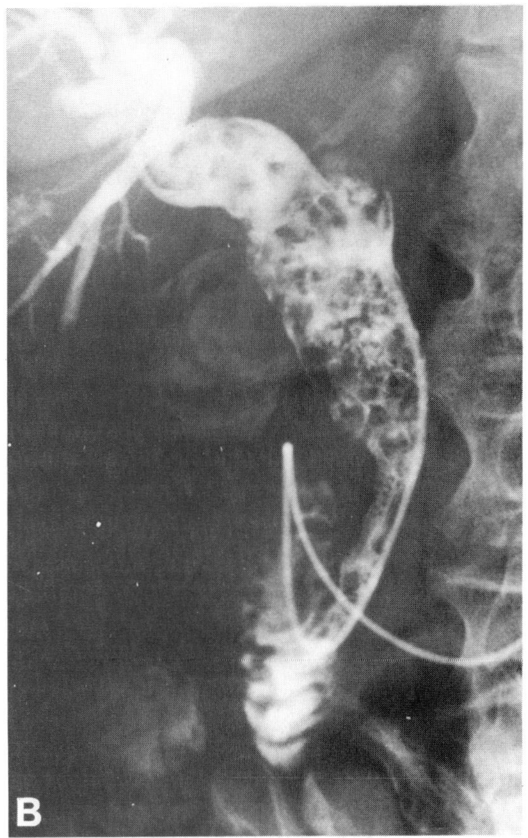

FIG 3.
Large stone burden in the common bile duct **(A)** before and **(B)** after shock wave lithotripsy. The patient developed acute cholecystitis as a result of an impaction of a large gallbladder stone after lithotripsy and underwent successful cholecystectomy with exploration of the common bile duct. We learned from several cases that septic complications may occur after ESL. Therefore, perioperative administration of antibiotics is advised. (From Sauerbruch T, Holl J, Sackmann M, et al: Treatment of bile duct stones by extracorporeal shock waves. *Semin Ultrasound*, CT, MR 1987; 8:155. Used by permission.)

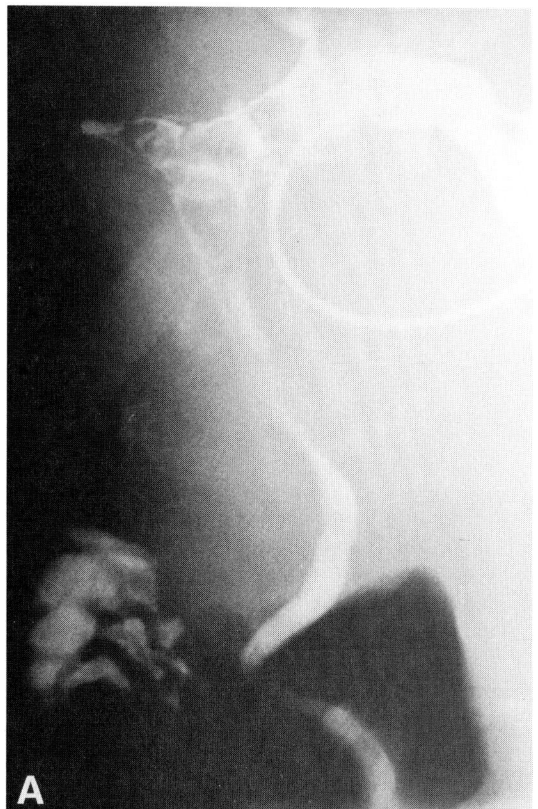

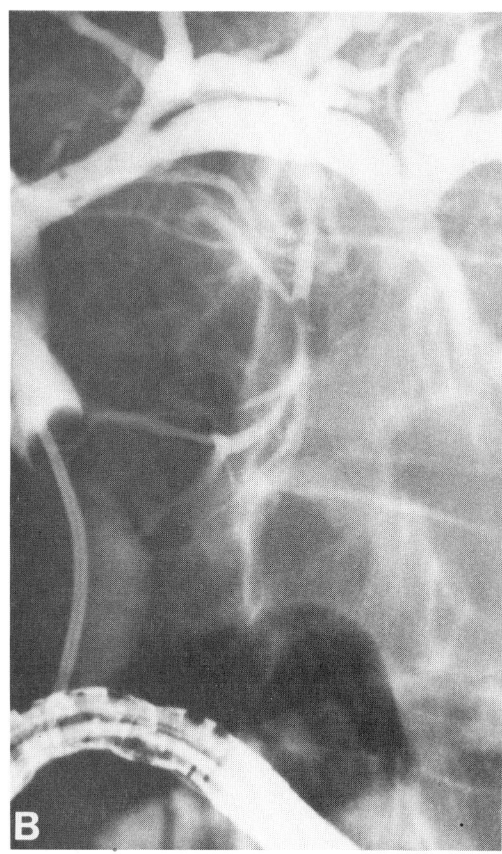

FIG 4.
Multiple impacted stones in the bifurcation of the bile ducts and resection of the right liver lobe owing to echinococciasis. Several surgical attempts to remove the stones had failed. After two ESL sessions, all fragments and stones could be successfully extracted with a Dormia basket, and the bile ducts were stone-free (**B,** retrograde cholangiogram with a balloon catheter). (From Sauerbruch, T: Behandlungen von Gallensteinen durch extrakorporale Stoßwellen. Erste Erfahrungen. *Akt Chir* 1988; 23:58. Used by permission.)

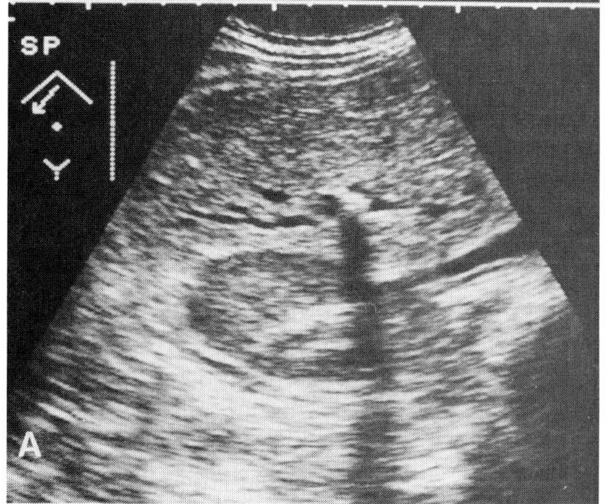

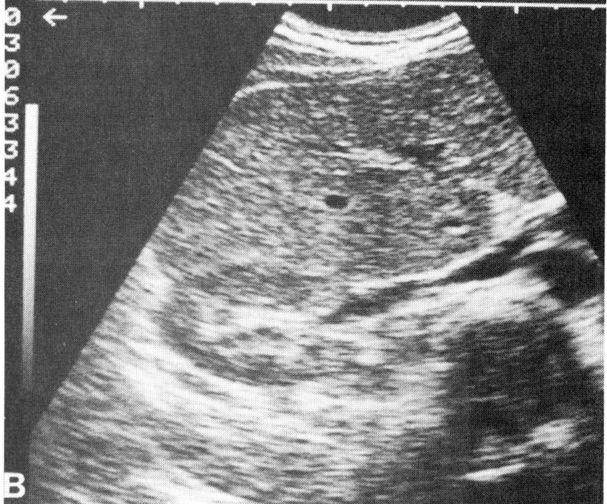

FIG 5.
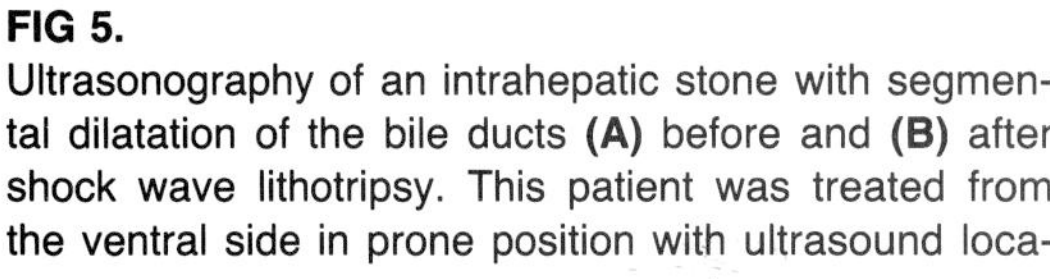
Ultrasonography of an intrahepatic stone with segmental dilatation of the bile ducts **(A)** before and **(B)** after shock wave lithotripsy. This patient was treated from the ventral side in prone position with ultrasound location of the stone. (From Sauerbruch T, Holl J, Sackmann M, et al: Treatment of bile duct stones by extracorporeal shock waves. *Semin Ultrasound, CT, MR* 1987; 8:155. Used by permission.)

Nonsurgical Therapy of Gallstones: Implications for Imaging

Joseph F. Simeone, M.D., Joseph T. Ferrucci, M.D.

The year 1988 represents a major landmark in the diagnosis and management of gallstone disease. First and most important is the virtual revolution in treatment, as several new nonsurgical modes of therapy are being introduced almost simultaneously to physicians in the United States. These include oral bile acids, extracorporeal shockwave lithotripsy (ESL), and contact dissolution with methyl tertiary butyl ether (MTBE). Paralleling these developments, gallstone imaging is undergoing a similar period of rapid transition. As these new therapeutic techniques become more widely available, diagnostic gallstone imaging will become a more rigorous and demanding exercise. Heretofore, the only therapy available was cholecystectomy and therefore the only issue for radiologic interpretation was binary. Are gallstones present or not? A positive or negative answer sufficed. However, because all the new nonsurgical modes of therapy are predicated on specific, objective morphologic characteristics of the gallstone burden and functional status of the gallbladder, there is a new need to quantify, characterize, and measure the gallbladder and its contents. Sonographic and cholecystographic techniques will necessarily become more refined. Correllation and comparison of unorganized data will become routine for final judgment as to size and number of gallstones. This discussion reviews some of these new requirements in the imaging diagnosis of gallstones.

UNTRASONOGRAPHIC TECHNIQUES

Special technical maneuvers for performing ultrasonographic studies of the gallbladder will assume new clinical importance (Fig 1). Sizing artifacts from reflective surfaces, axial versus lateral resolution meaurements, and magnification of hard copy images for measurements will now require attention. Optimal stone meaurements should be done in the axial (AP) diameter as resolution in this dimension is superior to lateral resolution. In addition, there will be a need to tailor patient positioning in order to separately count and meaure stones individually. Hard copy should be magnified for better depiction of stone details. Markers or cursor readouts of stone dimensions should also be clearly displayed. Transducer frequencies of at least 5 mHz will be required in order to obtain ideal image quality. It is anticipated that abdominal radiologists and ultrasonographers will find these new requirements readily mastered.

URSO ELIGIBILITY: IMAGING IMPLICATIONS (TABLE 1)

The principle morphologic criteria for primary treatment of cholesterol gallstones with the newly Federal Drug Administration–approved

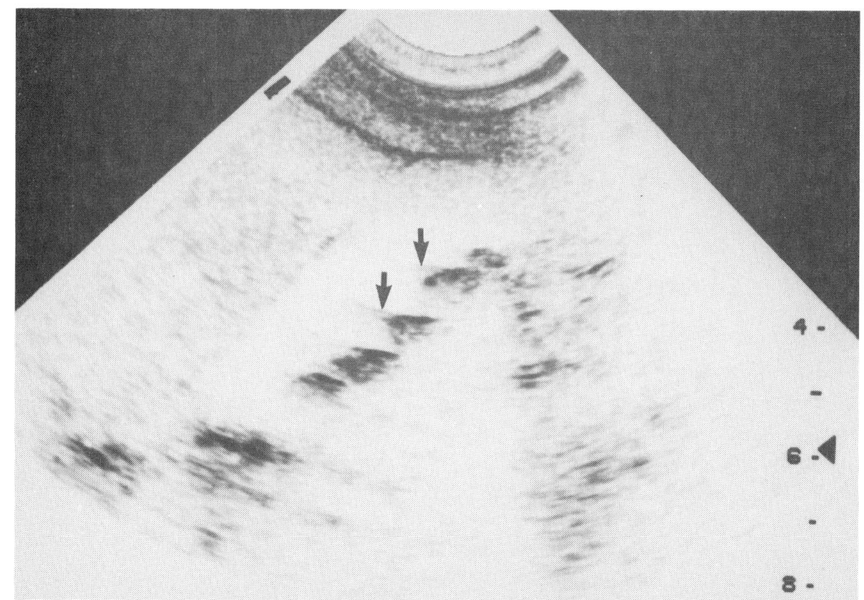
4 -
6 -
8 -

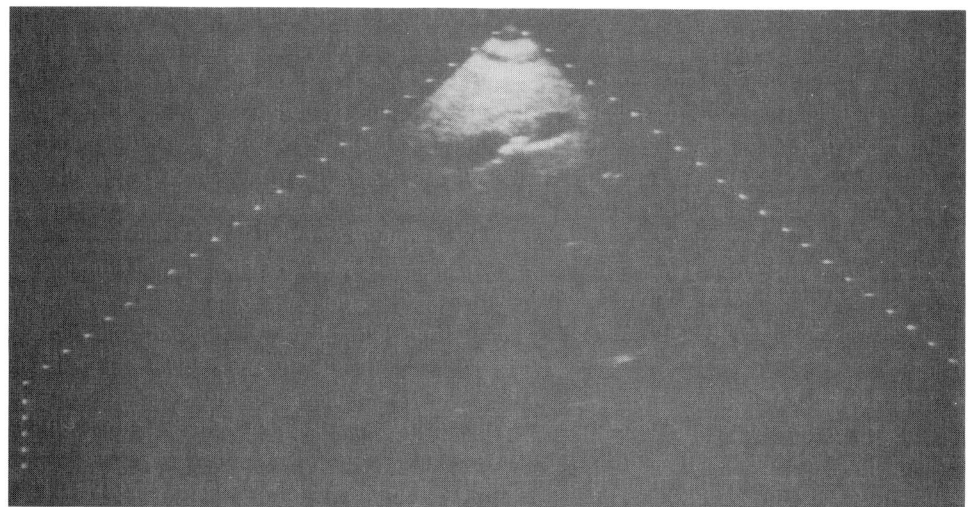

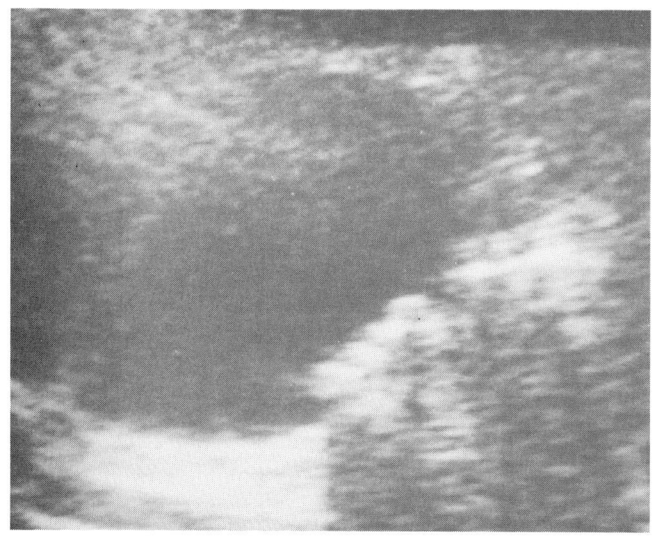

TABLE 1.
URSO Eligibility Imaging Criteria (Ciba-Geigy)

OCG	—Must function
Plain film	—Stones nonradiopaque (no Ca^{++} nidus> 3 mm)
US	—Size <20 mm (no limit on number)

oral bile acid, ursodeoxycholic acid (URSO) are listed above. These are adapted from the FDA Ciba-Geigy URSO clinical trial protocols. To what extent they may be liberalized in the future remains to be determined.

Assuming the patient has a diagnosis of gallstones established by some previous imaging technique, the size of the gallstones as measured on sonography must not exceed 20 mm in greatest diameter of the largest stone. However, at present there is no practical limit on the number of stones. The rationale for the limitation of 20 mm relates to the stone surface area available for dissolution. The smaller the stone, the larger the surface area and the more likely and more complete the ultimate dissolution.

On plain abdominal radiographs, stones must be nonradiopaque. Calcified stones or stones with a calcific rim will be excluded. However, gallstone with a small calcific nidus less than 3 mm would still be suitable for URSO therapy. As with sonography, radiographic technique must be optimized. Coned views of the right upper quadrant in the prone position will give the best results. Radiographic technique using low kvP and high mas will maximize calcium detectability.

Oral cholecystography must disclose that there is adequate gallbladder visualization. This assures that the cystic duct is patent, which is essential if URSO-rich hepatic bile is to flow into the gallbladder lumen to exert its local chemolytic effect. The gallstones also must be radiolucent when visualized during oral cholecystography. Because overlying bowel gas or stool or rib calcification might obscure right upper quadrant calcification, a more focused view of the stones provided by coned-down views during oral cholecystography often more precisely localized stone and nonstone calcifications than a full abdominal film. Small central foci of gallstone calcification may be invisible on the plain abdominal radiograph and may only be disclosed after the gallstone is contrasted against opacified bile in a functioning gallbladder (Fig 2). Right upper quadrant calcifications may be more specifically identified as being within or not within the gallbladder (Fig 3). The classic techniques for performing oral cholecystography should be once again implemented.[1] Measurement of stone size by oral cholecystography will assume a new importance because precise stone size determination by sonography will not always be possible. Optimal oral cholecystography technique should minimize the effects of radiographic magnification. Therefore, overhead radiographs should be made with the patient in the prone oblique position. Magnification factors for each individual radiographic unit should be calculated. Measurements of stone size determined on upright spot films should be individually corrected for magnification. Many younger physicians and radiologists will have to relearn the standard principles of patient preparation, oral cholecystographic contrast excretion pathways, and principles of cholecystographic interpretation.

ESL ELIGIBILITY: IMAGING IMPLICATIONS (TABLE 2)

The two major differences between patient eligibility for URSO therapy and eligibility for ex-

FIG 1.
Ultrasound scanning techniques. **A.** Side lobe artifact visible on the lateral aspect (*arrows*) of the gallstones makes precise determination of lateral stone diameter difficult. Exact anteroposterior dimensions are also imprecise because of sound beam absorption by the stone and the consequent inexact depiction of the posterior stone border. **B.** Minified image makes measurement of stones quite difficult. **C.** Magnified image of stones permits precise stone size diameter determination and accurate stone number assessment.

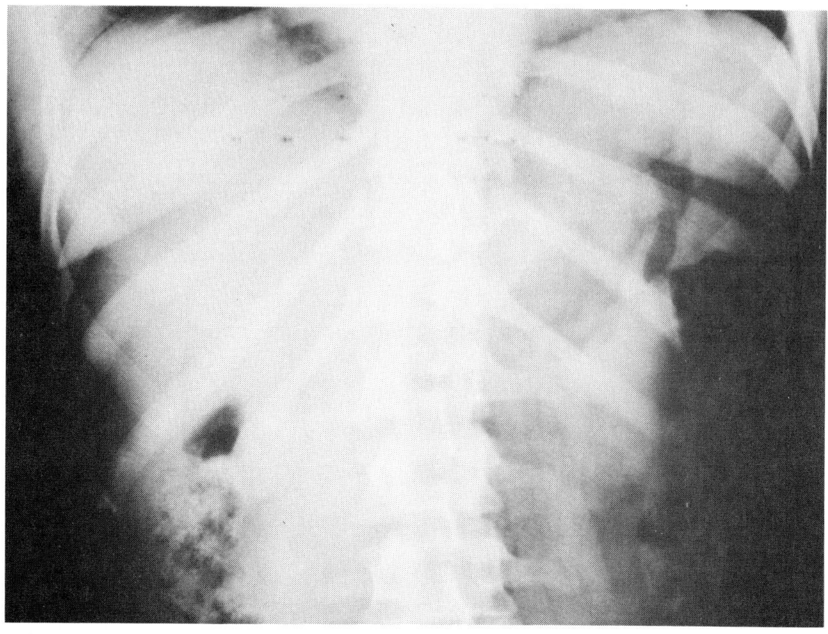

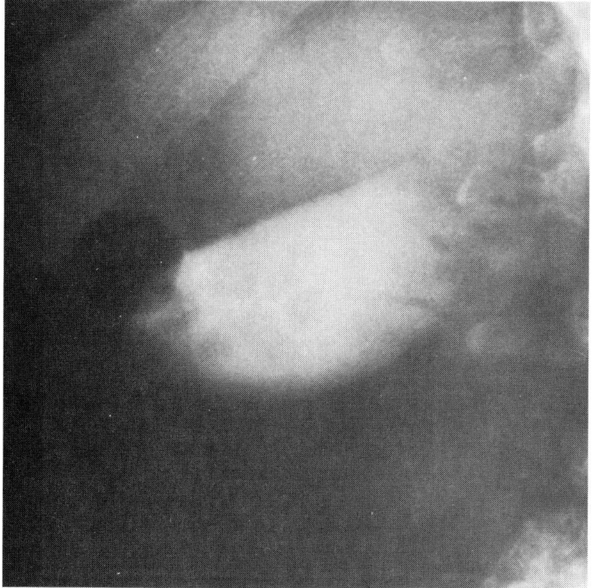

FIG 2.
Calcification not visible by plain film and only visible by OCG. **A.** Plain film of the abdomen demonstrates no right upper quadrant calcification. **B.** Coned down view of the gallbladder demonstrates multiple central calcifications within several gallstones.

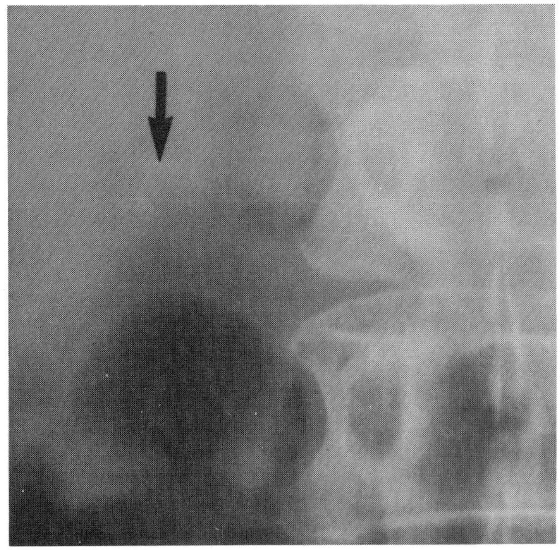

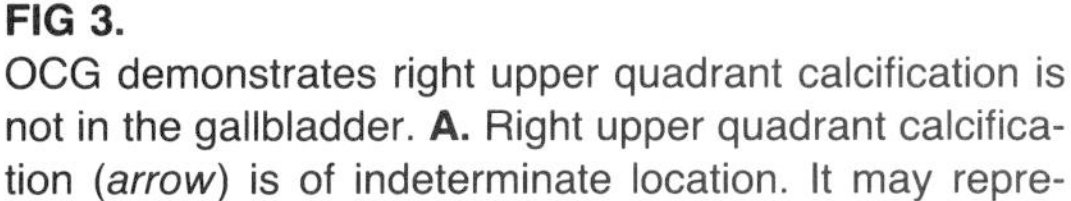

FIG 3.
OCG demonstrates right upper quadrant calcification is not in the gallbladder. **A.** Right upper quadrant calcification (*arrow*) is of indeterminate location. It may represent a calcified gallstone. **B.** OCG demonstrates that the calcification (*arrows*) is remote from the gallbladder.

TABLE 2.
ESL Eligibility Criteria (Dornier)

OCG	—Must function
Plain Film	—Stones nonradiopaque
US	—Size <30 mm
	—Less than three stones

tracorporeal shockwave lithotripsy (ESL) are the number of gallstones and size of gallstones. For URSO use, any number of stones may be present measuring 2.0 cm or less in diameter. In the FDA-approved clinical trial protocols for ESL, no more than 3 stones may be present, and no stone may exceed 3.0 cm. Thus the criteria for ESWL (at least with the Dornier and Medstone protocols approved to date) are more limited relative to stone number but more liberal relative to size than with oral bile acids.

Ultrasound will be used to examine patients after ESL procedure to check for stone fragments, sludge, or possible complications of ESL, such as biliary duct dilation, focal liver changes, pancreatitis, or gallbladder wall abnormalities. Standard sonographic techniques can be used to look for fragments or sludge. If small, nonshadowing fragments are seen, movement of the fragments with a change in position of the patient will confirm their presence. If sludge is present, stone fragments lying within the sludge will have to be searched for more carefully so they are not missed and the patient thus declared free of calculi. The highest resolution transducers will be required during post-ESL scanning to search for these fragments within the sludge.

CHOLECYSTOGRAPHIC-ULTRASONOGRAPHIC CORRELATIONS

One of the great stories of technologic obsolescence in modern medicine was the extraordinarily rapid demise of oral cholecystography when real-time sonography was introduced in the mid-1970s. The oral cholecystogram had served as the unchallenged gold standard for gallstone diagnosis for some 40 to 50 years, but within 3 to 4 years after the introduction of sonography it all but disappeared from clinical practice.

The now well-known advantages of sonography include speed, no need for ingestion of contrast medium, far greater sensitivity for detecting small stones, ability to survey other anatomic structures in the abdomen, lack of ionizing radiation, and ability to perform the study on an emergency or unscheduled basis. The common problem of the significance of a poorly visualized or nonvisualized gallbladder in a patient with undiagnosed abdominal symptoms was instantaneously resolved, and the well-known 10 to 30 percent incidence of unpleasant gastrointestinal side effects following oral contrast ingestion for oral cholecystography was eliminated.

Although sonography is widely accepted as being approximately 15 to 20 percent more sensitive than oral cholecystography in the detection of gallstones (Fig 4), emerging correlative experience when the two procedures are performed in conjunction with imaging workups for nonsurgical gallstone therapy discloses new insights into biliary calculus imaging. For example, ultrasound appears to be less accurate in counting stones than OCG, and direct correlation and comparison between ultrasound and OCG will be necessary for precise stone number determination in almost every patient (Fig 5). Moreover, measurements of gallstone size by sonography are quite accurate in the size range of <2 cm but are not so accurate when stones exceed 2 cm (Fig 6). This is due to the acoustic reflection and absorption of the ultrasound beam obscuring the deep and polar surfaces of the typical large oval calculus. Thus, the larger stones often under consideration for ESL may attenuate the ultrasound beam. The back wall of the stone may not be visible, and exact measurement in the axial plane will not be possible because all of the stone cannot be seen by sonography. Further, as stones increase in size to greater than 1 cm, they tend to become ovoid in shape. The diameters of an oval stone are better determined by OCG than by the lateral resolution of the ultrasound beam, which is the way an oval stone presents to the US beam with the patient in the supine position.

Some radiologists may not know that identification of the exact number of gallstones may be misleading by both sonography and oral cholecystography. Because of overlap and obscuration to the x-ray and/or ultrasound beam, however, tailored techniques using decubitus, upright, and prone positions will be increasingly utilized. Further, cross-checks between findings of oral cholecystography and sonography will be necessary. In general, the imaging studies showing the greatest number and largest stones should be considered the correct result. A strong revival of the once outmoded oral cholecystogram is a foregone conclusion.

PATIENT ELIGIBILITY (TABLES 3, 4)

Although the commonly quoted figure of 1 million new gallstone patients diagnosed annually in the United States is widely accepted, knowledgeable sonographers have long suspected that the number of gallstone patients that could be found on a careful sonographic population screening survey would be even higher.[2,3] Recent studies have confirmed this as discussed by Roda in chapter 10. Nevertheless, little data exist as to the proportion of such patients potentially suitable for the new nonsurgical forms of therapy, including oral bile acids, contact dissolution, and shockwave lithotripsy. Certain generalizations, however, apply. First, all patients being assessed for the nonsurgical approaches will require a functioning oral cholecystogram. The only available data in the literature pertinent

TABLE 3.
MTBE Eligibility Criteria

OCG	—No consensus yet
Plain film	—No stone calcification
US	—No limit on size or number
CT	—No dense calcification
	—Access route suitable

TABLE 4.
Eligibility for Nonsurgical Therapy (Estimated)

MTBE	—c. 60%
Oral bile acids	—c. 40%
EWL	—c. 20%

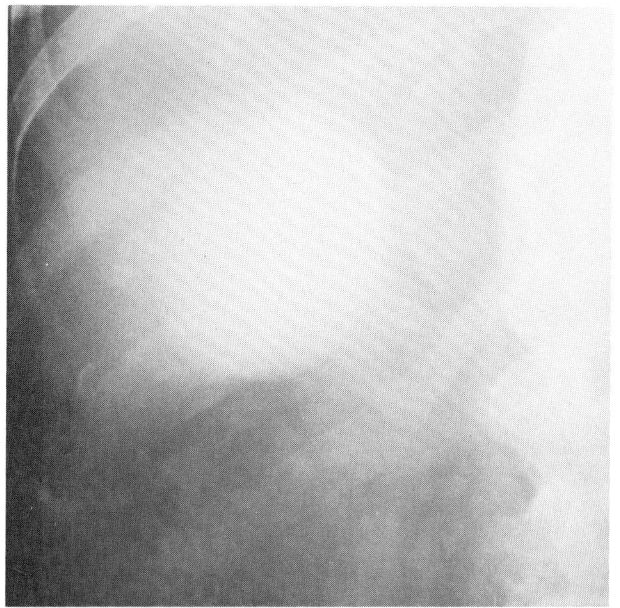

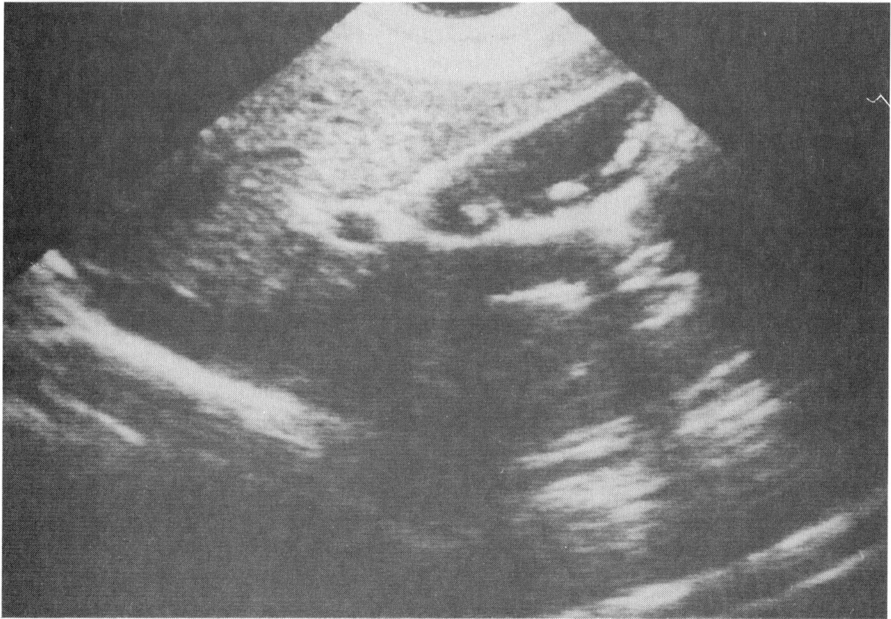

FIG 4.
OCG misses stones. **A.** An oral cholecystogram demonstrates a well-opacified gallbladder with no calculi visible. Several other spot films also did not demonstrate calculi. **B.** Ultrasound scan clearly demonstrates several small stones.

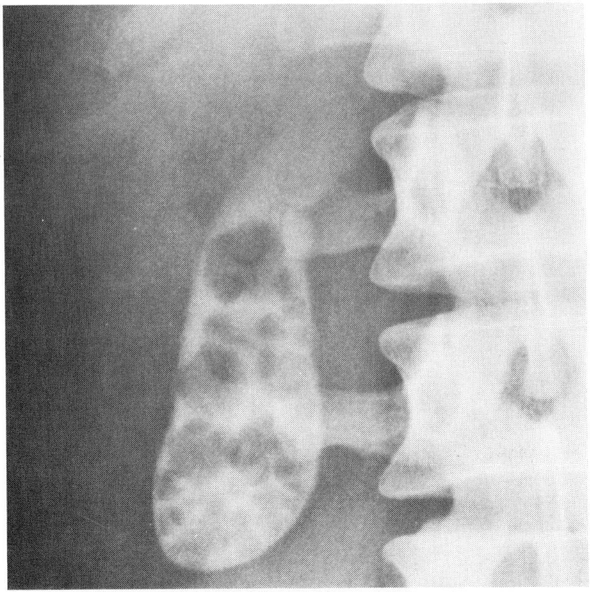

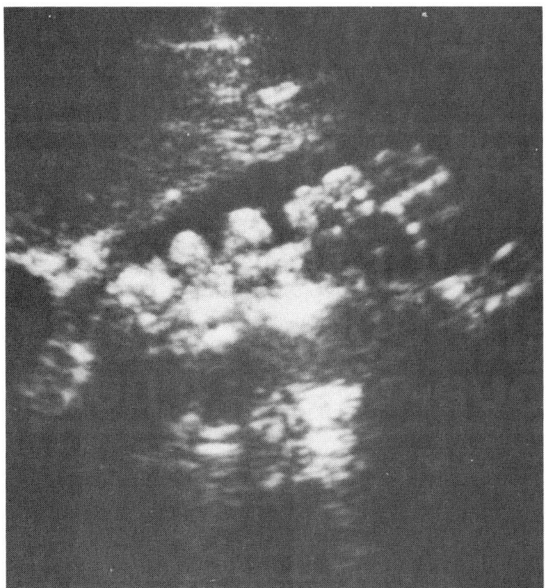

FIG 5.
OCG better demonstrates size, shape, and number of stones. **A.** OCG clearly demonstrates multiple stones, probably in two families. The largest stone contains curvilinear airlike densities characteristic of the "Mercedes Benz" sign. **B.** Ultrasound demonstrates a maximum of eight stones. Individual stone shape is indeterminate.

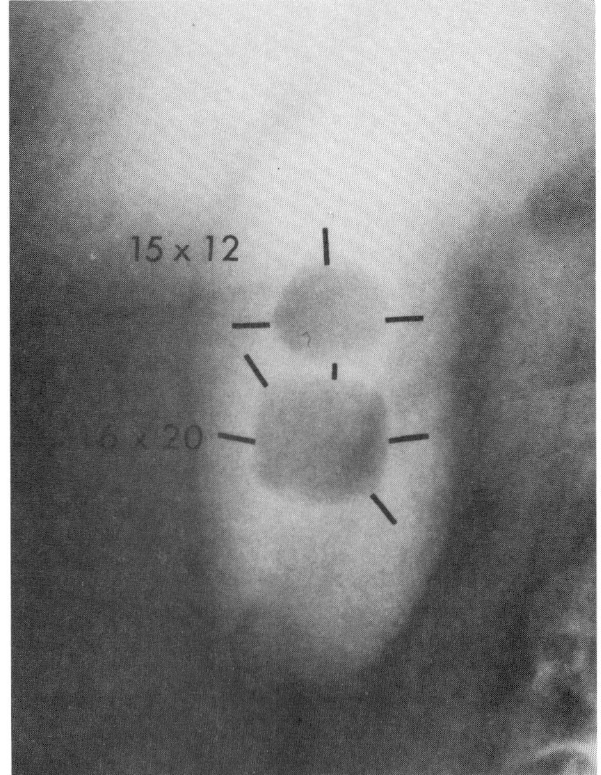

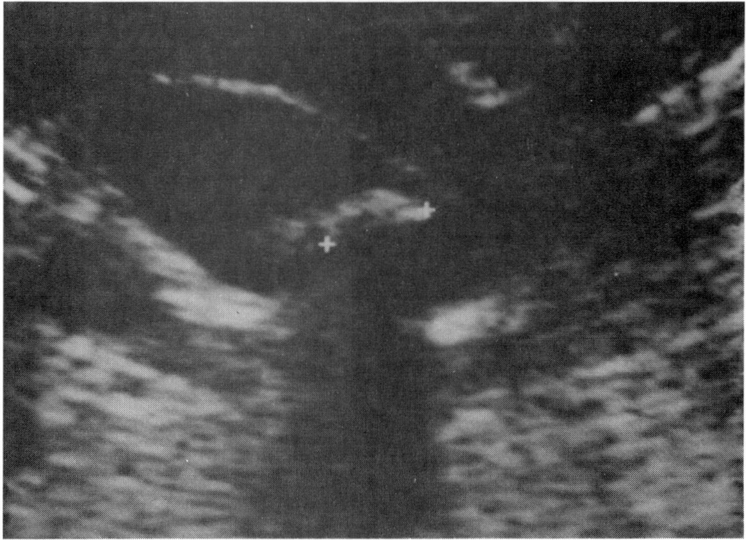

FIG 6.
OCG best demonstrates size and shape of stones. **A.** OCG demonstrates two stones present in the gallbladder. Corrected for magnification, these stones measure 16 × 20 mm and 15 × 12 mm. **B.** Maximal stone size that could be demonstrated was 13 mm on all of the ultrasound scans performed. The size of the stones prevents the sound beam from clearly delineating the back wall of the stone and makes measurement in the axial plane imprecise.

to this question come from the GREPCO study.[4] In this population survey of asymptomatic patients in Italy, individuals who had gallstones demonstrated by sonography were found to have a 28 percent incidence of a nonvisualizing oral cholecystography. Conventional wisdom holds that radiopaque gallstones are present in about 20 percent of all patients. The GREPCO data shows similar figures (18 percent). Analysis of 100 consecutive surgically removed gallstone-containing gallbladders at the Massachusetts General Hospital also showed 17 percent of patients to have heavily calcified stones.[5] Our data at MGH and the GREPCO data also carefully analyzed stone size and number. Both studies suggest that in toto about 50 percent of all gallstone patients would be currently suitable for oral bile acid therapy utilizing the FDA-sanctioned eligibility criteria. By the same token, the criteria currently in effect for extracorporeal lithotripsy are stricter, allowing approximately no more than 25 percent to be eligible for shockwave treatment.

CONCLUSION

Gallstone imaging is entering a period of renaissance. It is characterized by rehabilitation of the once obsolete oral cholecystogram, greater emphasis on quantification of gallstone morphology, and correlation of multiple-imaging methods, including sonography, oral cholecystography, and plain film roentgenography.

REFERENCES

1. Berk RN, Leopold G, Ferrucci JT: *Radiology of the Gallbladder and Bile Ducts: Diagnosis and Intervention*. Philadelphia, Saunders, 1983.
2. Barbara L, Sama C, Labate AMM, et al: A population study on the prevalence of gallstone disease: The Sirmione Study. *Hepatology* 1987; 7:913–917.
3. Jurgensen T: Prevalence of gallstones in a Danish population. *Am J Epidemiol* 1987; 126:912–921.
4. Rome Group for the Epidemiology and Prevention of Cholelithiasis (GREPCO): Radiologic appearance of gallstones and its relationship with biliary symptoms and awareness of having gallstones. Observations during epidemiologic studies. *DG DS SI* 1987; 32(4):349–353.
5. Brink JA, Simeone JF, Mueller PR, Richter JM, Prien E, Ferrucci JT: Morphologic characteristics of gallstones removed at cholecystectomy: Implications for shock wave lithotripsy. *AJR* (in press).

Implementation of a Biliary Lithotripsy Center: Logistics

William E. Torres and Harvey V. Steinberg

In these days of rising health care costs and increasing competition between hospitals as well as among groups of physicians, starting a biliary lithotripsy center requires a great deal of forethought. A variety of issues should be addressed and settled prior to beginning architectural planning. One of the primary issues to be dealt with is who is to run the center. Should biliary lithotripsy be under the domain of one group, as has occurred in renal lithotripsy; or would it be beneficial to draw from the skills of radiologists, gastroenterologists, and surgeons in order to most efficaciously manage the center and treat patients? The significant expenditures necessary to fund and implement a first-class center with an ever-tightening health care dollar is a serious consideration that threatens to become a critical issue in the times that lie ahead. In addition, questions with regard to the need for and role of, as well as the market for, biliary lithotripsy must be addressed.

THE BILIARY LITHOTRIPSY TEAM

At our institution, the approach has been to form a biliary lithotripsy team composed of radiologists, gastroenterologists, and surgeons; each group having its own special and, in the case of biliary lithotripsy, essential talents. The radiologist is responsible for coordinating and evaluating the radiological portion of the screening process as well as providing the ultrasound expertise vitally necessary to perform the procedure. The gastroenterologist and/or the surgeon is responsible for obtaining and evaluating the clinical and laboratory data as well as for jointly providing the treatment. Our experience in performing the procedure on 40 patients to date makes it quite clear that a working knowledge of ultrasound is essential to perform the procedure. Ultrasound plays a critical role both in the initial gallbladder localization as well as in the actual treatment. We believe that the responsibility for the treatment should rest with physicians and not with technologists. It was decided, therefore, not to add an ultrasound technologist to our staff.

THE RATIONALE FOR THE CENTER

Our institution decided that gallstone lithotripsy and its adjunct procedures should both attract and be attractive to physicians and their patients. Biliary lithotripsy will provide an alternative to those patients who are either unwilling or, owing to reasons of poor health, unable to undergo cholecystectomy.

The procedure currently requires a 2-night, 3-day hospital stay by FDA-approved protocol. This in all probability will soon be reduced to a mere overnight hospitalization, with the projected likelihood that this procedure can eventually be performed on an outpatient basis, with few exceptions. The ramifications of being able to treat gallstone disease as an outpatient procedure are clear and would be widely embraced by physicians, patients, and third-party carriers in a nation embattled with rapidly rising health care expenditures over the past decade. In 1983, for example, the annual increase in the rate of health care expenditure averaged 10 to 15 percent, with total expenditures of $313.3 billion.[1] The federal and state governments have taken a variety of cost-containment steps in an attempt to slow rising costs[1–3] and will certainly attempt to reduce costs even further in the future.

It has been estimated that 20 million people in the United States have gallstone disease and that well over $1 billion is spent annually on this problem; the vast majority of the cost arises from the 500,000 to 600,000 cholecystectomies performed yearly. It has been estimated that the average total cost (including hospitalization) for a cholecystectomy is approximately $10,000 per patient in 1988 and depends on the region of the country.[4] The average hospital stay in 1986 for cholecystectomy was 10.5 days. At this time, the exact cost of biliary lithotripsy is difficult to pinpoint, but it is expected to be approximately one half that of cholecystectomy. Using current criteria, it appears that approximately 30 percent of patients with gallstones will be candidates for biliary lithotripsy,[5] with a great many more patients potential candidates when the criteria are expanded to include, for example, more than three stones or calcified stones.

THE LITHOTRIPSY CENTER

With the aforementioned issues in mind, the planning of the biliary lithotripsy center began. From its initial conception to its complete fruition the center required approximately 1 year. The biliary lithotripsy center would be located on an outpatient surgical floor of the Isobel Fra-

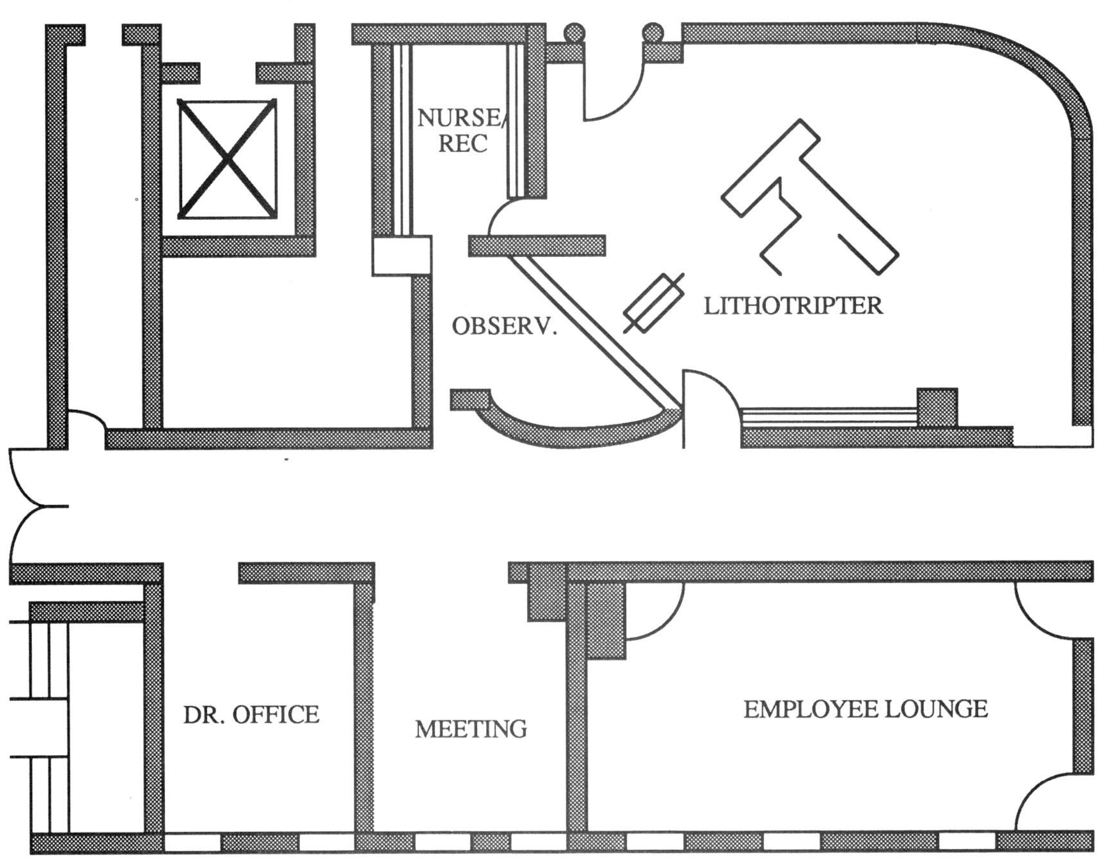

FIG 1.

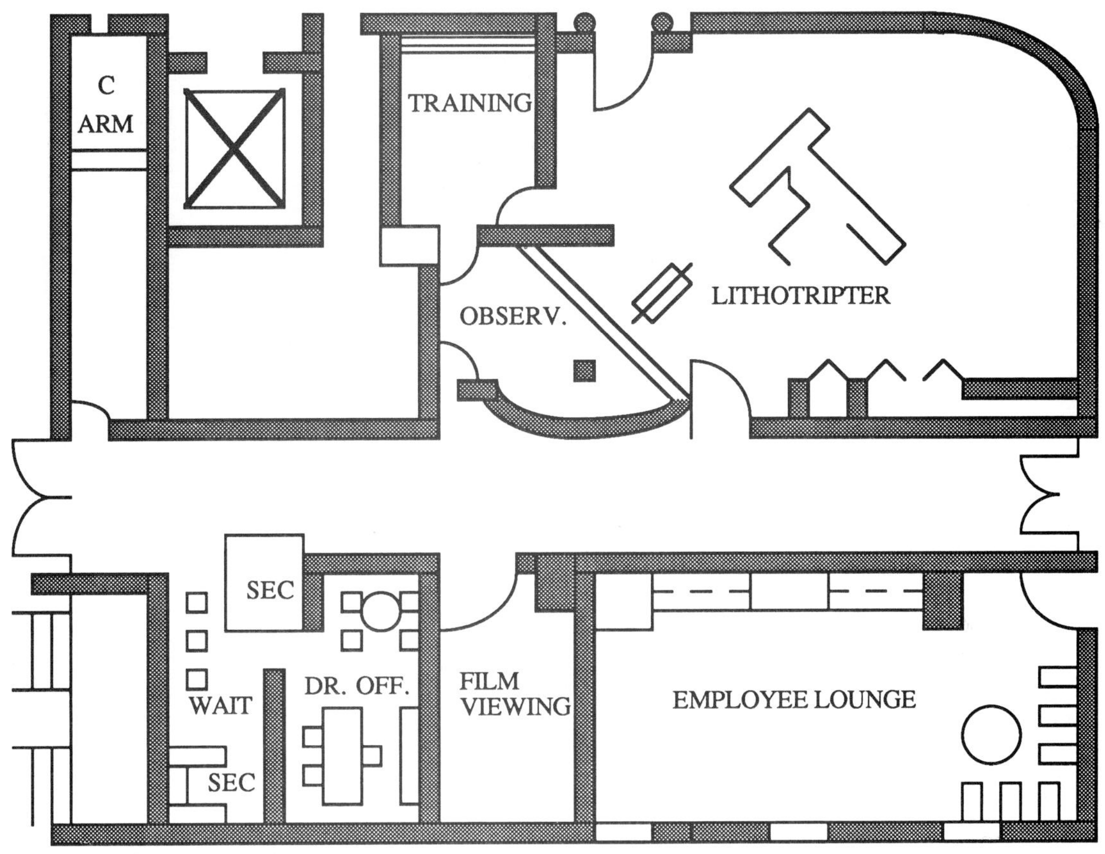

FIG 2.

zier outpatient center of Crawford W. Long Hospital of Emory University, occupying 2868 square feet of space. Outpatient surgery and the lithotripsy center would share a large, redecorated waiting area measuring 2100 square feet. Our patients would be processed through the outpatient surgical center before the procedure and afterward be transferred to a hospital room. The center itself, as originally envisioned by the architect and the hospital administration, contained space (Fig 1) for the lithotripsy suite, a separate observation area, nurse-record room, a doctors' office and a conference room (architect: Vance Cheatam—Nix, Mann and Company). It was readily apparent that additional space for support personnel and a reading room would be necessary (Fig 2); therefore, the conference room was incorporated into the doctors' office and with a small amount of space from an adjoining employees' lounge. The center also had its area for a lithotripsy coordinator, a secretary, and a reading room. It was also decided to convert the area initially allocated as a nurse-record room into a training center. Such a center, it was believed, targeted to the training of physicians, would be needed in the future.[6]

THE LITHOTRIPSY SUITE

The working area of the lithotripsy suite is basically a rectangle, measuring approximately 600 square feet, with a centrally placed lithotripter (Fig 3). The patient stretcher of the Dornier MPL-9000 was positioned so as to be easily accessible to the operating console. Periodic adjustments to both the table and water cushion as well as stone fragment assessment using the out-of-line transducer can thus be accomplished most readily. The central position of the patient

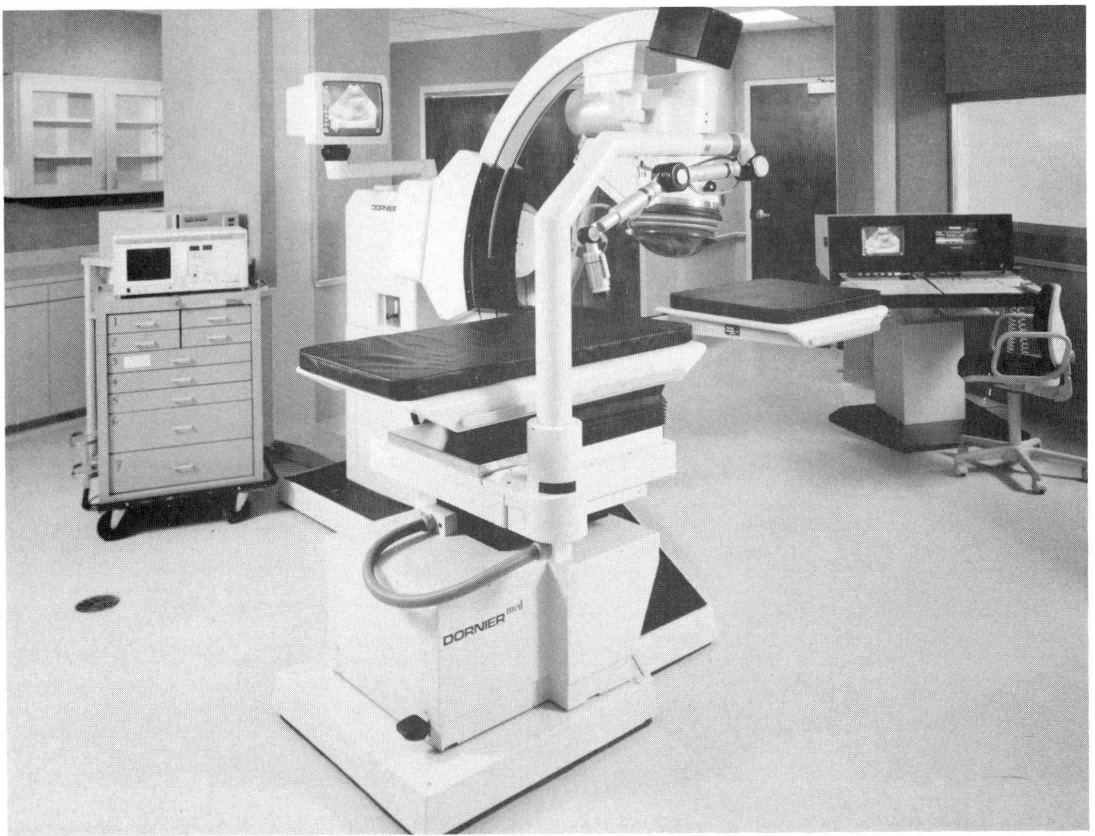

FIG 3.
Crawford Long Hospital Dornier MPL 9000 Biliary Lithotripsy Suite.

stretcher allows unencumbered movement of personnel around the table. Designated areas were developed for anesthesia, the operating console, storage for supplies, as well as a separate space for the control cabinet and the nitrogen gas necessary for the machine. The architectural design was created not only to optimize our space but to minimize sound transmission within and outside our room. A special sound-absorbing blanket was installed above the acoustical tile ceiling. The walls were designed to prevent sound transmission to areas adjacent to the lithotripter by staggering the wall studs and then interweaving a sound-absorbing blanket through the studs. The combination of the walls being covered in sound soak along with the shape of the room parlay into a decrease in noise volume during treatment. The machine has also been placed on a special platform by the manufacturer to diminish the transmission of sound. The room design allows the personnel in the room to perform the procedure in comfort without special ear coverings.

Anesthesia is located at the far end of the stretcher with sufficient room to maneuver whether the patient is positioned supine or prone. The vast majority of patients in the German experience have had lithotripsy in the prone position. To date we also have only performed lithotripsy in the prone position, but see no reason why the procedure cannot be performed supine. The Dornier MPL-9000 allows a great deal of flexibility in patient positioning which to date has not been fully explored and cultivated. Since all our patients have had the procedure using intravenous sedation, the customary positioning of the anesthesiologist at the patient's head has not been necessary. A special alcove was designed to accommodate anesthesia equipment, including an anesthesia cart, monitoring equipment, and anesthetic gases.

The room should have ample storage space. A series of cabinets line the far side of the room with glass inserts on the wall-hung units allowing for easy access. All material relevant to biliary lithotripsy including drugs, ultrasound gel, x-ray folders, and linen are readily available. The room is equipped with a standard stainless-steel sink built into the the counter top. A separate area with double hung doors is used to house the control cabinet and gases necessary for the lithotripter.

Two types of illumination are provided in the room. Multiple fluorescent lights serve as the major light source while incandescent lights are used both for background and for subdued light during the procedure. The latter lighting system is controlled by a rheostat switch.

The operating console contains two monitors. One monitor is for the ultrasound operating system while the second monitor displays patient data as well as information pertaining to patient positioning and the actual shock wave therapy. This console was positioned so as to allow for unimpinged viewing from an adjacent observation area. The physician operating the console can by means of a head set communicate with individuals in the observation area. An additional ultrasound monitor is positioned across the patient stretcher for use during the initial localization as well as for subsequent reevaluation during the procedure.

THE OBSERVATION AREA

The unique curvilinear shape of the observation area was adopted by the architect to help accent the importance of both the procedure and the space (Fig 2). This area is clearly the focal point when one first enters the lithotripsy center. The observation area, measuring 160 square feet, has room to accommodate 6 to 10 people and is separated from the lithotripter by two large panes of glass that can be closed off by horizontal blinds. The room has a fluorescent lighting system controlled by rheostat; when the light in the observation room is dampened neither the patient nor the staff can see into the observation area from the lithotripsy room. The patient, we believe, is more comfortable with this arrangement as opposed to a two-way mirror system. As mentioned earlier, communication between the lithotripsy suite and the observation area is possible through a telephone line via a special headset and speaker.

THE LITHOTRIPSY TRAINING ROOM

The training room, measuring 156 square feet, is rectangular in shape with built-in cabinets, book shelves, and space for projection screen. X-ray view boxes with a small shelf for radiographs are on an adjacent wall. The audiovisual equipment includes an overhead TV system and VCR, two caramate projectors, and two routine slide projectors. A variety of both VCR tapes and slide material covering gallbladder disease as well as basic and biliary ultrasound is available.

THE LITHOTRIPSY FILM VIEWING ROOM

The lithotripsy center also has a dedicated film viewing room that measures 136 square feet (Fig 2). It is equipped with a motorized viewer or alternator with 28 panels, each capable of holding up to four 14 × 17 radiographs. A film storage bin is adjacent capable of storing several hundred patient films.

THE PERSONNEL

The center began with the physicians of the biliary lithotripsy team and a secretary. It was soon apparent, however, that a separate administrative assistant or coordinator to run the center with a secretary for scheduling was necessary. A nurse was hired to assist in the lithotripsy room and to prepare the patients prior to lithotripsy. In addition a full-time PA has been hired to oversee the screening process. The coordinator runs the center on a day-to-day basis with a major responsibility being compilation of the vast amount of paperwork necessary for the FDA study. In addition, this person oversees the work of the secretary. This secretary is one of the most important people in the lithotripsy area, since it is with the secretary that the initial contact between the prospective patient and the center occurs. Preliminary screening is also an important function that can prove both cost-cutting and time-efficient when handled by a knowledgeable, articulate secretary.

EXTRA-LITHOTRIPSY DEPARTMENTAL RELATIONSHIPS

The lithotripsy center must coordinate activities with a variety of departments—radiology, laboratory, pharmacy, and the business office. Of these, one of the most important is the business office. Since the procedure is investigational, third-party payers are mixed in their coverage; this will be true until the cost-benefit of the procedure is proved. We believe that patients often base their decision on whether or not to have the procedure on the willingness of the hospital to work with their particular financial situation. The patients at our institution are not only told of the entire procedure cost but are provided with a variety of payment options.

PATIENT FLOW FOR SCREENING AND PROCEDURE

Once the referring physician or patient makes contact, the lithotripsy secretary offers to answer questions and will send out information on both biliary lithotripsy and the lithotripsy center. After filling out a questionnaire the patient, if he or she are felt to fit into the existing protocol, is scheduled for screening. Patients from outside our immediate area are asked to have a double-dose oral cholecystogram performed at their local hospital to allow the screening process to be performed at our center in one day. Once the patient arrives for screening, the PA coordinates all the activities and performs the initial physical exam. The screening material is reviewed, and the patient either is accepted for the procedure or is sent a letter explaining the reason for nonacceptance and is referred back to the primary physician. If the patient is accepted for the procedure there must be at least a 1-week delay prior to the procedure to allow for the medication, ursodeoxycholic acid, or placebo to be taken.

On the day of the procedure the patient reports to the admissions office of the outpatient center, is scheduled for admission to the hospital following the procedure, and is sent to the lithotripsy center for treatment.

SUMMARY

Biliary lithotripsy is simply the beginning of a new wave of procedures to treat patients with gallstones. The lithotripsy center should be used as a springboard for the evaluation of patients with gallbladder disease and for providing patients with the most current information on both existing and investigational treatments.

REFERENCES

1. Steinberg EP: The impact of regulation and payment innovations on acquisition of new imaging technologies. *Radiol Clin North Am* 1985; 23:381—389.
2. Linton OW: Radiology in the medical swirl. *AJR* 1985; 145:118–120.
3. Pickwick CE: Aspects of successful health care management—1984. *Radiographics* 1985: 5:503–505.
4. Medicare report. *Medical Economics Magazine* 1986.
5. Sackmann M, Delius M, Sauerbruch T, et al: Shock-wave lithotripsy of gallbladder stones: The first 175 patients. *New Engl J Med* 1988; 318:393–397.
6. Williams CO, Groce KA: The importance of appropriate suite design in the era of computerized imaging. *Radiol Clin North Am* 1986; 24:337–346.

Alternative Treatments for Gallstones: The Surgeon's View

R. A. Malt

Cholecystectomy is virtually a perfect operation in that it removes a diseased organ and its contents in exchange for a small, usually aesthetic scar, a modicum of discomfort, a short hospital stay, and no physiological impairment. Or, so it might be.

DRAWBACKS OF CHOLECYSTECTOMY

Only the surgeon thinks his or her scars are the ultimate, and patients perceive discomfort variably. In 1985, the average length of stay in American hospitals for patients under 65 years old was 7.5 days—for those over 65 years, 9.5 days.[1] The duration of sick leave from work after an uncomplicated operation can be 6 weeks. Furthermore, the mortality rate after cholecystectomy is 7.5 percent in patients over 65 years old.

Even when the operation is conducted by the finest of surgeons, the possibility of iatrogenic injury to the extrahepatic bile ducts exists because of myriad anatomical variations. Furthermore, unexpected functional abnormalities may occur unpredictably, lumped as the postcholecystectomy syndrome.[2,4] Although the results may not be generalizable, in Barcelona only 53 percent of patients were free of symptoms after cholecystectomy.[5] The rest complained of dyspepsia, flatulence, pain, diarrhea, or hernia: the longer the period of observation, the worse the apparent result. Because these results coincide well with those from a Swedish study three decades earlier,[6] they seem secure.

ADVANTAGES OF NONINVASIVE EXPULSION OF GALLSTONES

Despite costs, perhaps only 10 percent less than those of the average cholecystectomy ($7650, exclusive of professional fees: 1986 data), a noninvasive method of ridding a patient of gallstones has intrinsic merit. In this respect palms go to auricular pressure, because it costs almost nothing. Simply by applying pressure for 20 minutes three times a day after meals to hard seeds placed over the four locations on the external ear representing the points of reference for the biliary system, the liver, and the duodenum, gallstones that had been found by imaging methods in 326 Shanghai patients were propelled from the biliary system into the stools of 82 percent of them, as compared with only 7 percent of controls in a blinded trial.[7] Identity of the biliary stones as such was confirmed by assays of cholesterol and bilirubin and by infrared spectroscopy or scanning electron microscopy.

If these observations can be confirmed, other methods of clearing stones must fall before them. Until they are, extracorporeal shock wave lithotripsy will be the pre-eminent noninvasive method unless unexpected complications appear. After all, ESL of the gallbladder takes only an hour and is minimally and evanescently uncomfortable. It leaves no scar and injures no bile ducts. The greatest inconvenience may be that of taking ursodeoxycholic acid for an unpredictable period afterward to eliminate the calculous rubble.

IMPERMANENCE OF LITHOTOMY AND LITHOTRIPSY

Any treatment that leaves a physiologically abnormal gallbladder in place is impermanent. During 1954 and 1955, Swedish surgeons removed stones from the gallbladders of 53 patients whose gallbladders functioned normally on the basis of oral cholecystography; the gallbladders were retained.[8] The objective was to inflict a lesser operation than usual, to operate with less risk than usual, and to leave an ostensibly normal organ. Fifteen years later, however, when 74 percent of the patients, almost all of them women, could be reassessed, 69 percent had been reoperated upon for calculous disease. Of the remainder, half had symptoms of calculous disease, and others had discomfort of some kind. Between this and an earlier Swedish study, the estimates of recurrence rates were 25 to 50 percent within 3-to-4 years. These rates are compatible with estimates derived from radiocarbon dating of gallstone growth, which also identified a latent period of at least 2 years (mean 8.0 ± 5.1 years, standard deviation) after stone formation began until they became symptomatic; the growth rate of stones was about 2.6 mm/year.[9]

Although biliary sludge in the atonic gallbladders of patients receiving total parenteral nutrition is said to form stones in a matter of weeks, as determined by ultrasonography, direct confirmation by inspection of the excised gallbladder remains to be done.[10]

INDISPENSIBILITY OF CHOLECYSTECTOMY

Cholecystectomy is indispensible for the proper treatment of certain kinds of calculous disease: namely, gangrenous cholecystitis, acute cholecystitis refractory to antibiotic therapy, symptomatic stones in the gallbladder and common bile duct simultaneously, many cases of acalculous cholecystitis, huge stones, pigment stones, and cholesterol stones with an aggregate mass more than 3 cm in diameter.

APPROPRIATENESS OF ESL

Extracorporeal shock wave lithotripsy is appropriate therapy now for three or fewer cholesterol stones in the well-functioning gallbladder of a patient who is willing to take ursodeoxycholic acid for as long as is required, especially someone who wants to get back to normal life as soon as possible. It may come to be proper for disintegration of gallstones in patients with ascites or portal hypertension, who are fearsome surgical risks.[11] Most appealing is the possibility that ESL will come to be the treatment of choice for selected patients with asymptomatic gallstones who have recovered from one attack of nonalcoholic pancreatitis.[12] All these requirements are so limiting, however, that it is no wonder that only 25 percent of patients referred to Grosshadern Clinic, University of Munich, are suitable for biliary lithotripsy.[13]

RECOMMENDATIONS FOR THERAPY

For reasons of economy and efficiency, noninvasive lithotripsy should be managed by surgeons, just as all facets of the treatment of urinary calculi are managed by urologists. The dispassionate master of all modalities appropriate for the patient's benefit will recommend the best one in the least time.

Enough experience with the results of ESL has been gained for it to be confidently recommended as treatment for a typical patient. In the ripeness of middle age, if I were that patient and had the kind of gallstones suitable for lithotripsy, ESL is what I would want. I should prefer to lie on a table for an hour every 5-to-10 years than to have the discomfort of an operation, of being out of work for at least 2 weeks, and of knowing that I would almost certainly not be performing at peak efficiency for a while after returning—provided that I didn't have to take ursodeoxycholic acid (or any other medicine) too long. If my son had gallstones, he should have a cholecystectomy by a surgeon of my choice.

REFERENCES

1. National Center for Health Statistics; data, 1985.
2. Moody FG: Postcholecystectomy syndromes. *Surg Ann* 1987; 19:205–220.
3. Lasson Å: The postcholecystectomy syndrome: Diagnostic and therapeutic strategy. *Scand J Gastroenterol* 1987; 22:897–902.
4. Bar Meir S, Halpern Z, Bardan E, et al: Frequency of papillary dysfunction among cholecystectomized patients. *Hepatology* 1984; 4:328–330.
5. Ros E, Zambon D: Postcholecystectomy symptoms: A prospective study of gallstone patients before and two years after surgery. *Gut* 1987; 28:1500–1504.
6. Kjellgren K: Persistence of symptoms following biliary surgery. *Ann Surg* 1960; 152:1026–1036.
7. Chen PN, Dong SR, Chen K, et al: Auricular pressure in the treatment of gallstones: A randomized, clinical trial of traditional Chinese medicine. *China Acupunct Moxibust* 1985; 5:241–43, in *Hepatology* 1987; 7:781–783.
8. Norrby S, Schönebeck J: Long-term results with cholecystolithotomy. *Acta Chir Scand* 1970; 136:711–713.
9. Mok HYI, Druffel ERM, Rampone WM: Chronology of cholelithiasis: Dating gallstones from atmospheric radiocarbon produced by nuclear bomb explosions. *N Engl J Med* 1986; 314:1075–1077.
10. Messing B, Bories C, Kunstlinger F, et al: Does total parenteral nutrition induce gallbladder sludge formation and lithiasis? *Gastroenterology* 1983; 84:1012–1019.
11. Castaing D, Houssin D, Lemoine J, et al: Surgical management of gallstones in cirrhotic patients. *Am J Surg* 1983; 146:310–313.
12. Moreau JA, Zinsmeister AR, Melton LJ III, et al: Gallstone pancreatitis and the effect of cholecystectomy: A population-based cohort study. *Mayo Clin Proc* 1988; 63:466–473.
13. Heberer G, Paumgartner G, Sauerbruch T, et al: A retrospective analysis of 3-year's experience of an interdisciplinary approach to gallstone disease including shock waves. *Ann Surg* 1988; in press.

Introduction
Panel discussion: Assessing the Technology, the Market, and the Future

J. T. Ferrucci

The concluding panel discussion, entitled "Assessing the Technology, the Market, and the Future," is not intended to be a comprehensive wrap-up of such an immature, complex, and constantly changing subject. It is meant instead to provide an opportunity for selected nonphysician authorities to add their perspectives to the issues, especially as biliary lithotripsy is introduced into clinical practice here in the United States. We have assembled a highly distinguished group of health care executives representing a variety of different agencies and interests. They are critical, they are thoughtful, and whether they can forecast the future remains to be seen. They have been given a wide latitude of approaches to take in these remarks, including the opportunity to reflect on their own impressions or their own agencies' or constituencies' agenda, or to elaborate on the issues or concerns that are most important to them.

The order of speakers has no particular significance: Mr. Richard DiMonda, Director of Dornier Fund of the Cornier Medical Systems of Marietta, Georgia; Mr. Leonard Capuano of the Pharmaceutical Division of the Ciba-Geigy Corporation in Summit, New Jersey; Mr. Robert Britain, manager of the Diagnostic Imaging and Therapeutic Systems Division of the National Electrical Manufacturers Association; Ms. Halyna Breslawec, Director of the Division of Gastroenterology, Urology, and General Use Devices of the Food and Drug Administration, Mr. Henry Alder, Director, Division of clinical Services and technology at the American Hospital Association,and Mr. Philip Drew of Drew Consultants, a medical consulting firm.

Lessons from the Kidney ESWL Experience*

Richard Dimonda

Biliary lithotripsy, as compared to its predecessor, kidney lithotripsy, is in a early stage of development. Many questions are apparent and still more are hidden. When considering how this new technology will affect health care in the United States, it is helpful to look at the more mature yet closely related technology, specifically renal extracorporeal shockwave lithotripsy.*

Before the introduction of renal ESWL, therapy for patients with kidney stones—particularly surgical removal of the stones—was administered mostly in the larger institutions (Fig 1). There was, in effect, a natural centralization of therapy. The introduction of ESWL dramatically shifted the delivery of health care services in the United States to the sites having ESWL. A different but still centralized diffusion of the technology now exists.

If we look at similar statistics regarding cholecystectomy (Fig 2), we see that this surgical procedure is done in most every acute care hospital. This decentralized diffusion of existing technology (surgery) has a number of important implications for the impact biliary ESWL will have on health care services. Centers having biliary ESWL will not draw patients from just large hospitals but will attract patients from nearly all of the hospitals.

If a biliary lithotripter were owned by an individual hospital, we estimate that in order for the unit to break even about 80 percent of the patients will need to come from neighboring hospitals. If we assume that some years from now there will be several hundred lithotripters in the United States, this will create a very significant revenue shift, potentially from 6,000 hospitals to only several hundred ESWL sites.

Of course, not all cholecystectomy patients will switch to biliary ESWL. Many will not meet the ESWL selection criteria, and others will choose one of the several other dissolution alternatives that are emerging along with ESWL. But, on the basis of what we have heard at this meeting, it would appear that the most mature, developed, and soon to be available technology that is an alternative to surgery will be ESWL. So it will be the ESWL sites that first alter the referral patterns in a given health care provider market.

There are several strategies that hospitals probably ought to be thinking about in light of the impact that this technology could have on this shift in the delivery of health care. First, hospitals could consider forming partnerships among themselves to share an ESWL machine, especially if they are in a state governed by certificate of need. Another significant alternative is for institutions to set up mobile lithotripters.

Second, with all the adjuvant procedures discussed at this meeting, hospitals might consider doing more than just buying a lithotripter. They might establish a center that specializes in the management of biliary disease. Such a center

*ⓉDornier Medical Systems

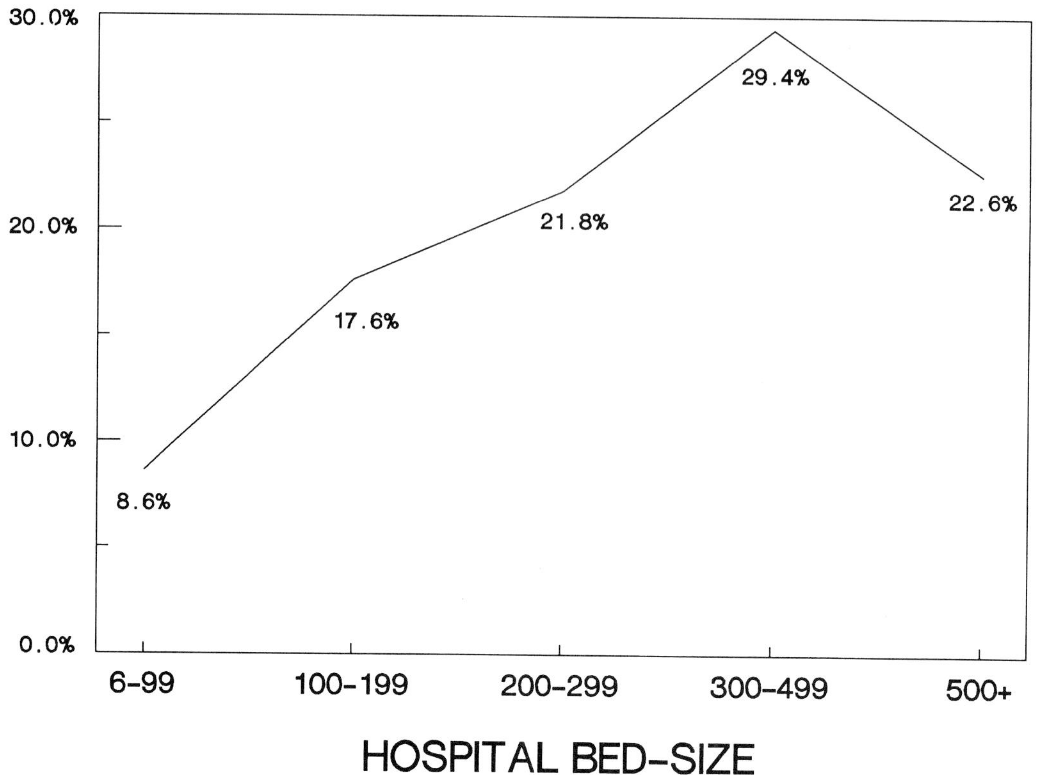

FIG 1.
Urinary Operations by Hospital Size

could be established as a free-standing clinic, as it appears that many of these procedures might ultimately be managed in an outpatient environment.

Aside from such planning and policy decisions, health care professionals are presented with other challenges associated with the technology itself. As I sat here these past 3 days, I had a sense of empathy for those of you who were trying to sort out the different lithotripter alternatives. One of the key problems in comparing the performance is the lack of uniformity in and, in some cases, lack of definitions for the concepts and key terms.

As my colleagues say, you don't have to be a rocket scientist to figure out that each system is producing a very different shockwave from the other. Not only is their method of generation different but the resulting shockwave is different. Some shockwave systems produce a very short rise time shockwave. Some also produce a very short pulse width on the shockwave; others have longer pulse widths. Different companies deliver energy into different focal volumes and at different pressures. And clinicians administer vastly different numbers of shocks to treat the same stone burden. Probably more important and basic than all of these concerns is the fact that the clinical results are different.

Differences in clinical outcome might not be that apparent at this meeting because we had very few comprehensive studies presented. If we take a lesson from the kidney stone experience, however, we might predict how these differences will appear for biliary systems. With greater experience in renal lithotripsy, we are now finding that some systems do not break larger stones as effectively as smaller ones. From Dornier's 8 years of research specifically on biliary stones we found that they are much harder to break than kidney stones. Some even more significant performance issues should be emerging in the biliary stone field than those that exist in the kidney ESWL field now. This may not be apparent right now in biliary ESWL, primarily because the data of some studies are so small and they are not grouped by stone size. There is a need to define carefully stone burden before treatment and group results by stone size so the results of the different machines can be meaningfully compared.

Something else I found to be striking was the varying definition of success. Some presenters said they achieved 96 percent fragmentation. What does that mean? How many fragments? How big?

Some people define success as a function of stone size. As we have seen during this meeting, ultrasound is not as exact as we would like it to be in measuring stone size and number. In some cases, it is difficult to tell whether we have one or seven stones in the gallbladder. So I have trouble understanding how some researchers claim their patients' gallbladders have fragments after ESWL of 0.5 millimeter diameter while others claim diameters of only 0.4 millimeters.

We can be certain, however, that ultrasound is sensitive in detecting whether a stone is present. Must we, therefore, assume that the only important determination is whether the patient is free of stones?

Given the uncertainities inherent in the field at this time, it is important to establish a set of clinical and technical measurement standards or at least common definitions by which we all present our information. If we can go to a clinical meeting someday and see researchers following a similar format with similar definitions, it would make the interpretation of these results much easier and more meaningful.

With these as reference points, we will be able to start figuring out which technology is producing the best results. This will not be a single parameter type of analysis. It will really

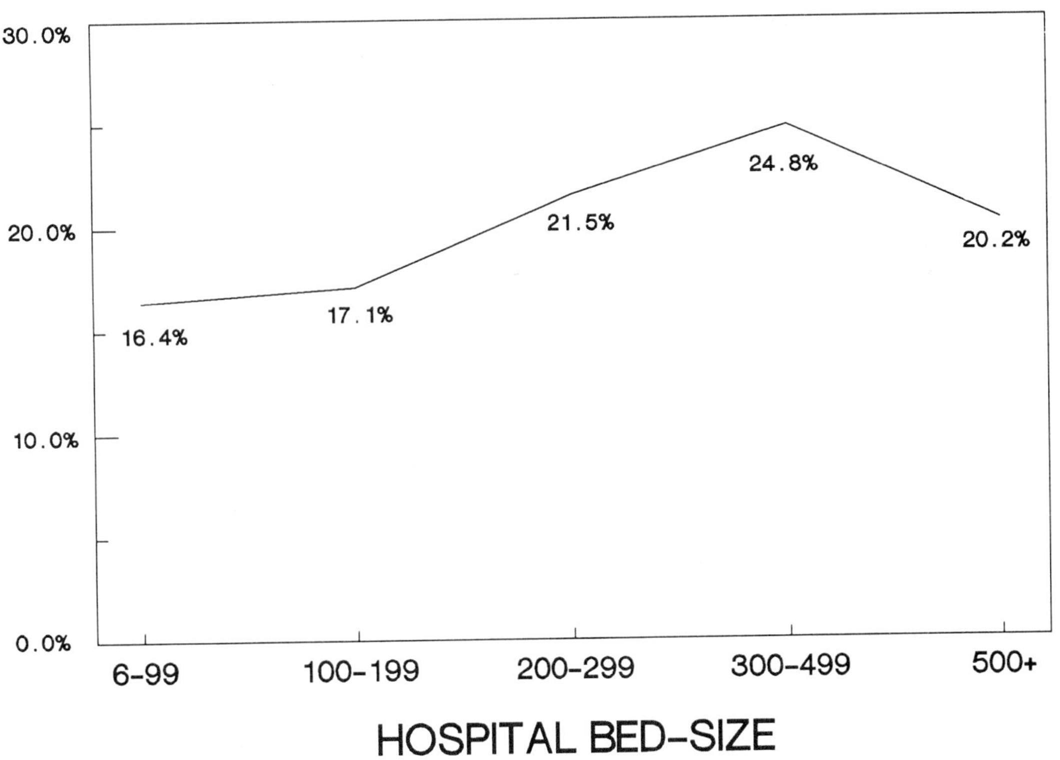

FIG 2.
Cholecystectomies by Hospital Size

be a matter of optimizing a variety of factors—imaging, focusing and targeting, as well as defining the best shockwave for fragmenting stones. We are not really in a position to compare those at the moment.

Just as there are uncertainities regarding biliary ESWL, so are there questions about what the future of gallstone therapy will hold. We see the future as having many therapeutic options. Right now, we are emphasizing noninvasive techniques, but this will probably be the tip of the iceberg in the management of gallstone disease.

There is a wide range of other effective and invasive procedures. Cholecystectomy is the gold standard against which lithotripsy, in many respects, is competing. Other invasive alternatives include direct dissolution, mechanical crushing and extraction, laser fragmentation, and mechanical and chemical ablation. Because of the sudden industry attention being focused on this area of gallstone therapy, other technologies will undoubtedly emerge, which will further influence these therapies.

Which of these will enter the clinical arena and what their indications will be depends on the safety of each one, its efficacy, the preference of the patient, when FDA approval is given and, therefore, when diffusion begins. Who pays and how much—the reimbursement question—must then be decided. All of these factors are going to influence the use of gallstone technologies in the real world as opposed to the manner in which we might like to think that they could be used.

My last comment is on the role of the physician in this area—the question of who will guide the patient through this maze of alternatives and who will then deliver the care. If it is the physician who is involved directly in any one of these procedures who does the guiding, then therapy selection cannot help but be biased. If it is not that physician, then who? Related questions are who will educate the referring physician about the options and how this education will be done.

In deciding who is to administer gallstone therapy, we must consider the qualifications necessary to deliver that care, especially in regard to biliary ESWL. Each of the interested physician groups should move ahead to develop credentialing programs as soon as possible.

Dornier has taken a number of steps to work with each of these groups, but it is very important that they each take their own initiative. This might best be done through meetings that bring each of the different physician specialty groups together for the purpose of reaching some agreement about the standards for care and the physician's qualifications. It does little good to have each of the interested physician groups develop separate and possibly conflicting or at least self-serving standards.

In conclusion, let me just say that over the next 5 years we think that there are going to be many treatment options combining different technologies in this field, and from these will emerge three important challenges, one for each of three major groups involved in biliary ESWL. Industry will need to develop better definitions or better frames of reference so that the consumers and clinicians can facilitate product and performance comparisons. Hospitals need to develop strategies to suit the competitive demands of their local marketplace and also to form the right kinds of partnerships so their place in the delivery of gallstone therapy is ensured. Lastly, physicians have to reach agreement on the kind of qualifications and credentialing programs to ensure that biliary ESWL patients receive the best possible care.

Cost Comparison of Gallstone Therapies

Leonard R. Capuano

Traditionally, management of gallstones consisted of cholecystectomy or a "wait and see" approach in which nothing was done in the hope that symptoms would not become more frequent or severe. Recently, the bile acid ursodiol, to be marketed as Actigall by Ciba Pharmaceuticals, was approved for the treatment of gallstones in patients at high risk for surgery and in patients who refuse surgery. In addition, extracorporeal shockwave lithotripsy coupled with dissolution therapy, although still experimental, may soon constitute yet another option for gallstone management. With the availability of ursodiol therapy and biliary lithotripsy, patients diagnosed as having gallstones can be given a much broader range of alternatives for management of their gallstones.

Physicians will be able to offer surgery, pharmacologic dissolution, and lithotripsy combined with dissolution therapy as therapeutic choices. With more choices, however, comes the question of how to select the best option. Is one option consistently the correct choice for all patients or will the best option vary from patient to patient so that each case must be evaluated individually and a selection made on the basis of the unique characteristics of each patient?

The most obvious factors involved in the choice of a treatment strategy include its safety and its efficacy. If these factors are more or less equal among treatment options, in today's economic climate the cost of the various alternatives will be an important consideration. As long as the end result, gallstone elimination, is the same, then the alternatives can be compared in economic terms.

The decision tree in Figure 1 will be used to examine and compare the three treatment options—surgery, pharmaceutical dissolution (ursodiol), and lithotripsy plus ursodiol—from an economic standpoint.

DECISION TREE ANALYSIS

The probability values on the decision tree are based on the incidence of the various occurrences reported in the literature. The published information on cholecystectomy indicates that mortality occurs in roughly 1 percent of cholecystectomy patients,[1-5] retained stones occur in about 1 percent [6] and postcholecystectomy syndrome occurs chronically in approximately 20 percent.[7] Thus, cholecystectomy is unsuccessful in about 22 percent of patients. It can be assumed that the remaining 78 percent of patients have successful surgery.

The success rate of pharmaceutical dissolution depends largely on the size and type (whether stones are floating or nonfloating) of gallstones. Fromm and Malavolti recently estimated the dissolution rates for gallstones of various sizes and types[8]; these data are shown in Table 1. Using this information and data on the relative frequency of occurrence of the different gallstone types in 598 patients in an ongoing clinical trial

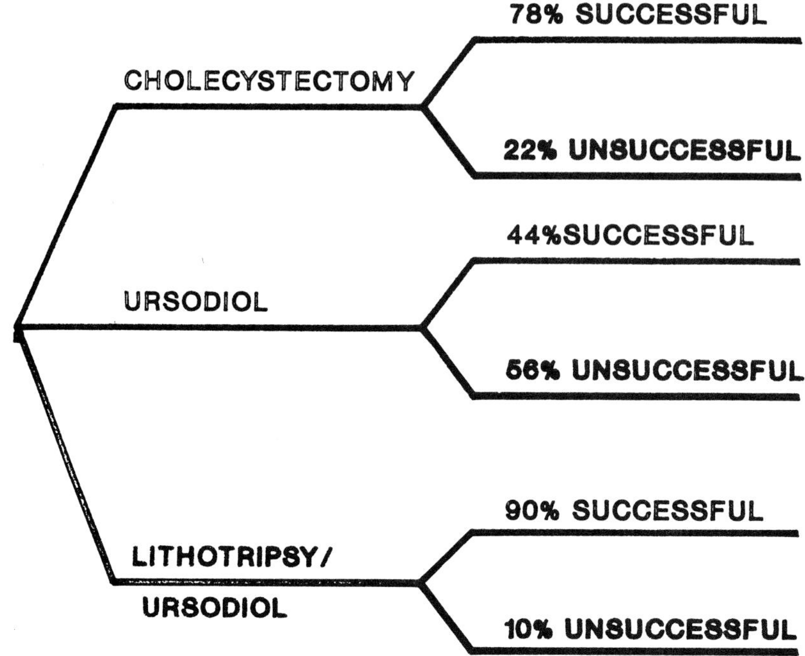

FIG 1.
Decision tree for gallstone therapy.

by Ciba-Geigy, also shown in Table 1, one can calculate the weighted average rate of successful dissolution for all types of gallstones to be 44 percent. The remaining 56 percent of patients in whom dissolution is unsuccessful are assumed to undergo cholecystectomy following their unsuccessful ursodiol treatment.

Lithotripsy plus an ursodiol-chenodiol combination has been shown to result in successful dissolution in 90 percent of patients when the dissolution agents are given for one year.[9] The 10 percent of patients for whom lithotripsy is unsuccessful are assumed to undergo subsequent cholecystectomy.

One can now examine the costs of each alternative. In assigning costs to the various options, we used only the cost of the therapy itself; that is, we did not include diagnostic or follow-up costs, which are assumed to be similar for all of the treatment options. Hospital costs are the average charges per hospital bill for particular DRG categories for 1986.[10] Professionals' fees

TABLE 1.
Outcome of Ursodiol Treatment in Patients with Three Types of Gallstones*

DIAMETER OF STONE	OTHER FEATURES	% OF PATIENTS WITH DISSOLUTION	TIME REQUIRED FOR COMPLETE DISSOLUTION	RELATIVE OCCURRENCE†
<15mm	Floating	90	1 Year	3%
<5mm	Nonfloating	60	1 Year	14%
5–15mm	Nonfloating	40	1.5 Years	83%

*Based on estimates by Fromm H, and Malavolti M: *Adv Int Med* 1988, 33;409.
†Based on relative frequency of occurrence in population of 598 patients in an ongoing clinical trial.

TABLE 2.
One-Year Costs

PROCEDURE	HOSPITAL CHARGE	+	PROFESSIONALS' FEES	+	URSODIOL COST	=	TOTAL COST OF PROCEDURE
Cholecystectomy without CBE:							
DRG #198: <70 yr w/o CC	$ 4,444		$2,100		–		$ 6,544
DRG #197: ≥70 yr and/or CC	$ 7,493		$2,100		–		$ 9,593
Cholecystectomy with CBE:							
DRG #196: <70 yr w/o CC	$ 6,494		$2,800		–		$ 9,294
DRG #195: ≥70 yr and/or CC	$10,529		$2,800		–		$13,329
Lithotripsy for urinary stones:							
DRG #324: <70 yr w/o CC	$ 2,143		$1,800		$1,700		$ 5,643
DRG #323: ≥70 yr and/or CC	$ 2,865		$1,800		$1,700		$ 6,365
Ursodiol Treatment							One-Year Cost
Physician's visits at 1, 3, 6, 9, and 12 mos. @ $45 per visit					$ 225		
Liver enzyme tests at 1, 3, and 9 mos. @ $50 per test					$ 150		
Ultrasound every 6 mos. @ $125 per ultrasonogram					$ 250		
Ursodiol @ $90 per month					$1,075		
Total					$1,700		

CC = Complications or comorbidity; CBE = Common bile duct exploration.

are the combined fees for the surgeon, the assistant surgeon, and the anesthesiologist. Surgeons' fees are the midpoint of the fiftieth percentile of surgeons' fees from a nationwide data base of 1987 surgeons' fees, in which fees from New York City were the highest and fees from Rochester, New York, were the lowest.[11]

The cost of cholecystectomy, shown in Table 2, is the sum of the hospital charge plus the costs of professionals' fees. If we assume, on the basis of what is reported in the literature,[5] that 25 percent of cholecystectomies include common bile duct exploration, we can estimate that the weighted average cost of surgery for patients under 70 and without complications or comorbidity (CC) is $7,232, and that the cost for those 70 or older and/or with a CC is $10,527.

Table 2 also presents the costs of ursodiol therapy. Patients undergoing treatment take two 300 mg capsules of ursodiol per day. During the first year, they should visit their physician 1, 3, 6, 9, and 12 months after treatment is initiated and undergo liver enzyme tests at 1, 3, and 9 months and ultrasound at 6-month intervals. The total costs of ursodiol therapy are $900 after 6 months and $1,700 after one year.

The cost of lithotripsy plus ursodiol consists of the sum of the costs of the hospital charge, professionals' fees, and ursodiol therapy (Table 2). For this analysis, it is assumed that only one lithotripsy procedure is required for successful elimination of stones. As yet, DRG costs have not been assigned for lithotripsy. Because biliary lithotripters are modest modifications of renal lithotripters, and the personnel and the length of hospitalization are presumably similar for the two procedures, DRG hospital costs for renal lithotripsy can be used to approximate the cost of biliary lithotripsy. To these costs must be added the costs of professionals' fees, also based on those for renal lithotripsy, and the cost of 12 months of ursodiol treatment. Although the research on which our probability values for lithotripsy are based was done with an ursodiol-chenodiol combination, there is no such combination available commercially. As a result, the cost of ursodiol alone is applied for these analyses.

CALCULATION OF EXPECTED COSTS OF THE THREE TREATMENT OPTIONS

The expected cost for each treatment option is the probability of the occurrence of each possible outcome times the annual cost of that outcome summed for all possible eventualities.

These calculations are shown in Table 3. In calculating the expected costs of cholecystectomy, we did not include any of the expenses associated with mortality, retained stones, or postcholecystectomy syndrome, primarily because there is insufficient information on the costs of these eventualities. As a result, the expected costs of cholecystectomy are the same as the one-year weighted average costs.

For ursodiol treatment, it is necessary to calculate the expected costs associated with treating each of the three different types of gallstones (Table 3). The probability of success is multiplied by the annual cost of ursodiol treatment and added to the probability of failure times the cost of treatment failure. It is assumed that patients who do not have partial gallstone dissolution after 6 months of treatment are treatment failures and will undergo cholecystectomy. The cost of failure, therefore, is assumed to be the cost of 6 months of ursodiol treatment plus the cost of cholecystectomy. In reality, at least some of the patients whose treatment fails will not undergo cholecystectomy because they are poor risks for surgery or they refuse surgery. Nevertheless, to simplify the analyses, it is assumed that all treatment failures will undergo cholecystectomy, a worst-case scenario. When the weighted-average expected cost for all gallstone types is calculated using the relative frequency of occurrence of the different stone types, the cost for patients under 70 and without a CC is $7,118 and the cost for patients 70 or over and/or with a CC is $5,282.

The expected cost of lithotripsy plus ursodiol is calculated by multiplying the one-year cost of lithotripsy treatment by the 90 percent success rate of lithotripsy and then adding the cost of failed lithotripsy (Table 3). The cost of failed lithotripsy is calculated by adding the hospital costs and professionals' fees for lithotripsy, the cost of 6 months of ursodiol therapy, and the cost of cholecystectomy, and then multiplying this sum by the 10 percent rate of failure.

COMPARISON OF EXPECTED COSTS

Figures 2 and 3 compare the expected costs of the various treatment options in each of the two patient populations. The relative costs of the different options are generally similar for the two populations. Surgery is clearly most expensive. Figures 4 and 5 show the differences in cost between surgery and the other treatment options, or the cost savings that result when other options are chosen instead of surgery. In patients younger than 70 without a CC, the cost of ursodiol treatment is less than that of surgery for all

TABLE 3.
Expected Costs

PROCEDURE	PROBABILITY OF SUCCESS × ANNUAL COST	+	PROBABILITY OF FAILURE × ANNUAL COST	=	TOTAL EXPECTED COST
Cholecystectomy					
<70 yr w/o CC	0.78 ($ 7,232)	+	0.22($ 7,232)	=	$ 7,232
≥70 yr and/or CC	0.78 ($10,527)	+	0.22 ($10,527)	=	$10,527
Ursodiol					
Floating stones <15 mm					
<70 yr w/o CC	0.9 ($ 1,700)	+	0.1 ($900+$ 7,232)	=	$ 2,343
≥70 yr and/or CC	0.9 ($ 1,700)	+	0.1 ($900+$10,527)	=	$ 2,673
Nonfloating stones <5 mm					
<70 yr w/o CC	0.6 ($ 1,700)	+	0.4 ($900+$ 7,232)	=	$ 4,273
≥70 yr and/or CC	0.6 ($ 1,700)	+	0.4 ($900+$10,527)	=	$ 5,591
Nonfloating stones 5–15 mm					
<70 yr w/o CC	0.4 ($ 1,700)	+	0.6 ($900+$ 7,232)	=	$ 5,559
≥70 yr and/or CC	0.4 ($ 1,700)	+	0.6 ($900+$10,527)	=	$ 7,536
Lithotripsy Plus Ursodiol					
<70 yr w/o CC	0.9 ($ 5,643)	+	0.1 ($2,143+$1,800+$900+$ 7,232)	=	$ 6,286
≥70 yr and/or CC	0.9 ($ 6,365)	+	0.1 ($2,865+$1,800+$900+$10,527)	=	$ 7,338

CC = Complications or comorbidity.

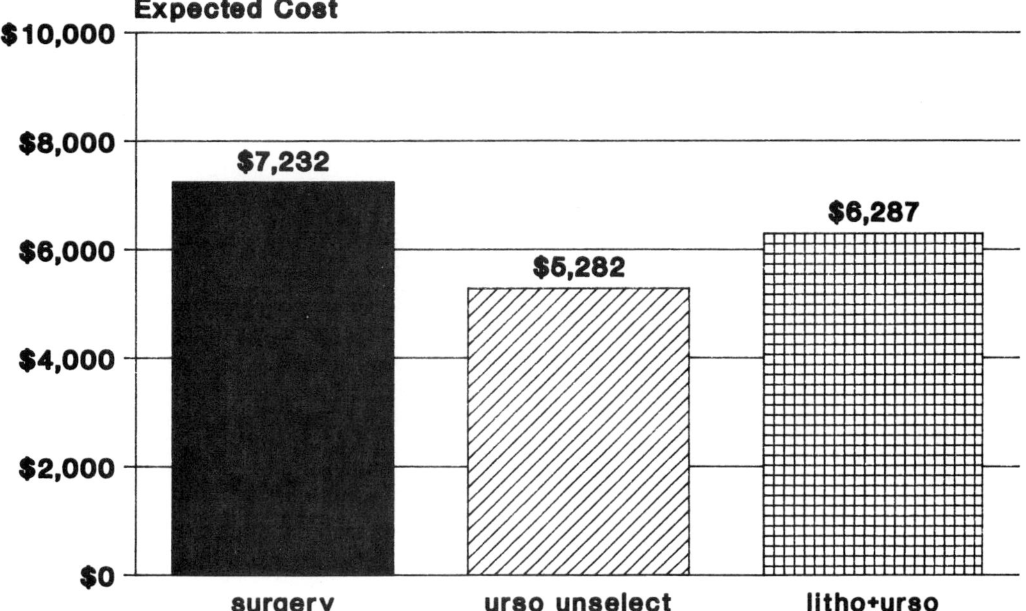

FIG 2.
Comparison of expected costs of treatment options: Patients <70 without CC; F = floating stone; NF = non-floating stone; CC = complications and comorbidities.

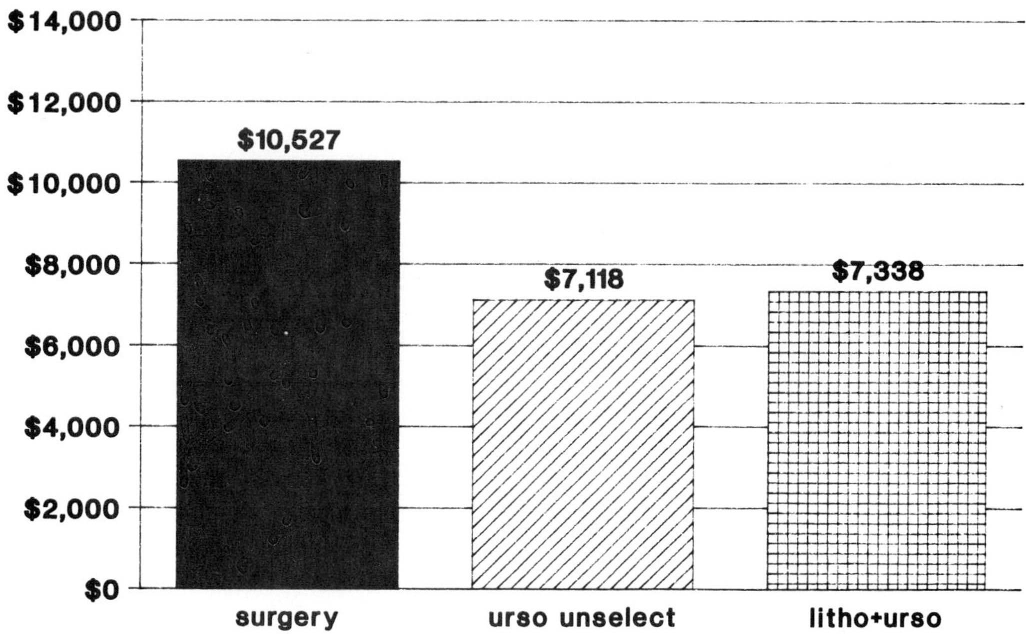

FIG 3.
Expected cost comparison of ursodiol vs. surgery vs. lithotripsy: Patients <70 without cc; cc = complications and comorbidities.

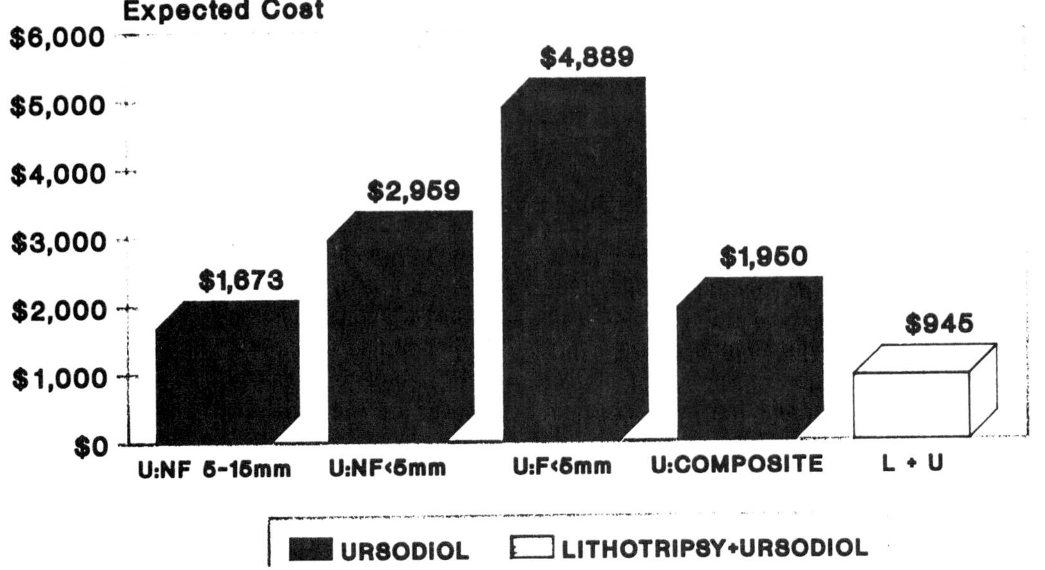

FIG 4.
Differences in expected costs of surgery and other treatment options: patients < 70 without cc; CC = Complications and Comorbidities; F = Floating Stones; NF = Nonfloating Stones.

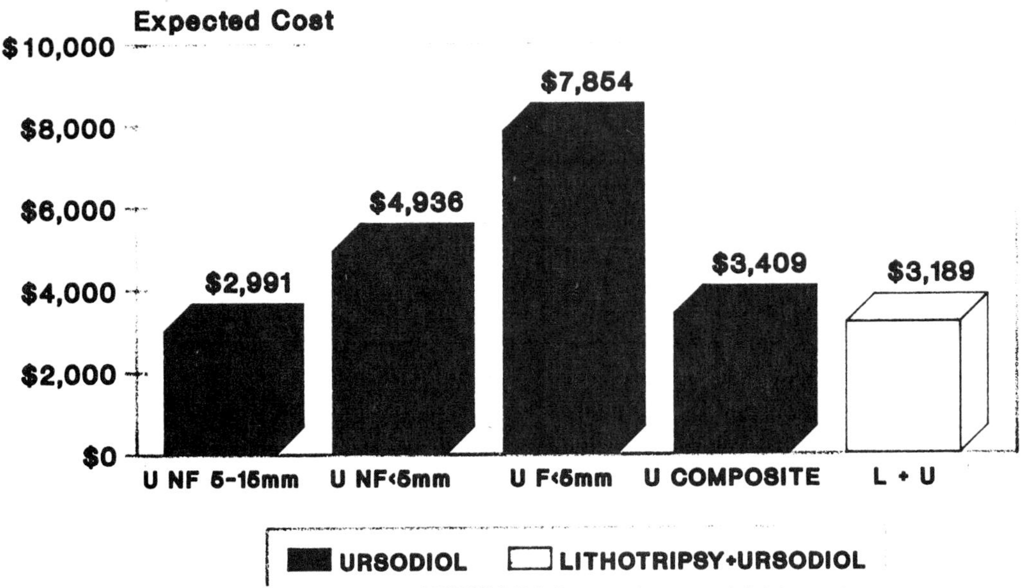

FIG 5.
Differences in expected costs of surgery and other treatment options: patient >= 70 and/or with cc; CC = Complications and Comorbidities; F = Floating Stones; NF = Nonfloating Stones.

stone types, including the weighted average cost, by at least $1,673 (23 percent of the cost of surgery) and by as much as $4,889 (68 percent). In patients 70 or older or with a CC, savings are at least $2,991 (28 percent) and as much as $7,854 (75 percent). Lithotripsy plus ursodiol treatment also costs less than surgery, costing $946 (13 percent) less than surgery in patients younger than 70 without a CC and $3,189 (30 percent) less than surgery for patients 70 or older or with a CC.

Comparison of lithotripsy plus ursodiol treatment with ursodiol treatment alone reveals that in patients under 70 without a CC, ursodiol treatment alone is less expensive in all cases by at least $727 (12 percent of the cost of lithotripsy plus ursodiol) and by as much as $3,943 (63 percent). For the other population, lithotripsy plus ursodiol is less expensive than ursodiol alone for patients with nonfloating stones from 5 to 15 mm in diameter by $198 (3 percent of the cost of lithotripsy plus ursodiol) but more expensive for patients with nonfloating stones less than 5 mm in diameter by $1,747 (24 percent) and for patients with floating stones less than 15 mm by $4,665 (64 percent).

LIMITATIONS OF THE ANALYSIS

The decision tree analysis used here provides a simple and straightforward means of determining and comparing the outcomes and costs of the three treatment options we wished to analyze. As such, this means of analysis contains some oversimplifications that must be addressed.

The most serious criticism of this analysis is that it considers only the costs incurred during the first year of treatment and does not take into account costs that could occur in subsequent years, such as the expenses associated with stone recurrence and the need for retreatment. These costs would apply to treatment with ursodiol alone and to lithotripsy plus ursodiol. According to information in the published literature, gallstones recur following dissolution in about 50 percent of patients within 5 years,[8,12,13] or about 13 percent per year. Although this is a considerable proportion of patients, we should note that the rate of successful redissolution among these patients is substantially higher than the initial dissolution rate.[12] It is not possible to comment on the frequency or significance of retreatment after lithotripsy treatment because as yet no data exist on the incidence of stone recurrence following this therapeutic option.

As mentioned before, the estimations of the cost of cholecystectomy do not take into account the costs of surgical failures. The costs assigned to cholecystectomy, therefore, may be somewhat conservative. Thus, cost estimates were probably underestimated for ursodiol treatment, for lithotripsy, and for cholecystectomy, or for all treatment options considered here.

The costs used for biliary lithotripsy were approximations based on the cost of renal lithotripsy and may therefore not be correct. Certainly the anatomy and physiology of the kidney differ significantly from those of the gallbladder. Until lithotripters become regular hospital equipment and a standard therapeutic regimen is established for biliary lithotripsy and adjuvant ursodiol treatment, however, estimation of the costs of this treatment strategy will remain difficult to verify.

In this analysis, we have stratified the patient population according to the DRG classifications. This stratification is arbitrary and may be misleading, but reimbursement systems follow this classification system and our cost analysis must follow it as well.

Our decision tree does not take into account any quality of life considerations. This analysis was based solely on economic considerations of treatment options that have been shown to be effective. Considerations such as quality of life, patient preference, and medical considerations certainly cannot be ignored.

Finally, costs vary widely throughout the United States. Thus, the results of this cost analysis may change in magnitude and direction when costs from different geographic locations are used in the calculations. The arithmetic calculations presented here, therefore, imply a degree of accuracy that is not warranted.

CONCLUSION

Surgery is clearly the most expensive treatment option. Treatment with ursodiol, in most cases, is the least expensive of the three treatment strategies evaluated here. Lithotripsy plus ursodiol therapy may be less costly than ursodiol treatment alone for some patients 70 or older or with a CC, but apparently not for the patients under 70 without a CC. Thus, the age and health of each individual patient should be evaluated and a treatment alternative selected on the basis of each particular case. Additional data will be needed before we can draw further conclusions concerning the relative cost-effectiveness of these treatment options.

REFERENCES

1. Weckesser EC: Surgery for gallbladder disease in Ohio: A survey of 3,085 operations. *Am J Surg* 1964; 103:695.
2. Boquist L, Bergdahl L, Andersson A: Mortality following gallbladder surgery: A study of 3,257 cholecystectomies. *Surgery* 1972; 71(4):616.
3. McSherry CK, Glenn F: The incidence and causes of death following surgery for nonmalignant biliary tract disease. *Ann Surg* 1980; 191(3):271.
4. Seltzer MH, Steiger E, Rosato FE: Mortality following cholecystectomy. *Surg Gynecol Obstet* 1970; 130:64.
5. Meyer KA, Capos NJ, Mittelpunkt AI: Personal experiences with 1,261 cases of acute and chronic cholecystitis and cholelithiasis. *Surgery* 1967; 61(5):661.
6. Dempsey DT, Rosato EF: Surgical management of cholelithiasis, in Cohen S, Soloway RD (eds): *Gallstones*. New York, Churchill Livingstone, 1985, p 191.
7. Rusticali AG, Labate AMM, Sama C, et al: Specific and non-specific symptoms before and after cholecystectomy. Proceedings of the International Meeting of Pathochemistry, Pathophysiology, and Pathomechanics of the Biliary System, Policlinico S. Orsola-Nuove Patologie. Bologna, Italy. March 14–16, 1988, p 147.
8. Fromm H, Malavolti M: Dissolving gallstones. *Adv Intern Med* 1988; 33:409.
9. Sackmann M, Delius M, Sauerbruch T, et al: Shock-wave lithotripsy of gallbladder stones. *New Engl J Med* 1988; 318(7):393.
10. Medicare data: All inpatient hospital bills—fiscal year 1986. Health Care Financing Administration, Bureau of Data Management and Strategy, U.S. Department of Health and Human Services, Baltimore, MD, 1987.
11. HIAA data base, Health Insurance Association of America, Washington DC, 1987.
12. Ruppin DC, Dowling RH: Is recurrence inevitable after gallstone dissolution by bile-acid treatment? *Lancet* 1982; 1:181.
13. Lirussi F, Iemmolo Rm, Orlando R, et al: Gallstone recurrence and redissolution: An eight-year follow-up study. Proceedings of the International Meeting on Pathochemistry, Pathophysiology, and Pathomechanics of the Biliary System, Policlinico S. Orsola-Nuove Patologie. Bologna, Italy. March 14–16, 1988 p 55.

A Trade Association's View on the Future of Lithotripsy

Robert G. Britain

I would like to tell you how a trade association could help the advancement of lithotripsy.

The National Electrical Manufacturers Association is a trade association based in Washington, D.C., that represents more than 600 manufacturers of electrical products. One division of the association, called the Diagnostic Imaging and Therapy Systems Division, specifically is focused on medical devices used in diagnostic imaging and therapy.

This division has six sections that individually address x-ray, ultrasound, nuclear therapy, magnetic resonance, and picture archiving and communications systems.

A few years ago, lithotripters were incorporated into NEMA's product scope. A lithotripsy section was not established at that time, however, because there was only one lithotripter manufacturer on the market.

Times have now changed. There are about 10 manufacturers actively carrying out investigations under FDA purview for renal and/or biliary, and two manufacturers have FDA approval for renal lithotripters.

My board of directors has asked me to investigate the possibility of organizing a lithotripsy section because of this increased activity.

Throughout this meeting I have had conversations with most of the lithotripter manufacturers, and I believe there is enough interest to continue to pursue the organization of a new section.

What is it that NEMA can do for the industry? We can facilitate discussions within the industrial community with some freedom of antitrust worries. We can also facilitate communication between industry and the medical profession. Further, we can facilitate discussion with industry and the Food and Drug Administration. At the present time, all of these types of discussions seem to be on a one-on-one basis.

Let me give you some examples of this interaction and communication. For quite a number of years now, we have had a standing committee comprised of members of NEMA companies and the American Institute of Ultrasound in Medicine. The focus of this committee has been the safety and safe use of diagnostic ultrasound equipment. Two outputs of this committee have been a safety consideration document and test methodology guidance. FDA personnel attend almost all of the meetings.

Our ties are also strong with the American College of Radiology. NEMA and ACR have a number of combined working groups addressing many aspects of picture archiving and communications systems at a time when this technology is still developing. NEMA routinely interacts with committees of the American College of Radiology, for example, its Oncology Committee.

NEMA spearheaded a move to reclassify magnetic resonance imaging devices from FDA's premarket approval class III to a lower regulatory class II. This reclassification was found acceptable by FDA's advisory panel and FDA's final action is now imminent. The industry may wish to consider reclassification a few years hence for lithotripters, perhaps in 3 or 4 years when we find the FDA review pipeline completely plugged up with PMA supplements.

Now you have heard examples of what we have done in some nonlithotripter areas. For the near future for lithotripters, NEMA will plan to continue discussions with manufacturers to compile a list of concerns related to FDA's premarket approval reequirements. We will also meet with FDA staff to better understand FDA's concerns with lithotripters. When this is accomplished, we would hope to provide a forum whereby both FDA and the industry can exchange their points of view.

After 3 days of listening and talking to attendees at this conference, I fear that this list of concerns might be 3 miles long.

As a trade association, we have worked with the Food and Drug Administration for more than 15 years and know too well about FDA's preoccupation about the safety of diagnostic ultrasound. In the opinion of many people in industry, diagnostic ultrasound is regulated to a greater degree than other devices we consider to have greater risk. Why? FDA points to insufficient long-term studies for bioeffects.

The point here is that we would not want a similar situation to manifest itself for lithotripters. For this reason, the industry may want to discuss the appropriateness of sponsoring or in some other way initiating long-term biologic effect studies.

Biliary lithotripsy will probably prove to be as important an advance as renal lithotripsy was in the early 1980s. However, I would like to leave you with this caveat: the FDA process itself is like a sporting event. In the area of renal lithotripsy, it was probably like running a mile-long event. Due to the complexities associated with biliary lithotripsy, it will be more like a marathon. Don't get discouraged, though. During the course of the clinical trials, the medical community will gain valuable information on the use of lithotripsy and the potential patient populations who could benefit from biliary lithotripsy will become better defined. I think I can safely say that the best of lithotripsy is yet to come.

In September my board of directors will meet to decide whether or not NEMA should establish the Lithotripsy Section. I don't think there is any question but that they will.

A trade association must be able to show accomplishments and I would hope to be able to report on our work at your next meeting in Vancouver.

I save the most important item until last. All of the previous examples of NEMA's activities I presented in some way involved the medical profession. It is vitally important that we have access to *your* knowledge base. I want to assure you that in some way you will have input into important decisions in the lithotripsy area that are initiated by NEMA.

FDA Approval of Extracorporeal Shock Wave Lithotripsy for Biliary Indications

Halyna P. Breslawec Ph.D.

The Food and Drug Asministration (FDA) is responsible for the review and approval of medical devices, including extracorporeal shockwave lithotripters, for investigation and for marketing. The regulatory device evaluation process is by necessity a reactive one. FDA's approval decision for a device must follow the completion of a significant amount of research. This research provides the basis for the evaluation of the safe and effective use of a device in a clinical setting much like the one in which it will be used when it is marketed.

The history of the approval process dates back to 1938, when the Federal Food, Drug, and Cosmetic Act of 1938, the 50th anniversary of which we are commemorating this year, authorized the Food and Drug Administration to regulate medical devices in order to assure their safety. The passage of the 1976 Medical Device Amendments to the Act further provided FDA with the mandate and authority to ensure that medical devices are safe and effective and to regulate devices during most phases of their development, testing, production, distribution, and use.

FDA review and approval mechanisms focus on specific devices, not generic categories of devices. Approval, therefore, is granted by FDA for a particular device, a particular manufacturer, and a particular indication. The Amendments provide a mechanism for the regulatory review and approval of medical devices dependent on the degree of regulatory control necessary to achieve safety and effectiveness. Those devices presenting higher risks are subject to greater regulatory control. Three categories of devices were established. Class I devices are subject to general controls, including registration, premarket notification, and adherence to good manufacturing practices. In addition to the general controls, Class II and Class III devices are also subject to incremental requirements. Class II devices are those whose safety and effectiveness cannot be reasonably assured through general controls alone, but for which enough information is known to allow for development of performance standards that would provide such assurance. Class III is the most stringent category and is reserved for devices that are life-supporting or life-sustaining, or of substantial importance in preventing impairment of human health. All new devices (those unlike any device marketed before 1976) are also considered Class III devices. FDA must grant premarket approval before Class III devices can be marketed. Extracorporeal shockwave lithotripters for all indications, including renal or biliary uses, are considered Class III devices. The approval mechanism provides that each device is approved for a specific indication.

Two mechanisms for reaching the marketplace are available under the regulations. The nature of the device determines whether premarket notification or premarket approval procedures apply. The first, the premarket notification process, considered by many a grandfathering provision, is called the 510(k) process after the section of the Medical Device Amendments (510(k)) outlining this provision. Under this mechanism, devices are evaluated to determine if they are substantially equivalent to devices that were in commercial distribution prior to the enactment of the medical device amendments. Examples of these devices currently include mechanical or ultrasonic lithotripters, endoscopes, and catheters. Most devices in distribution today enter on the market through this mechanism.

The second mechanism for reaching the marketplace is the PMA, or premarket approval application process. The PMA process is reserved for new devices that require an evaluation of their safety and effectiveness and are therefore subject to the highest degree of regulatory control. Extracorporeal shockwave lithotripters are currently being evaluated through this mechanism. The applications for such devices (PMAs) are evaluated to assess if a reasonable assurance of safety and effectiveness for the use of a device for a specific indication exists. The PMA review process is far more stringent than the 510(k) process and occurs during the statutorily mandated 180-day review period. After the PMA is submitted to FDA, a filing review is performed to determine if a PMA is administratively complete. The review process takes 45 days. If so, a PMA is filed, meaning that a comprehensive, thorough review process will begin.

During its substantive review, FDA reviews, among other things, who the device is intended for, the conditions under which it is to be used, the risks and benefits of using the device in a given indication, and the reliability of the device. To assess the safety and effectiveness of a device, FDA relies on valid scientific evidence. This is defined by the regulations as evidenced from well-controlled studies, partially controlled studies, and depending on the type of device, some studies and objective trails without matched controls, well-documented case histories conducted by qualified experts, and reports of significant human experience with a marketed device. This last category is important because lithotripters for renal and biliary indications may currently be used more widely overseas than in the United States. These data then provide a basis from which FDA, in conjunction with qualified experts, can conclude that there is reasonable assurance of the safety and effectiveness of a device under its conditions of use.

The agency does not rely exclusively on internal reviews of PMAs. In fact, FDA relies on a panel of outside clinical experts to provide an additional technical and clinical review and an approval or disapproval recommendation for a PMA. PMAs for extracorporeal shockwave lithotripters for biliary lithotripsy will be reviewed by a panel that evaluates the data presented, discusses the data in open session, and makes a recommendation, continues its internal deliberations, summarizes information pertaining to the safety and effectiveness of the particular device, and concludes, based on all of the above, whether to approve the device.

The standards that are used by FDA regarding the approval of a device are actually reverse standards. We can deny approval for any of several reasons. One is a lack of reasonable assurance of the safety or effectiveness of a device. Another is deficiency of the manufacturer in the processing, packing, or installation. A third is false or misleading labeling of the device. There are other grounds for disapproval, but these are the most pertinent.

Investigations involving medical devices are also regulated by FDA under the investigational device exemption or IDE provisions. An IDE enables a firm to involve investigators in clinical trials of a particular medical device.

Lithotripter manufacturers have done well in this process so far. Two have received premarket approvals—PMAs—for machines indicated for renal and urinary stone applications. Another PMA is partially through the process; the firm has applied to FDA, the application has been filed, the panel has recommended approval, and the final review is underway. Other firms have also made submissions to FDA.

In the investigational arena, ten applications (IDEs) to conduct gallstone investigations in the United States have been submitted to FDA. Eight, involving six firms, have been approved. These applications differ in a number of respects, including the application, for example, common duct stones versus gallbladder stones. A number of the investigations involve pretreatment with litholytic drugs or concomitant drug use.

One of the issues that needs regulatory attention and that we are working to resolve is how to evaluate regimens that use drugs in conjunction with lithotripsy. We are working very closely with our FDA colleagues in the Center for Drug Evaluation and Research to develop a method that will ensure a fair and expeditious resolution of any scientific or regulatory concerns that might arise in this area.

We have further acted to facilitate the approval process by allowing each manufacturer of each device a very reasonable number of sites in the United States for studying biliary indications. We think that this provides an adequate opportunity for the collection of good clinical data. To paraphrase a comment made earlier at this symposium, this approach will permit widespread evaluation before widespread application.

FDA's evaluation of biliary lithotripters is by necessity a slow process. Although much can be learned by comparing this review and approval process to that involving renal lithotripsy, some distinctions should be made. The first lithotripter for kidney indications received relatively rapid PMA approval primarily because a good application was submitted and because it offered a superior treatment modality in an area where the alternatives were much riskier.

There are different risks, different issues, and different alternatives in biliary lithotripsy. We therefore are taking a very deliberate approach in our review of approval applications. Although we are *not* waiting for a consensus to develop on how this particular treatment modality fits into the therapeutic armamentarium against gallstone disease, we are waiting for the submission of complete safety and effectiveness data on each of the separate devices that is being investigated.

The Hospital's Perspective

Henry C. Alder

It is now quite evident that cholelithotripsy will have a significant impact on the treatment of gallstones. In considering the impact of this new form of therapy on hospital operations, these are three areas where important effects may occur. These are:

1. Impact of cholelithotripsy on present inpatient gallstone procedures, namely cholecystectomy
2. New patterns in the clinical management of the gallstone patient
3. Cholelithotripsy coverage and reimbursement

IMPACT OF CHOLELITHOTRIPSY ON CHOLECYSTECTOMY

From 1981 to 1986 an average of 487,000 cholecystectomies were performed each year in acute care hospitals in the United States. The volume of procedures varied from year to year in an unpredictable fashion. However, the prevalence of cholecystectomy has remained constant during these years at 2 procedures per 1,000 population.

The American College of Surgeons has identified cholecystectomy as one of the top ten surgical procedures in the United States, but its ranking has remained either 9 or 10 since 1975. Although cholecystectomy is a relatively prevalent procedure, it actually only accounts for 2 percent of *all* hospital surgical procedures. In view of the present expectations for the role of lithotripsy, it is evident that there will be a *shift* of hospital finances and resources from surgery to other clinical departments.

In a 1983 survey of gallbladder surgery in the United States conducted by the Metropolitan Life Insurance Company, the average hospital charge for cholecystectomy was $4,070. Assuming this equates to approximately $5,500 per procedure in 1988 dollars, the financial impact of 487,000 cholecystectomies on acute care hospital revenue is approximately $2.8 billion per year. If 25 percent of cholecystectomies are replaced by cholelithotripsy, $700 million in surgery revenue would be redistributed to shockwave lithotripsy or partially eliminated because of lower lithotripsy charges. For example, one cholelithotripsy IDE site charges $4,300 for the procedure, of which $2,650 are hospital charges. Although these charges may not reflect actual hospital charges after clinical trials have concluded, they do suggest hospitals may experience up to a $2,800 reduction in revenue for every cholecystectomy that is replaced by cholelithotripsy.

CLINICAL MANAGEMENT OF THE GALLSTONE PATIENT

One of the most perplexing issues regarding cholelithotripsy is the coordination and management of the gallstone patient. Although this is strictly a physician-driven issue, hospital management will invariably become involved in allocating the resources to initiate the new service.

Before cholelithotripsy was introduced earlier this year, the treatment of gallstones in the United States involved a number of different specialties. Patients suspected to be affected with gallstones are referred by an internist or general practitioner to a radiologist to perform and interpret a cholecystogram or an ultrasound scan, and, if diagnosed, to a general surgeon for cholecystectomy. General surgeons, internists, and GPs may refer complicated cases to a gastroenterologist for follow-up.

Similarly, cholelithotripsy appears to be a multispecialty procedure, not unlike percutaneous transluminal angioplasty. A team approach to patient management is necessary to capitalize on the strengths in managing the patient's response to treatment.

The current clinical investigation of gallstone lithotripsy offers a glimpse into the posssible multifaceted approaches to patient management. In Europe, cholelithotripsy studies are directed by gastroenterologists who have experience with ultrasound imaging techniques. In the United States, trials are often conducted by two or more specialists, including radiologists, gastroenterologists, and general surgeons. For example, in an effort to create consensus early on in their cholelithotripsy service, Baylor University Medical Center (which is the first Medstone site) took the initiative to involve the chiefs of medicine, radiology, and surgery in the planning, deliberation, site visits, and presentations associated with the acquisition and operation of the gallstone lithotripter. The results to date have been satisfying. An ongoing effort is required on the part of hospital management to encourage the positive spirit of cooperation among the multispecialty groups.

At another investigation site, the radiologist and gastroenterologist jointly manage patients to the extent that they see all patients together and treat them together. At a third site, the gallstone lithotripter is managed by the chief of surgery with consultation from radiology. At this time it is difficult, if not inappropriate, to arbitrate who should or should not manage gallstone patients when cholelithotripsy is available. A prescribed protocol for patient management is best left to each facility based on the interests, skills, and experience of the medical staff. Obviously, the major issue must be centered around the provision of high-quality care to the patient.

COVERAGE AND REIMBURSEMENT

Coverage and reimbursement are major concerns for hospitals as they are for physicians in the present era of shrinking payments. One of the issues associated with the evaluation of a new clinical service is to determine to what extent the hospital's expenses can be recovered by payment from third-party payers. As many of you realize, during FDA-sponsored trials of drugs and devices, coverage policy typically is not established by most payers. As a result, payment must be handled on a case-by-case basis.

During cholelithotripsy clinical trials, several IDE sites have required patients to assume full responsibility for payment. The patients must negotiate with their own health insurance company to receive reimbursement for their out-of-pocket expenses. Another IDE site has assumed the role of patient advocate and will directly negotiate with the insurance company to provide patient coverage. One of the clinical investigation sites has obtained a positive response from the third-party payers in their region; they have obtained payment from two-thirds of their major payers to cover 90 percent of the FDA, major payers such as Medicare and Blue Cross/Blue Shield are expected to establish a coverage and reimbursement policy.

One salient aspect of cholelithotripsy that is expected to generate debate among payers is whether lithotripsy plus bile acid therapy is as effective as cholecystectomy. According to the National Gallstone Study, 25 percent of patients whose gallstones were dissolved by cheno formed stones again within five years. If similar results occur following cholelithotripsy, a significant number of patients will require further treatment. Although a lithotripsy procedure every five years may be innocuous to the patient, financially it compares unfavorably to cholecystectomy, which results in the total elimination of the gallstones. Payers may argue that cholelithotripsy increases costs. It is too soon to determine in what direction this issue may develop.

In conclusion, cholelithotripsy will not only impact medical practice but also alter the hospital's role. As partners in progress, medical staff and hospitals should look forward to working together constructively to bring about high-quality patient care for all.

The Future of Biliary Lithotripsy

Philip Drew

Biliary lithotripsy looks like a winner among medical technologies, and I believe it has an assured future. Making such a statement implies that the technology performs effectively and reliably and that clinical, operational, regulatory, and economic considerations all support its use.

With regard to the technology, it is obvious from this meeting that biliary lithotripters work very well, although patients have to be carefully selected. From the clinical point of view, the technology is important because gallstone disease is a very common ailment, creating widespread need for therapy. Lithotripsy is less invasive than any alternative except oral chemotherapy, and it's much faster and more definitive than chemotherapy. Finally, lithotripsy is less dangerous than some of the alternatives, particularly surgery, and one really has to take seriously the evidence that 10 percent of patients older than 65 die in the course of cholecystectomy.

From an operational point of view, biliary lithotripsy is certainly feasible. It does not require long and arduous training and is well within the scope of many clinicians and surgeons. From a regulatory point of view, it seems to me that there will be ample evidence to convince the FDA of its safety and its efficacy.

Finally, economic motivations will get clearer as the technique develops. It has been shown in some of the talks at this symposium that lithotripsy is less expensive than surgery, and it may even be cost-competitive with chemotherapy.

It is not apparent to me that any of the approaches taken by the different companies is definitely superior. Some data indicate that shockwaves generated by spark-gap lithotripters are more reliably effective than those by the piezo-electric devices, but as an engineer I am not prepared to stop there and say that it is proven. These devices are still under development, and there is much room for technical improvement. The very fact that so many companies have entered the field and taken so many different approaches are indications of the richness of the technical lode being mined.

That richness extends beyond lithotripsy to the other techniques. In fact, it seems very clear that lithotripsy is only one of several promising new approaches for treating gallstones. Many of the modes of treatment discussed here are going to turn out to be part of an armamentarium against gallstones. Lithotripsy is clearly in the picture; lysis clearly for some patients; endoscopy for others; and then there are alternatives including mechanical destruction, direct injection of solvents, and laser ablation.

One final consideration is the turf battle that seems to be shaping up among various specialists. We've heard pleas from radiologists who believe lithotripsy should belong to them because, after all, imaging is the key to this technique, and the real skill comes in recognizing the presence of stones, their location, and the degree of fragmentation. The gastroenterologists say the real skill lies in selecting patients, combining lithotripsy with chemotherapy, and taking full responsibility for management with chemotherapy; the imaging is merely incidental. The surgeons say that they undertook the definitive treatment in the past and should continue to do it.

Those are all convincing arguments from one point of view or another. In fact, one surmises that any one of these specialists could become adequately competent at the other aspects of the treatment and perform this technique without help. This is one of the chief reasons why I believe the proposed team approach is not going to emerge.

The right to perform biliary lithotripsy will not be awarded to any one profession, because there is no one to do the awarding. Instead, different specialists will grab this ball and run with it. The people who have come to this meeting are those who probably have that ambition. Those who learn how to perform this technique, learn the ins and outs and pros and cons, and learn to do it effectively will be the experts in the field to whom their colleagues will refer patients.

APPENDIX

EDITORS' NOTE

THE FOLLOWING SELECTED TECHNICAL SUMMARIES OF COMMERCIALLY AVAILABLE LITHOTRIPTER SYSTEMS ARE SUBMITTED BY COMPANY REPRESENTATIVES

DORNIER: MPL 9000 MULTIPURPOSE LITHOTRIPTER

B. Forssman
S. Schneider
B. Smith

HISTORICAL CONSIDERATIONS

The basic principles of ESWL®* evolved from Dornier's investigations into the causes of surface pitting often seen on the outer shell of its developmental spacecraft and supersonic airplanes. Studies revealed that when these craft collided wtih micrometeorites or raindrops at high speeds, shock waves were produced. These shock waves were found to create stresses inside material structures of the aircraft.

Further investigations demonstrated that a destructive effect occurred when these shock waves traveled through materials of varying acoustical properties, such as a fluid versus a brittle solid. If the resulting tensile or pressure forces were higher than the solid's strength, a mechanical breakdown of the brittle material would take place.

Basic research into the shock wave phenomenon revealed a principle of physics that has since become of decisive importance to medicine: shock waves can pass through organic tissues without harming them.

Next, Dornier researchers turned to methods of focusing light to solve the problem of aiming and concentrating the shock wave to a force that would be useful in a medical setting. This gave rise to the use of the semi-ellipsoid dish to focus shock waves to a fixed point.

Dornier's inquiries into the usefulness of shock waves for the destruction of kidney stones began in the late 1960s. The first in vitro experiments began in 1972. In 1974, a project initiated by Dornier engineers and physicians from the University of Munich to continue to test the concept in the laboratory was funded by the German government. Lithotripsy experiments with laboratory animals began in 1975. The world's first kidney stone lithotripsy treatment was conducted 5 years later on the Dornier Kidney Lithotripter prototype, the HM1.

By May 1982, 220 patient treatments had been conducted on the HM1; and the company's second prototype, the HM2, was installed at Grosshadern.

In October 1983, the HM3, which would eventually be the first commercially available lithotripter in the world, was made operational in the Katharinen Hospital in Stuttgart.

The HM3, in December 1984, was the first lithotripter to be granted FDA approval. Since water and living soft tissues have similar acoustical properties, shock waves are generated and transmitted through a water medium. The first lithotripters used a water tub, in which the patient was partially submerged.

In May 1987, the FDA granted marketing approval to the Dornier HM4, the first lithotripter to do away with the water bath and instead conduct the shock wave through a water cushion held against the patient's body. The HM4 also incorporated innovations in computerized partient positioning.

COMPARISON OF DIFFERENT SHOCK WAVE TECHNOLOGIES

The first consideration in evaluating a lithotripter should be the method of shock wave generation. This is the single most important component of a lithotripter directly affecting stone disintegration. Currently, there are three types of extracorporeal shock wave sources in practical use.

SHOCK WAVE SOURCES

Spark Gap

A comprehensive shock wave is formed by the electrical discharge of a capacitor between two electrode tips that are submerged in water. The expansion of gases at supersonic speed creates the shock wave. From the onset, this shock wave has a very steep wave front which corresponds to a fast rise time. The wave front is not influenced by either intensity or amplitude and does not change shape as it propagates along its path.

*ESWL® is a Dornier registered trademark.

TABLE 1.

Technical Parameters of the Three Different Shock Wave Sources

System	Aperture	Rise Time, t_R (ns)	Pulse Width, t_W (ns)	Pressure range, Bar	Focus: Axial, mm	Focus: Lateral mm
MPL 9000*	40°	<10	200	750–1300	20	3
Electromagnetic	26°	50–400	360	200–600	95	10
Piezoelectric	44°	200–500	330	500–1000	17	<3

The amplitude of the shock wave can be adjusted by varying the voltage across the capacitor. Focusing is accomplished with minimal transmission loss via a reflecting ellipsoid. Proper geometrical ellipsoid dimensions lead to an optimal focus, allowing for efficient stone disintegration while avoiding harmful side effects (including those caused by anesthesia).

Electromagnetic

This pressure wave is formed when an electrical impulse is applied through a slab coil placed in close proximity to an isolated metal membrane. The electromagnetic field induced by the coil causes the membrane to repel. The membrane moves at subsonic speeds owing to the inertia of the membrane in water, and as a result of the coil's effect on slowing the rise and fall times of the electrical pulse. This produces an initial pressure wave with a gradual inclining wave front and of long duration. Only later, after traveling a finite distance, does the wave front steepen. The steepening is dependent on both the intensity of the pressure wave and the propagation distance.

The amplitude of the pressure wave can be adjusted by varying either the current or the voltage. A lens is used for focusing and causes a measurable transmission loss. The system's aperture size is limited because the metal membrane diameter must be kept small for technical reasons. Therefore, the therapeutic focus is much larger than other methods of shock wave generation.

Piezoelectric

By applying a voltage impulse, a piezoelectric cystal will expand, creating a pressure wave in the surrounding water. Because this method is inefficient, either a single large crystal or many small crystals are required. This still produces a low-energy pressure wave with a slow rise time or gradual, inclining wave front.

To focus the pressure wave, the crystals are positioned in a concave, spherical arrangement. The diameter (and therefore, the aperture) of this system is large, producing a sharp focal point. The energy density in the focal point is high, but the total energy is low, owing to the small focal volume.

In its endeavor to remain the technological leader, Dornier has designed and built working prototypes of all three shock wave generation systems. As of this point, based on our experiences and clinical comparisons, alternative shock wave techniques have not duplicated the performance of spark-gap technology. The following discusses Dornier experience with each type of system.

System Results

Spark Gap Results

Dornier introduced the first extracorporeal shock wave lithotripter in 1983: and the performance, safety, and reliability are still considered the gold standard. Consequently, spark-gap technology and ellipsoid geometry have been improved to make stone destruction with low impulse energy a reality.

Dornier's new product, the Multipurpose Lithotripter 9000 (MPL 9000*), was designed to further improve stone disintegration by decreasing the focal size and increasing the pressure amplitudes. It produces the highest energy density in the focal point of all known systems.

Spark-gap systems produce shock waves with the fastest rise times and of the shortest durations. Measurement of these rise times is difficult with the currently available hydrophones because of their slow response times. The rise times shown in Table 1, therefore, can be used only as upper limits.

New hydrophones are being developed that have extremely fast response times, but they cannot be calibrated for absolute pressure measurements. However, with the aid of these new hydrophones and through theoretical calculations, it is estimated that the actual rise time for spark-gap induced shock waves is in the 1- to 10-nanosecond range.

In Figure 1, a typical MPL 9000* pressure wave profile

*CAUTION: Investigational device limited by federal law to investigational use. Not commercially available.

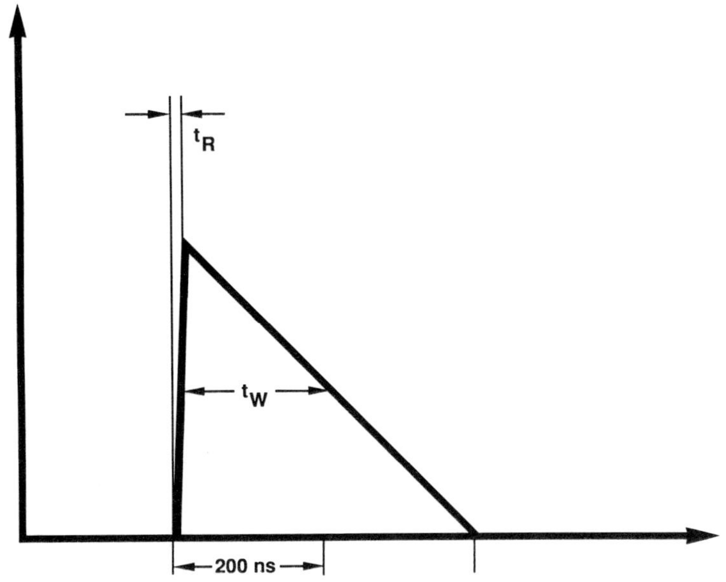

FIG 1.
A, ideal shock wave with 1 nanosecond rise time, 200 nanosecond half width, and minimal or no tensile waves (negative pressure). **B**, typical shock wave produced by the MPL 9000. (CAUTION: Investigational device, limited by Federal Law to investigational use. Not commercially available.)

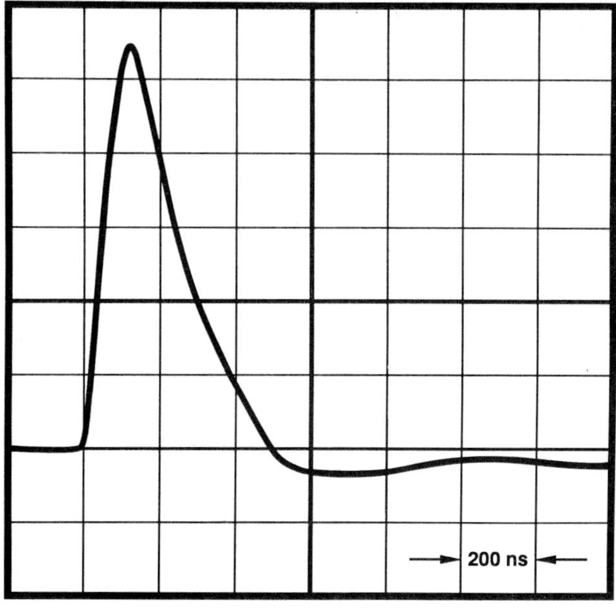

is compared to an ideal pressure wave as measured in the focal point. For the MPL 9000,* the rise time is not resolved because of the response time of the hydrophone, but it does demonstrate the short pulse width and low tensile wave component.

Electromagnetic Results

Dornier has built and tested several electromagnetic systems in its laboratory. The best prototype system has produced shock waves with pressure amplitudes of only 600 bar and with rise times and pulse widths of 50 and 360 nanoseconds, respectively. Although these results are superior to any other electromagnetic system available today, the significantly slower rise times and longer pulse duration of electromagnetic technology has proved inferior when compared with spark-gap designs.

Piezoelectric Results

In a piezoelectric system built for experimentation, Dornier employed a spherical arrangement of many crystals, a design comparable to other systems currently available. The therapeutic focus is concentrated in an area smaller than a 3-mm diameter circle. This area exceeds the resolution limits afforded by the current hydrophone. The pressure pulse produced is symmetrical in shape with a long rise and fall time. Because of low pressure amplitudes, further steepening is not realized as the wave propagates. Because of the sharp focusing, this system produces very high pressure amplitudes in a small area: but in relation to other systems, the total energy delivered is small.

Measurements and observations on the propagaion effects of shock waves were conducted in water, which represents an ideal medium. It can be assumed that as a piezoelectric-induced shock wave propagates through an inhomogeneous medium such as organic tissue of varying densities, further degradation of the shock wave will occur. Slower rise times and defocusing can be expected. Because the spark gap produces an immediate shock wave of high intensity, it does not require a finite distance to form its steep wave front and it is not affected by the tissue layer differences.

FRAGMENTATION DYNAMICS

From a physical point of view, several factors affect the stone disintegration process:

1. Time parameters of shock waves
   rise time (t_R)
   impulse width (t_W)

These times determine the pressure gradient in the direction of the stone and also the fragment size caused by the spalling or Hopkinson effect.

2. Energy parameters of shock waves
   impulse energy (Ep)
   energy density (ϵ)
   pressure amplitude (P)
   focal size; 6-db line of pressure distribution

Pressure amplitude and energy density are related by;

$$\epsilon \text{-} P^2/Z$$

where Z refers to sound impedance.

The fracturing process is complex and made up of multiple effects. Disintegration is caused by pressure and tensile waves produced in the stone and shear forces and cavitation on the stone surface. The first step in this process occurs at the stone/tissue interface where the shock wave first impinges. At this point, tensile waves arise, causing cavitation, and could result in fine erosion. At the same time, shear stresses are produced at the entry point and spread over the stone surface.

Tensile and shear stresses are also produced as the shock wave travels through the stone and hits the back wall. The tensile waves produced here travel back into the stone.

The dynamics of fracturing must also take into consideration the size of the focal area relative to the stone's size and its composition. For the MPL 9000,* a 3-mm focal width was chosen so that it would lie within even the smallest treatable gallstone. This ensures that the pressure wave produced perpendicular to the shock wave direction is used to its fullest potential in the fragmentation process.

As gallstones are generally larger and more difficult to break than kidney stones, each phase of the fragmentation process must be optimized. Because spark-gap technology creates pressure waves with the shortest rise times and pulse widths, it was the technology chosen to incorporate in the MPL 9000.* Both high pressure and tensile gradients are produced in the direction of the stone and high energy density is developed within the stone. This should lead to improved stone fragmentation. Electromagnetic and piezoelectric sources, owing to longer rise times, produce gradients much lower than spark-gap sources.

An important side issue is the tensile waves produced along the shock path at tissue layer interfaces. This can result in harmful cavitation effects. However, tensile waves can be minimized if the shock wave has a steep wave front and a short pulse width.

DEVICE CONSIDERATIONS

The rapid acceptance of ESWL® and the attempt by several manufacturers to gain regulatory approval of lithotripter devices, brings to light the necessity for objective criteria with which to evaluate technological alternatives. Clinical experience in Europe has shown that systems vary in the treatment of gallbladder stones. The appropriateness of a lithotripter is an equation which takes into account many factors including:

1. The imaging component

2. The stone targeting system
3. The patient handling system
4. The shock wave applicator
5. Aneshesia requirements
6. The user interface

The MPL 9000* (Fig 2) is a product incorporating Dornier's 20 years of ESWL® experience, and is designed to meet the specific requirements of biliary lithotripsy.

In the following sections, we will take a more detailed look at the MPL 9000* as it relates to the evaluation criteria listed above.

THE IMAGING COMPONENT

Owing to the radiolucent nature of gallstones, ultrasound imaging is the diagnostic technique of choice. Ultrasound systems, however, vary in their resolution capabilities. Conventional ultrasound transducer technology has a fixed focal zone within which the best resolution occurs and outside of which the beam diverges and the image quality degrades.

It is well known that ultrasound technology varies in performance in different clinical situations. Of the various transducer designs today, the optimal technology for balancing between resolution and focal length is multiple arrays. The MPL 9000* (Fig 3), will incorporate this state-of-the-art array imaging concept. A fully integrated, dual ultrasound system is used; one in the therapy head and another on an articulated arm. The arm-mounted transducer is designed to expedite stone localization and provide alternate angle monitoring throughout the fragmentation process. In this manner, the progress of fragmentation is monitored in real time, which should allow the physician to accurately ascertain when the therapy is complete and thus minimize the number of shocks delivered.

THE STONE TARGETING SYSTEM

An accurate method of targeting the stone is critical to the effectiveness of lithotripters and to reducing the need for retreatment. With ultrasound imaging, a pulse (sound beam) is directed into the body. The path traveled by the ultrasound

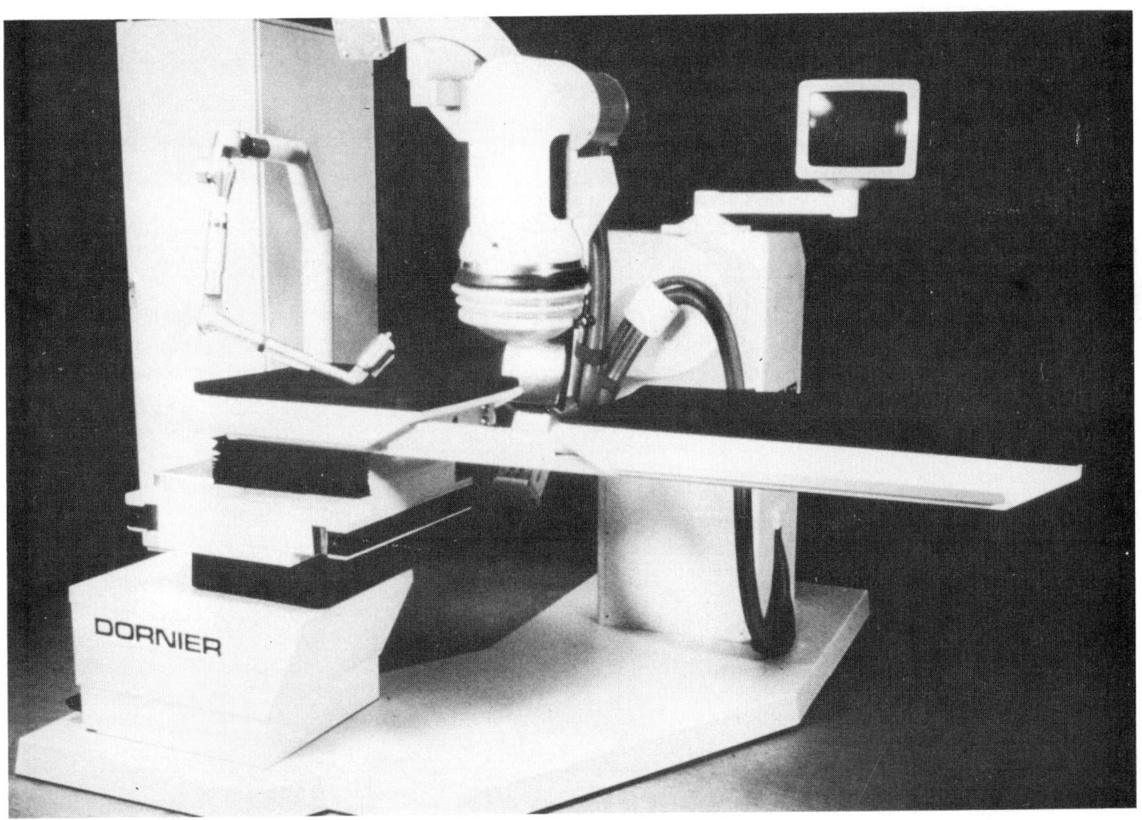

FIG 2.
Dornier's MPL 9000 lithotripter. (CAUTION: Investigational device, limited by federal law to investigational use. Not commercially available.)

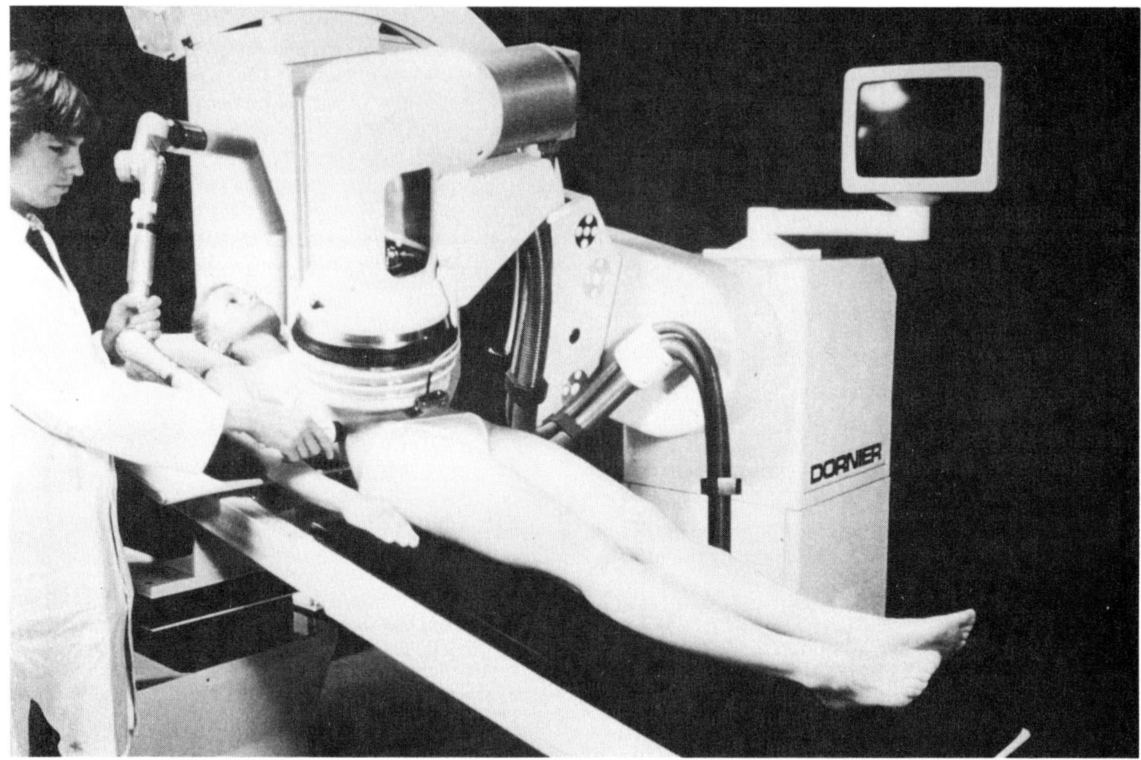

FIG 3.
Integrated dual ultrasound system with imaging probes mounted inside therapeutic head and on articulated arm.

beam will be bent slightly at each tissue layer interface, owing to refraction. If ultrasound imaging is not "in-line" with the shock wave path, it may lead to the mistargeting of the pressure pulse to the stone. Consequently, systems that have not incorporated in-line imaging have, to date, demonstrated a higher clinical re-treatment rate.

Biplanar imaging is made possible with the MPL 9000's* dual ultrasound system. This multiple view concept was designed to enhance the stone localization, targeting, and disintegration processes (Fig 4). Utilizing the out-line transducer, the gallbladder and gallstone are surveyed. Then, based upon computer calculations of respective angles from the articulated arm, the patient is automatically moved into the treatment position.

The in-line transducer is used to monitor the stone disintegration process in real time, without interrupting the procedure. It can also be used to retarget the stone if the patient moves. Another advantage of the MPL 9000's* dual ultrasound system is that it is designed to allow detection of hidden stone fragments during the treatment. Often, as fragmentation occurs, a layer of sludge forms between the remaining stone elements and the shock wave source (Fig 5). This sludge can cause excessive attenuation of the in-line ultrasound beam and, more important, the shock wave. In this case, the transducer on the articulated arm is used for monitoring and retargeting, since its viewing path is unobstructed.

THE PATIENT-HANDLING SYSTEM

Patient positioning is of key importance in treating gallstones, owing to the many anatomical variations that exist. This is further complicated by the fact that most gallstones are cholesterol in composition and tend to float in the gallbladder. As a result, optimal positioning is difficult.

FIG 4.
Illustration of biplane imaging used for targeting and monitoring the disintegration process.

FIG 5.
Example of how imaging probe mounted on articulated arm can be used to visualize fragments that are hidden from the in-line probe.

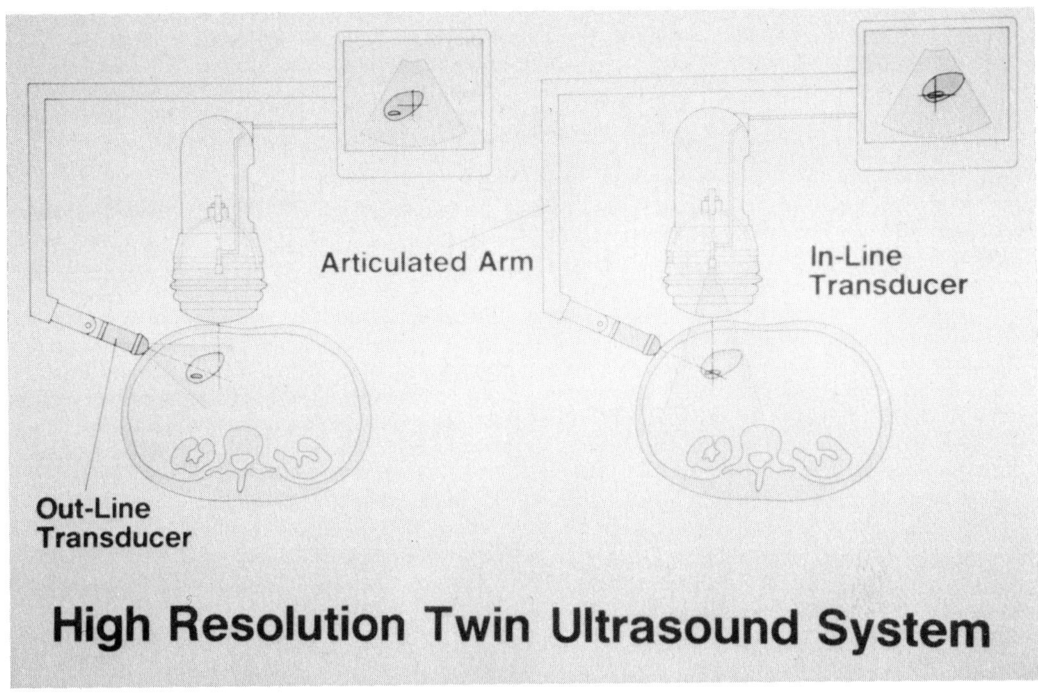
Articulated Arm
In-Line
Transducer
Out-Line
Transducer
High Resolution Twin Ultrasound System

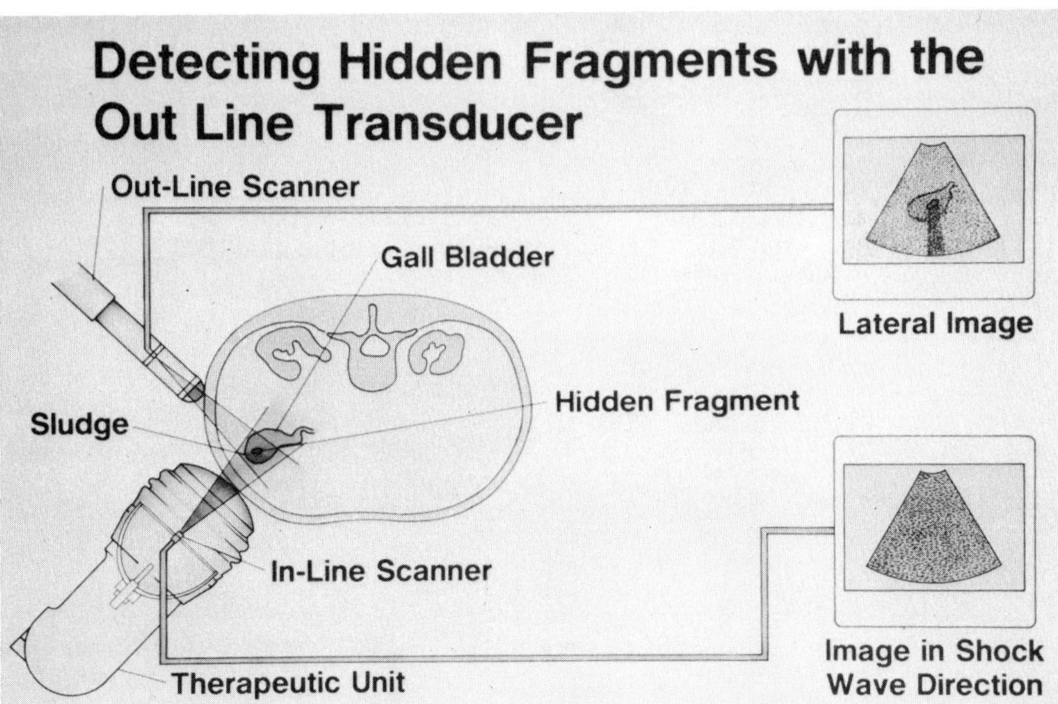
Detecting Hidden Fragments with the
Out Line Transducer
Out-Line Scanner
Gall Bladder
Lateral Image
Hidden Fragment
Sludge
In-Line Scanner
Therapeutic Unit
Image in Shock
Wave Direction

Consequently, a gallbladder stone lithotripter must enable treatments to be performed in the prone, supine, or lateral position, depending on the clinical presentation. The device must also allow variable table movement and tilt capabilities so that the stones can be positioned in the fundus or infundibulum.

The MPL 9000* employs a patient-handling system designed to afford the physician virtually unlimited lithotripsy treatment options (Fig 6). The patient table has longitudinal and transverse travel capabilities, as well as height, head up/head down angulation, and side-to-side tilt. The longitudinal and transverse motions are used to move the gallbladder into position. Table tilt and angulation are designed to allow the physician to compensate for anatomical variations and present the gallbladder in an optimum treatment position. The therapy head is mounted on a C-arm that accommodates overtable or undertable shock wave entry. Isocentric orbital rotation in either the overtable or undertable postion allows for treatment in axial oblique angles, enabling the physician to choose a shock wave path that avoids the spine and other sensitive tissue. The entire C-arm assembly can be tilted to further refine the entry angle of the shock wave.

During the treatment, several of these positioning variations are computer-controlled, based upon the ultrasound stone localization parameters. Positioning adjustments to compensate for patient movement or displacement of large stone fragments are made using in-line or out-line ultrasound guidance.

THE SHOCK WAVE APPLICATOR

Dornier's extensive research and clinical experience led to the conclusion that spark-gap technology was far superior to alternative shock wave methods. As previously discussed, a highly specialized therapeutic unit was developed for the MPL 9000* that balanced all critical shock wave parameters (Fig 7). In addition, in-line ultrasound monitoring provided by the transducer mounted in the therapeutic unit allows for real time viewing in the treatment axis while the out-line transducer provides an oblique viewing perspective. This feature is of particular value given that respiration, heart beat, and voluntary patient motion can cause mistargeting. Synchronized EKG triggering of the shock wave is also available to time the shock wave coincident with the refractory period of the heart cycle.

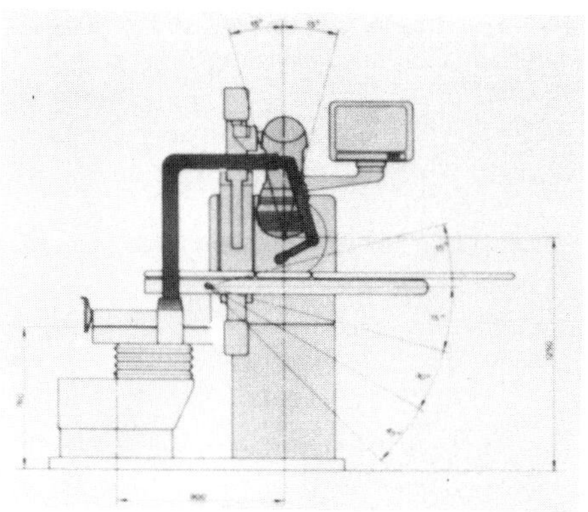

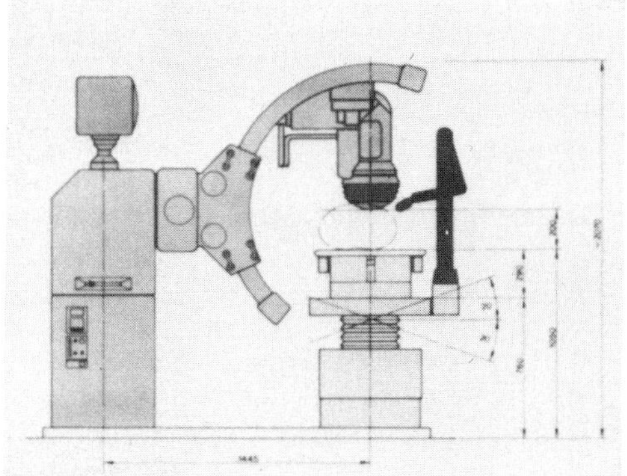

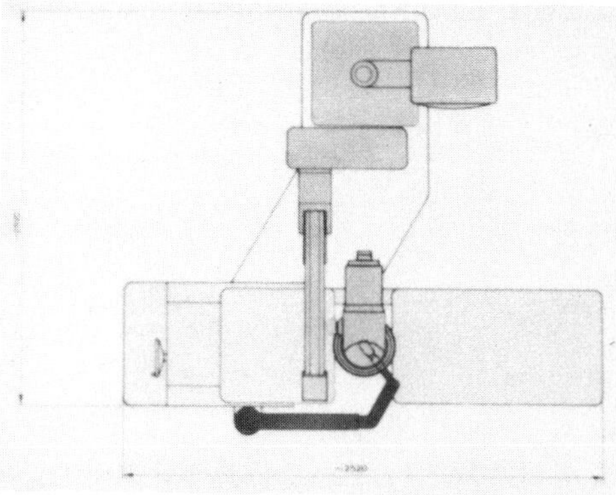

FIG 6.
Front, side, and top view of MPL 9000 illustrating flexibility in patient table and therapy unit positioning. (CAUTION: Investigational device, limited by federal law to investigational use. Not commercially available.)

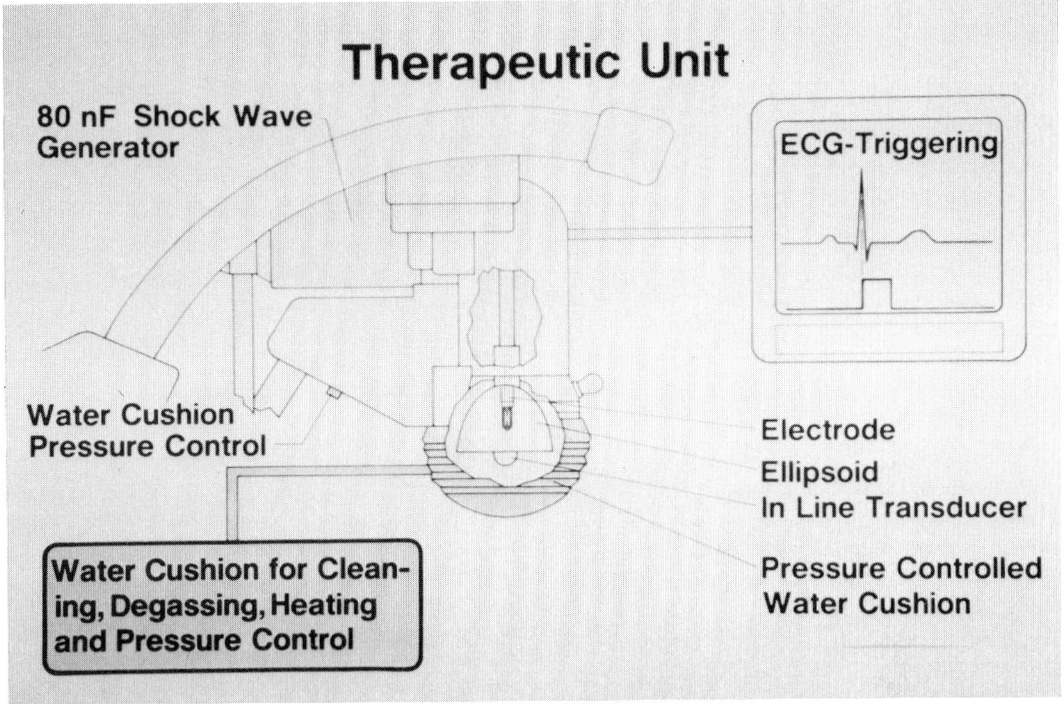

FIG 7.
Major components of the MPL 9000 therapeutic unit. (CAUTION: Investigational device, limited by federal law to investigational use. Not commercially available.)

Anesthesia requirements

An issue that dramatically differentiates shock wave sources is the difference in entrance pressures they exert on the body surface. This intensity directly influences the level of pain induced when the shock wave is applied. The painful or pain-free effect of a system is determined by the total energy of the shock wave, the maximum focal pressure, and the energy distribution in the transmission path leading to the stone. Although the total energy and the focal pressure can be reduced, it can be done only at the expense of disintegration effectiveness. Only through proper ellipse design can the energy distribution be optimized in such a way that the pressure at the therapeutic focus will be the highest and the pressure elsewhere will be kept to a minimum (Fig 8).

In the MPL 9000*, Dornier combined the proven, effective spark-gap technology with a wide aperture ellipsoid. The wider aperture is designed to spread the shock wave entrance pressure over a larger area in order to minimize the assocated pain. Another benefit of the wide aperture is the generation of a more highly focused pressure volume. The MPL 9000* also employs a variable voltage power supply that allows the physician to customize the treatment according to patient body habitus, stone size, and stone composition. Clinical experience with the MPL 9000* in Germany has shown that up to 30 percent of patients can be treated with no pain medication, with the balance (70 percent) requiring only the use of IV analgesics.

The User Interface

Essential to the efficiency of an ESWL® unit is the degree to which it relates to the physician. Systems that comprise several nonintegrated components can complicate therapy and lengthen overall procedure time. The ideal system provides fast and simple user interaction by presenting all primary controls in an organized and systematic fashion.

In the MPL 9000*, a modern and comprehensive control console acts as the center of operation (Fig 9). A dedicated

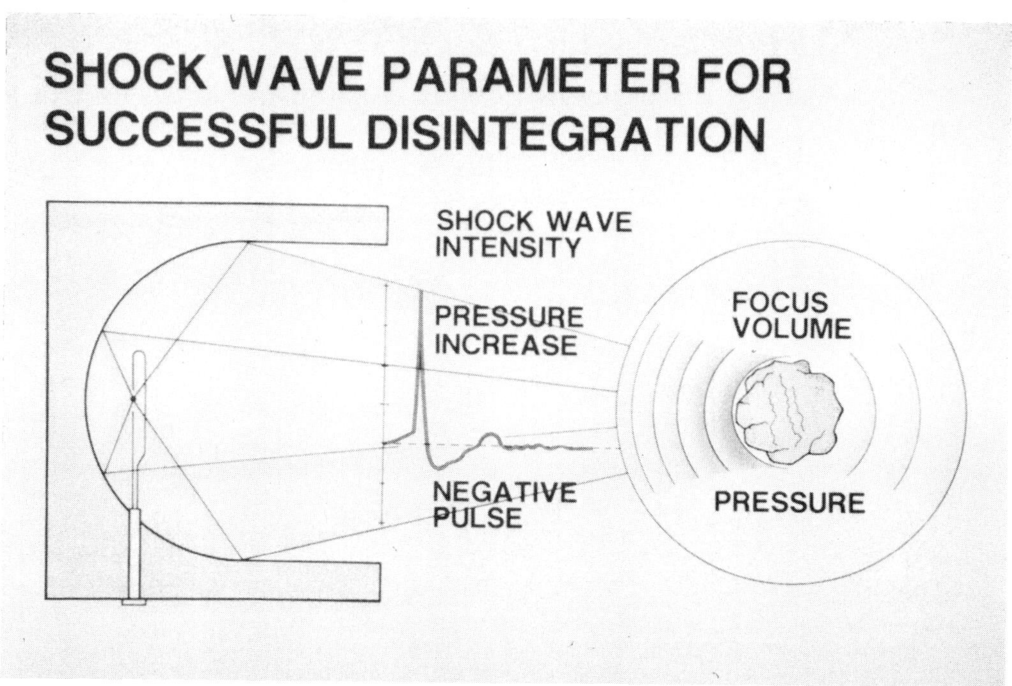
SHOCK WAVE PARAMETER FOR
SUCCESSFUL DISINTEGRATION
SHOCK WAVE
INTENSITY
PRESSURE
INCREASE
NEGATIVE
PULSE
FOCUS
VOLUME
PRESSURE

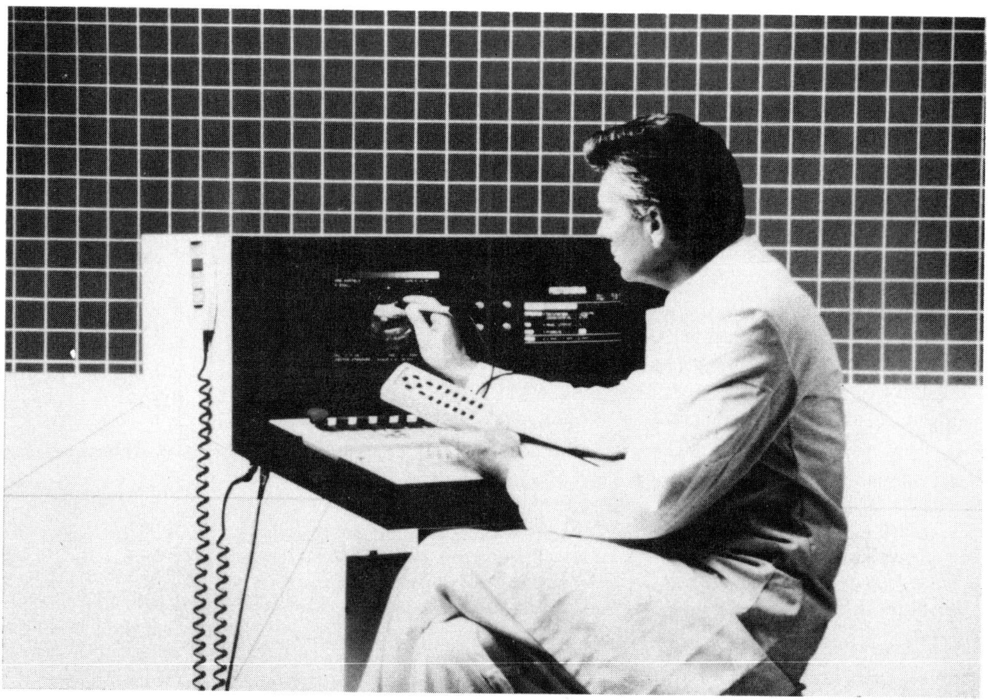

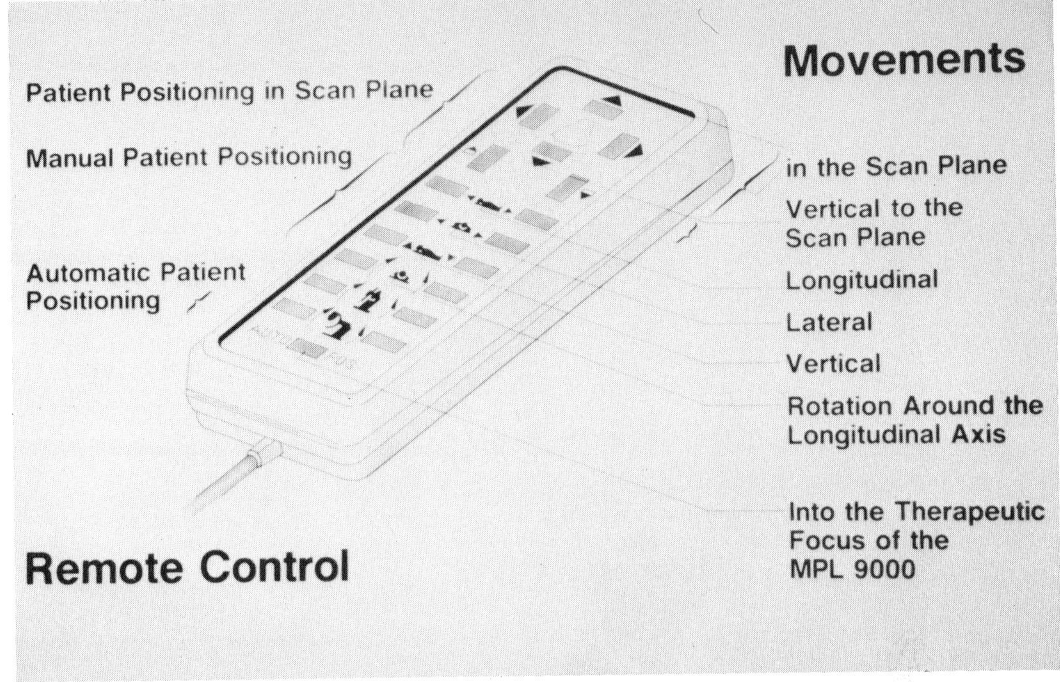

FIG 10.
Remote control unit allows operator to manipulate patient table and C-arm while standing close to patient.

text display provides the user with menu-prompted control function choices and allows the input of vital patient and procedure information. A second video monitor is used to view either the in-line or out-line ultrasound image during stone localization, targeting, and treatment. A light pen is used for computer-controlled positioning of the stone, and a full set of controls are available for optimizing the ultrasound image.

FIG 8.
Optimal ellipsoid design results in low entrance pressure and concentrated energy deposition on targeted stone.

FIG 9.
MPL 9000 control console designed for fast and simple user interaction. (CAUTION: Investigational device, limited by federal law to investigational use. Not commercially available.)

Adjustments in the patient-handling systems are made using the MPL 9000* remote control seen in Figure 10. The remote control unit allows manipulation of all patient table and C-arm motions. It is normally located at the operator's console but can be carried to table-side for closer monitoring of the patient during equipment positioning.

The MPL 9000* was designed in close collaboration with the world's leading experts in ESWL® therapy. Their input resulted in the incorporation of many features, designed specifically to facilitate gallstone treatments. Because of this book's focus on gallstone lithotripsy, those important aspects have been emphasized in this chapter. However, the MPL 9000* is a multipurpose lithotripter designed for both gallstone and kidney stone therapy.

In April 1988, Dornier initiated installation of 10 MPL 9000* units in the United States for the disintegration of gallstones. Clinical investigations are being conducted under a United States IDE protocol. Similar trials are scheduled to begin in the fourth quarter of 1988, on kidney stones and for the use of the MPL 9000* mobile lithotripter.

TECHNOMED INTERNATIONAL—SONOLITH 3000

Ms. Sarah Sorrel

Summary

Since its introduction in 1980, extracorporeal lithotripsy by focused shockwaves has become widely accepted as the method of choice in the treatment of urolithiasis.[2,7] Preliminary studies using lithotripsy to fragment biliary calculi are promising; however, important clinical differences between urolithiasis and cholelithiasis will ultimately determine the applicability of this technique to the treatment of biliary stones.

The Sonolith extracorporeal lithotripter introduced by Technomed International in 1986 is based on research begun in 1978 by the French National Institute for Medical Research (INSERM) in collaboration with the Department of Urology at the Edouard Herriot Hospital in Lyon, France. The Sonolith combines electrohydraulically produced shockwaves with ultrasound for stone localization. Clinical studies initiated in 1985 concluded that ultrasound localization was effective for extracorporeal destruction of kidney stones.[4] Further studies aimed at determining the Sonolith's effectiveness in the treatment of biliary calculi has yielded promising preliminary data.[10] This article provides an overview of the Sonolith describing the technological choices that were made in the course of its development and how these choices provided the opportunity for the Sonolith's subsequent evolution into both a clinically effective and cost-effective dual-purpose lithotripter.

Lithotripter Description

The key parameters which must be taken into consideratin for lithotripter design include the energy source, focusing system, and the stone location system. In the Sonolith, electrohydraulic shockwaves focused by an ellipsoidal reflector are used to fragment stones after localization with ultrasound. The shockwave focusing assembly is positioned with respect to the patient under computer control.

SHOCKWAVE GENERATOR

The majority of commercially available lithotripters use focused shock waves to fragment stones.[8] A shockwave is characterized by an extremely rapid rise time and an exponential decay time followed by a return to equilibrium. Absence of significant negative pressures considerably reduces the risk of tissue damage.[9]

Physical Principles of the Electrohydraulic Shockwave Generator

Based on safety and effectiveness considerations, electrohydraulic shockwave generation was chosen by our research group for the Sonolith.[5] The shockwave is produced by the underwater discharge of a capacitor between two electrodes situated at the first focus of an ellipsoidal reflector. The equivalent circuit of the electrical discharge is shown in Figure 1.

The energy discharge creates a plasma in the water at the first focus of the elipsoidal reflector, generating a spherical pressure wave with a very steep wavefront. Several centimeters away from the first focus, the laws governing the propagation of pressure waves approach those of classical acoustics. Reflection of the spherical wave by the ellipsoidal reflector results in a partially spherical wave centered at the outer focus of the reflector, as shown in Figure 2. A stone made to coincide with this point undergoes complex stress fields and possible cavitation phenomena, ultimately resulting in structural breakdown of the stone.

An experimental configuration developed in 1984 included a 2.4 μ F capacitor charged between 12 kV and 15 kV. However, high line inductance occurred when the capacitor was placed at a distance from the ellipsoidal reflector, resulting in considerable energy absorption at the time of discharge. By placing the capacitor as close as possible to

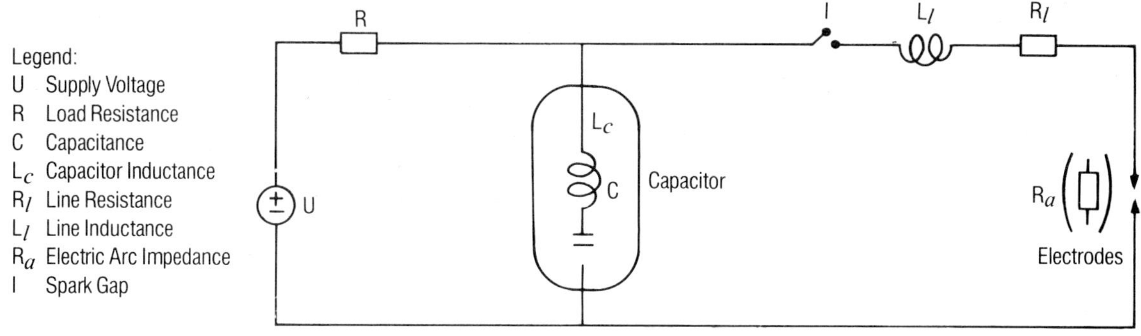

FIG 1.
Equivalent circuit diagram of the electrohydraulic generator.

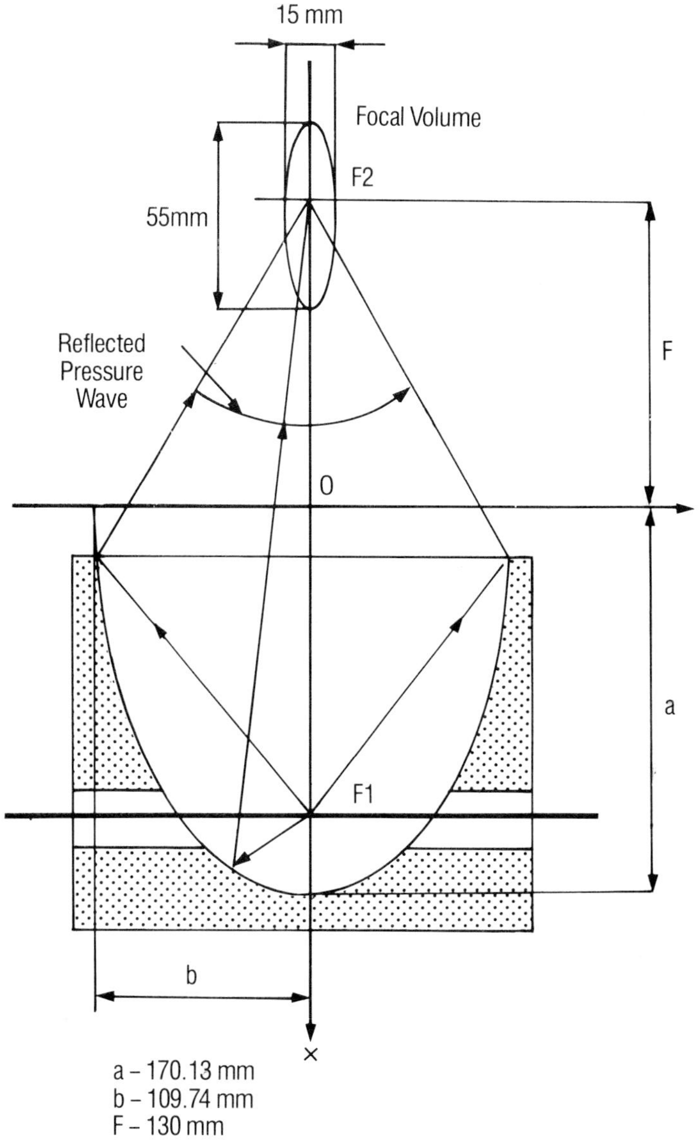

15 mm
Focal Volume
F2
55mm
Reflected Pressure Wave
F
0
a
F1
b
x

a – 170.13 mm
b – 109.74 mm
F – 130 mm

FIG 2.
Ellipsoidal reflector and focal volume.

the reflector, a capacitor of 500 nF could then be used to obtain the same peak pressures at the outer focus while using less energy.[11] Further improvements in the ellipsoidal reflector geometry enabled this energy to be decreased even further, while maintaining adequate pressures for effective stone destruction.[6] A consequence of this latest generator design is the ability to perform treatments without epidural or general anesthesia.

Medium of Shockwave Propagation

Water provides the medium in which shockwaves are generated and transmitted. It follows that the water will also provide the most superior coupling since the acoustic properties of soft tissue and water are very similar.

The first lithotripter design recognized the advantage of direct water contact for shockwave transmission. However, the water bath design required immersion of the patient and complicated patient handling and positioning. This led to the development of so-called dry systems in which the shockwave generator is contained in a closed system and contact with the patient is through a membrane.

Unfortunately, the membrane represents a barrier in the acoustic path at which energy losses can occur. Coupling difficulties resulting in bruising occur in cases where the patient's anatomy does not conform to the membrane surface. Further, the membrane requires the use of viscous coupling media, which the patient may find unpleasant.

For these reasons, the Sonolith shockwave generator is mounted in a small, mobile water basin located beneath an aperture in the treatment table top. The aperture is just large enough to allow direct water contact with the shockwave entry area. The patient remains dry during treatment, and yet the shockwave travels along an unobstructed path. A water-processing system mixes the water to a comfortable temperature. The water is then degassed to minimize energy losses by bubbles created when the shockwaves are generated and by the formation of a gaseous bubble layer at the water-tissue interface during treatment. This is achieved by applying a vacuum (approximately 100 mbar) to the water as it fills an auxiliary storage tank. The basin draining and filling procedure takes place after each patient treatment and requires not more than 15 minutes.

Characterization of the Shock Wave

A polyvinylidene fluoride (PVDF) hydrophone developed by Technomed International with a pressure-sensitive area of 2 mm in diameter and a response time faster than the shockwave rise time was used to measure the shockwave pressures produced by the Diatron generator. The Diatron includes a 200 nF capacitor charged at 14 kV and an automatic electrode adjustment mechanism which maintains an electrode interspace of 0.8 mm.

The PVDF hydrophone used for the characterization was calibrated against another PVDF hydrophone developed by Medicoteknisk Institut (Denmark). The calibration procedure repeated after the measurements showed no significant change in the sensor's sensitivity.

The time domain hydrophone response to the Diatron shockwave (obtained from a Tektronix 2430A oscilloscope trace) is represented in Figure 3. The average measured rise time of the shockwave is 200 ns, and the pulse duration is 0.40 μs. The peak pressure is expressed as a percentage relative to the peak pressure measured at the geometric second focus, P max.

The optimum relationship between rise time, shockwave duration, and positive and negative pressures is not known since the mechanism of lithotripsy is still poorly understood. However, there appears to be a logarithmic relationship between probability of stone fracture and pressure amplitude,[12] i.e., above a certain point, increasing pressure does not significantly increase efficiency. On the other hand, decreasing pressures even slightly will significantly decrease the probability of stone fracture.

What does appear important is the reproducibility of the shockwave. If the average shockwave provides effective lithotripsy, any outlying shockwaves may be painful. The Diatron's Computed Plasma Aperture System (COMPAS) automatically adjusts the electrode gap throughout treatment.

COMPAS consists of two pneumatic devices, each associated with an electrode and driven by the technical computer. Its purpose is to compensate automatically for increases in separation distance between the electrodes due to electrode wear during operation. After each treatment, a gauge driven by the computer measures the distance between the electrode tips. The computer then readjusts the electrode separation distance. This has resulted in standard deviations of pressure on the order of +/− 20 percent.

This minimum variation allows the average working pressure to be much higher than that of a machine with a much higher deviation, even for the same pain level.

Some variation may be desirable, however; assuming each solid structure has its own resonant frequencies, the probability of breaking the stone should increase if the pressure waveform is not absolutely consistent from shock to shock. For example, hitting a stone with a hammer in exactly the same way may be less effective than hitting it a little differently each time.

Clinical results with the Diatron generator[5] have demonstrated that the same clinical effectiveness as that achieved with the previous generator model can now be obtained without general or epidural anesthesia.

Another important parameter, the focal volume, is defined as the useful area of the pressure concentrated around F_2. It is often calculated as the volume in which the pressure is greater than 50% of P max. The focal volume of the Diatron shown in Figure 4 was determined from pressure field

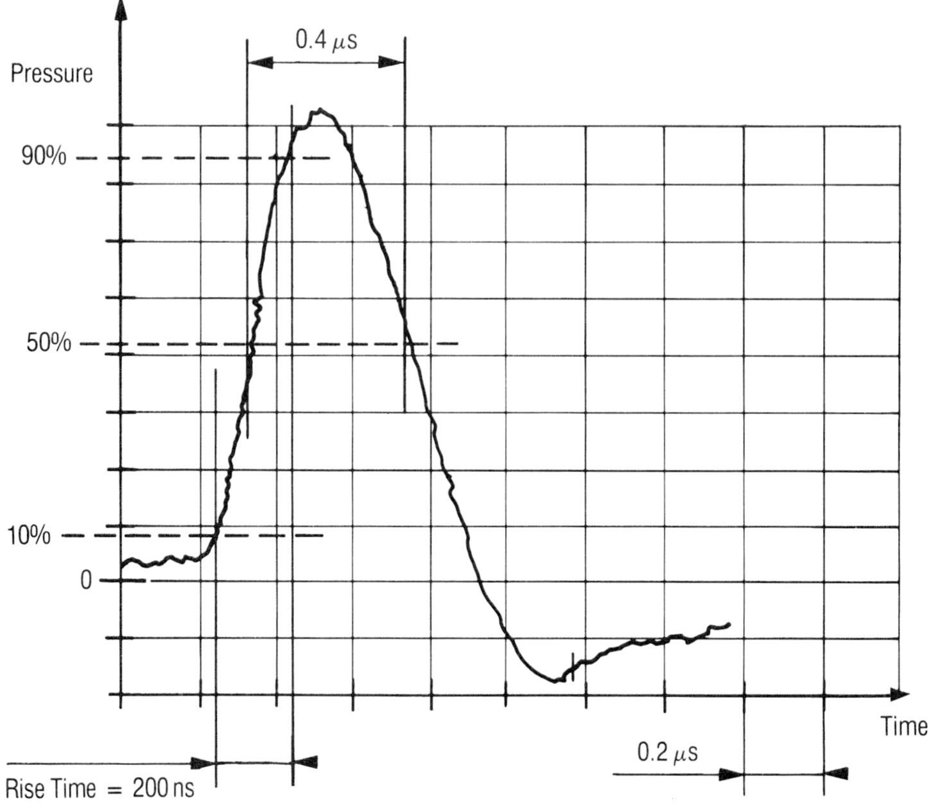

FIG 3.
Shockwave hydrophone response at focus.

plots in three orthogonal planes through the geometric second focus of the reflector. Three-dimensional plots of the relative positive and negative pressure fields in the X • Y plane are shown in Figure 5. Figure 6 shows how these planes are defined with respect to the ellipsoid.

The geometry of the Diatron was selected to optimize focal volume. Large focal volumes have been linked to pain and trauma to adjacent organs with reports of pancreatitis, renal failure, perirenal hematoma, unintended gallstone fracturing, and cardiac arrhythmias.[1] Reduction in focal size can result in large reductions of volume energy and thus pain.

On the other hand, too small a focus increases targeting accuracy requirements, length of procedure, and retreatment rates. The Diatron generator eliminates the need for anesthesia while maintaining clinical effectiveness by both increasing the entry area of the shock waves and reducing focal size.

IN SITU LOCALIZATION OF STONE

Principle

Although X-ray has been widely used in earlier lithotripters designed to treat kidney stones,[8] it is poorly suited to locating gallstones. On the contrary, ultrasound can be used to visualize all types of stones regardless of their X-ray density. Ultrasound is safe and easy to use and provides economic incentives by lowering capital equipment expenditures and installation costs.

Ultrasound loses much of its clinical and technical flexibility, however, when integrated into the lithotripter. This observation led Technomed to develop a unique locating system in which a free-standing ultrasound unit is coupled to a multi-articulated locating arm. The design enables the use of virtually any commercially available ultrasound unit and transducer type according to the imaging requirements. Moreover, this configuration enables the ultrasound unit to be readily upgraded as improved technology becomes available, easily repaired in the event of failure, and used for diagnostic purposes when the lithotripter is not in use.

The ultrasound transducer encased in a customized, water-proof sheath, attached to the extremity of the locating arm, allows free hand use of the transducer in a manner similar to diagnostic ultrasound. By virtue of its 6 degrees of freedom, the locating arm allows visualization of the gallstone or kidney stone in an infinite number of two-dimensional planes. At the moment the image of the stone is frozen, data from the encoders in each of the arm's articulations is recorded by the lithotripter's technical computer. The two-dimensional coordinates of the stone with respect to the ultrasound image (Fig 7) are then transmitted to the same computer, enabling a calculation of the spatial coordinates of the stone with respect to a coordinate system defined by the shockwave generator movement.

Locating Arm (Fig 8)

The theoretical deviation of the locating arm in any one of three orthogonal planes does not exceed +/− 0.9 mm. This value was determined from the sensitivities of the analog encoders in each of the arm's articulations. The magnitude of the error in localization is therefore largely depen-

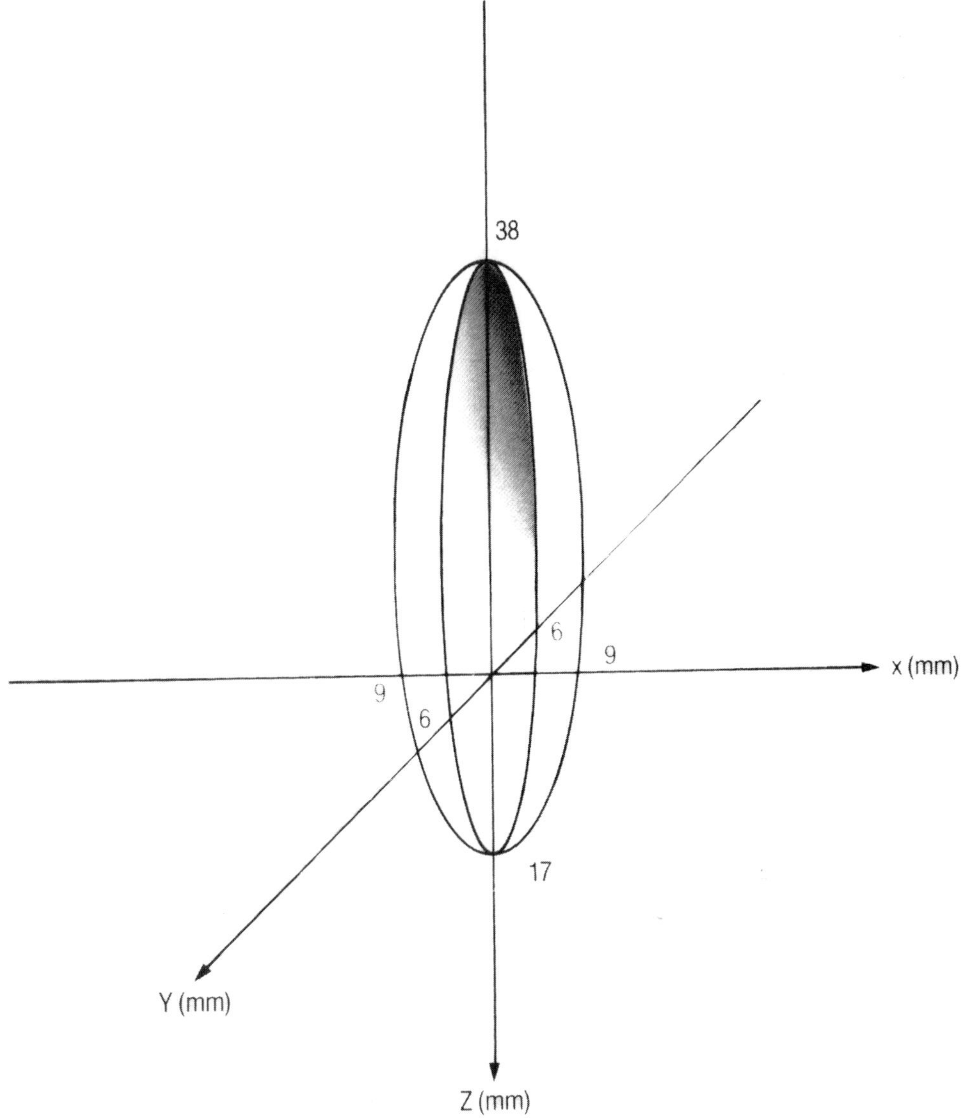

FIG 4.
Focal Volume at −6dB

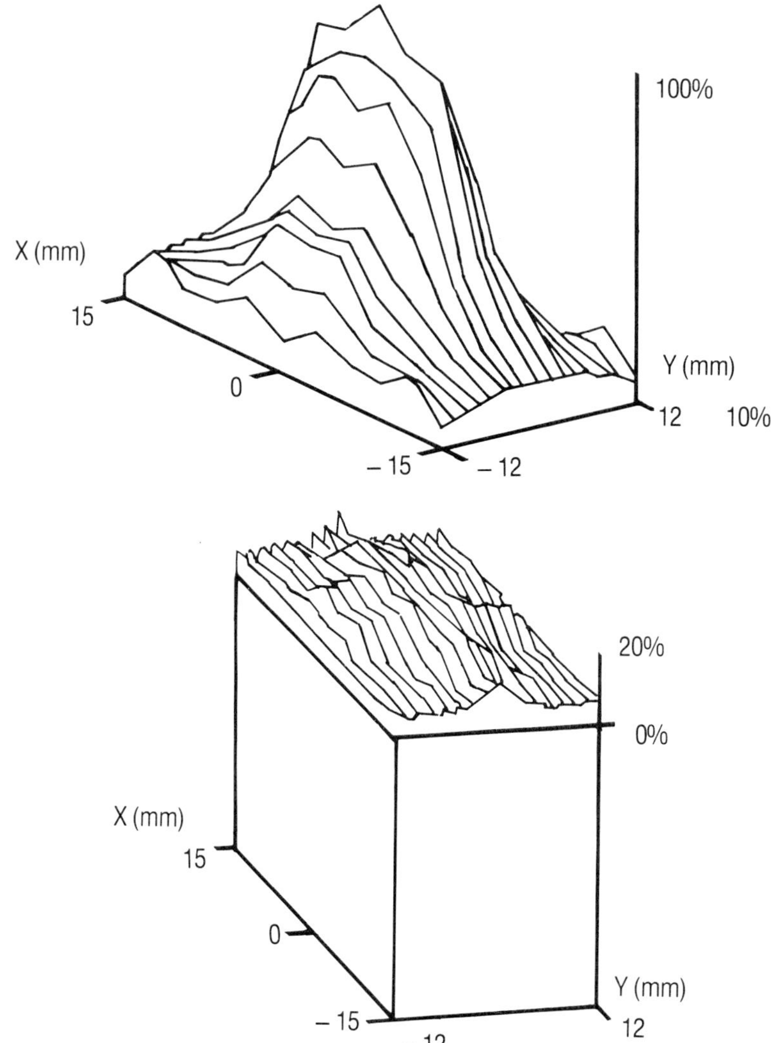

FIG 5.
3D plot of the pressure field in the X • Y plan; **A** positive pressure; **B** negative pressure.

dent upon the ultrasound image. Usually the coordinates of the stone as calculated on the ultrasound image are determined by superimposed grids. An uncertainty on the order of 1 mm will increase the maximum deviation by +/− 0.5 mm. The overall error in stone localization with this system can then be estimated on the order of +/− 2 mm.[5]

GENERATOR POSITIONING

After locating the stone, either the patient[8] or the generator is moved to focus the shockwave energy. In the Sonolith, the shockwave generator is displaced so that the focus coincides with the stone. The entire water basin subassembly moves along the two horizontal axis. The generator, consisting of the ellipsoidal reflector and high-voltage parts, is built into a metallic cylinder specially designed to allow movement along the vertical axis independent of the coupling basin.

The maximum deviation between the true position of the stone and the position of the reflector's outer focus can be calculated by taking into account the errors in stone localization due to ultrasound image, errors in the locating arm's position, and errors in the positioning of the shockwave generator. This error does not exceed +/− 1.6 mm in any one of the orthogonal axis in a volume 10 × 10 × 10 cubic centimeters.[5]

OPERATING SYSTEMS MANAGEMENT

The Sonolith 3000 dual purpose lithotripter shown in Figure 9 includes a treatment module and a control module which are used with a free-standing ultrasound scanner. Figure 10 shows how the various functions are allocated between the two modules. During treatment the patient lies on the treatment module, which contains the mobile shockwave generator and coupling basin, water-processing system, high-voltage power supply, and the locating arm. The operator interfaces with the lithotripter primarily through the control module, which contains the main computer, the technical computer, and a color TV monitor with interactive soft keys. The operating software (in compiled Pascal) is presented in the form of a series of step-by-step menus and instructions appearing on the screen. The software also includes maintenance functions. Patient treatment records and data on machine performance can be stored and printed. A telediagnostic program currently under development will provide a direct link between clinical installations and Technomed facilities for remote testing and malfunction analysis of the Sonolith.

Treatment Procedure

ANESTHESIA REQUIREMENTS

The Sonolith 3000 does not require epidural or general anesthesia; however, IV sedation is necessary for most patients.

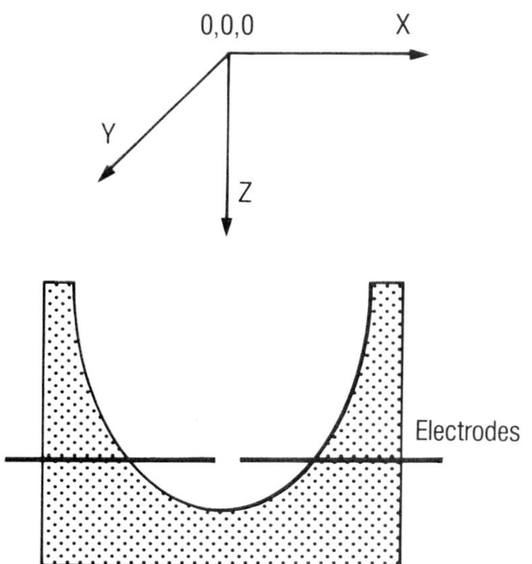

FIG 6.
Definition of the X,Y,Z axes.

PATIENT POSITIONING ON THE TREATMENT MODULE

The patient lies comfortably on the treatment module in either the prone or supine position for biliary treatments and in the supine position for renal treatments. The patient is positioned so that the contact area of the entering shockwave is above the aperture in the treatment module. Degassed warm water is in contact with only this area of the patient's body for purposes of coupling the shockwave.

STONE LOCALIZATION AND GENERATOR POSITIONING

A single localization procedure yielding one set of (x,y,z) coordinates is sufficient to position the shockwave generator for treatment, although it is possible to perform additional measurements (using different scanning planes, for example) in order to check the reproducibility of the results or to eliminate a possible error in manipulation (moving the probe at the moment the image is frozen, for example.)

During localization, the stone should be targeted at the appropriate distance from the bright spot on the image which actually represents the leading edge of the stone. During treatment, the ultrasound probe can be removed from the arm and mounted on the ellipsoid in such a way as to monitor the treatment in real time. After each series of 200 shockwaves, it is possible to perform a new localization procedure.

SHOCKWAVE GENERATION

The capacitor discharge which generates the shockwave is gated to the R wave of the patient's electrocardiogram. This ensures patient safety by preventing extrasystoles due to the pressure wave[8] and/or the electric field created in the generator during the discharge.

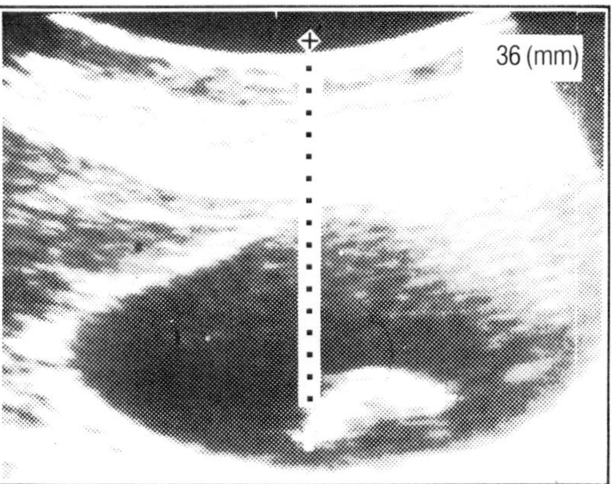

FIG 7.
Ultrasound image before treatment showing depth of the stone.

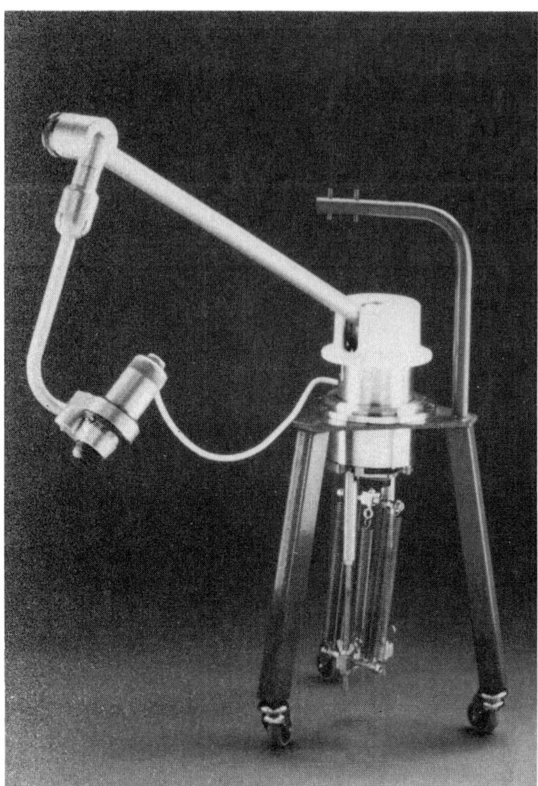

FIG 8.
Ultrasound locating arm.

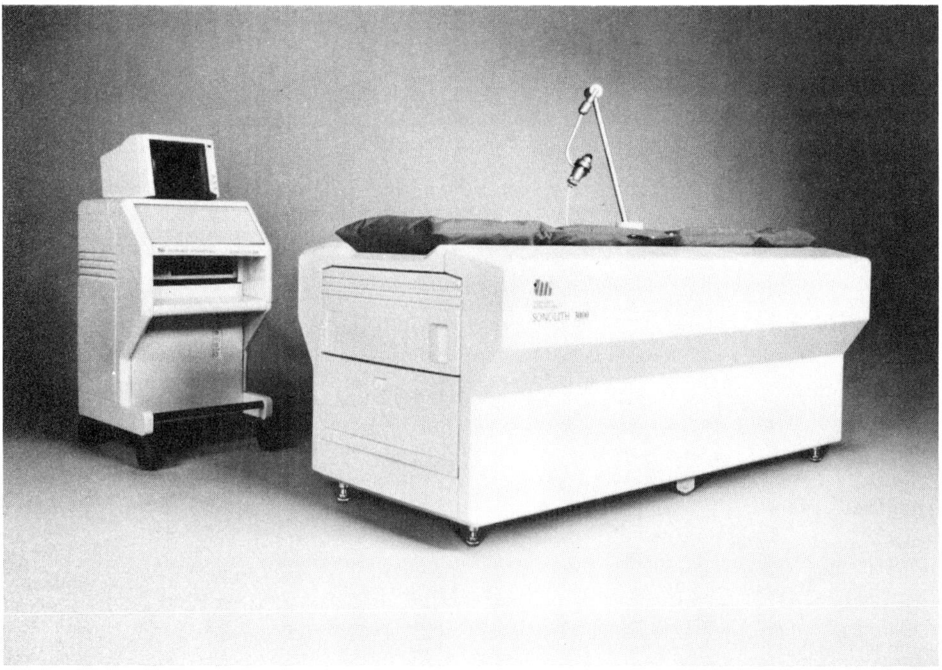

FIG 9.
Sonalith 3000 system.

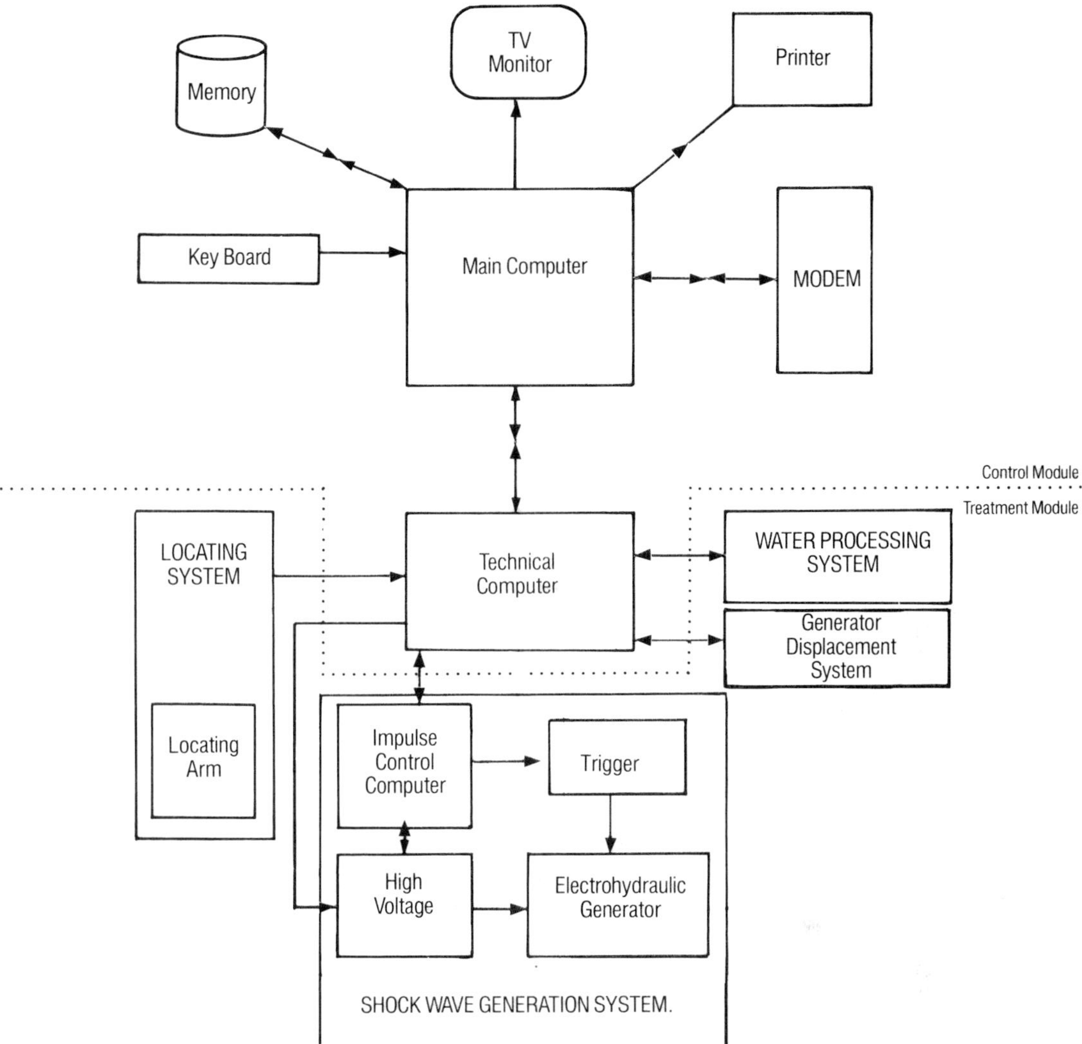

FIG 10.
Sonolith 3000 system architecture.

Clinical Results

Table 1 compares clinical results for urinary stones using the original generator model requiring epidural anesthesia and the Diatron generator requiring IV sedation. This comparison illustrates that the improved Diatron generator design, i.e., the change in ellipsoid geometry focus size and aperture have eliminated the need for general anesthesia without compromising treatment effectiveness. Furthermore, the mean number of shockwaves is not increased in the Diatron, and the retreatment rate is still on the order of 12 percent.

Although preliminary studies show that cholesterol gallstones may be more difficult to fragment than kidney stones, preliminary data with the Sonolith indicates a fragmentation rate greater than 85 percent for single stones less than 20 mm.[3] Unfortunately, long-term results are not yet available in order to evaluate clinical effectiveness in the treatment of gallstones.

Conclusion

In summary, the Sonolith provides a unique combination of technological features:

1. *The electrohydraulic shockwave generator,* universally recognized for its clinical effectiveness, *has been optimized to provide similar clinical results* without the need for either general or epidural anesthesia. A patented long-life

TABLE 1.
Sonolith Clinical Results for Extracorporeal Lithotripsy of Kidney Stones. Comparison of Early Generator Model and New Diatron Generator.

	SONOLITH 2000	SONOLITH 3000
Treatment time	45–60 min.	45–60 min.
Mean number of shocks	1750	1700
Successful fragmentation after one session	87%	85%
Failure to fragment after two sessions	6%	6%
Auxiliary procedures	8%	6%
Stone-free rate at 3 months	82%	85%
Number of patients	161	280

electrode configuration enables over 100 patients to be treated without hardware changes.

2. *The ultrasound locating system,* incorporating a multi-articulated arm and a free-standing ultrasound imager, allows accurate targeting of both renal and biliary calculi and continous real-time imaging during treatment.

3. *Computerized systems operation and management* increase ease of equipment use and broaden the possibility of system upgrades.

Finally, the compact and cost-effective design of the Sonolith makes it uniquely suited for operation as a transportable system. In this new concept, the lithotripter is transported to a hospital in a simple, inexpensive van. It is then brought inside the institution and set up for operation in approximately 45 minutes. Patients are then treated in the familiar surrounding of their own institution. Two transportable units have been in operation in France since October 1987 and have performed over 3,000 renal treatments with success equivalent to permanently installed Sonoliths. Technomed will be the first manufacturer to test such a concept for gallstones in the United States.

REFERENCES

1. AUA Committee on Percutaneous Lithotripsy and Noninvasive Lithotripsy. May 16, 1985.
2. Chaussy C, Schmiedt E, Jochan D, Brendel W, Forssmann B, Walther V: First clinical experience with extracorporally induced destruction of kidney stones by shock waves. *J Urol* 1982; 127:417.
3. Chaussy C: *Extracorporeal Shock Wave Lithotripsy. New Aspects in the Treatment of Kidney Stone Disease.* 1982. ISBN 3-8055-3620-8.
4. Martin X, Mestas JC, Cathignol D, Dubernard JM: Ultrasound Localization for Shock Wave Lithotripsy: *Lancet* 1985; Vol II No 8462-1005.
5. Martin X: Modified spark gap ellipsoidal reflector for anesthesia free extracorporeal shock wave lithotripsy. American Urological Association Meeting, Boston, 1988.
6. Mestas JL, Chapelon JY, Lenz P, Cathignol D, Dubernard JM: Realization d'un generateur D'ondes de Choc: Application a la Destruction des Calculs Renaux In Vitro. *Innov Tech Biol Med,* 1982; 3:573–581
7. Mestas JL, Martin X, Theillere Y, Dubernard JM, Cathignol D: Onde de choc et localisation ultrasone en lithotritie extracorporelle. *Jemu* 1987; No 6 2/9–28.
8. Ponchon T, Martin X, Mestas JL, Cathignol D, Lambert RP: Extracorporeal Lithotripsy of Gallstones. *Lancet* 1987; II:448.
9. Ponchon T: Public Communication, First International Symposium on Biliary Lithotripsy, Boston, July 1988.
10. Report of the American Urological Association Ad Hoc Committee to Study the Safety and Clinical Efficacy of Current Technology in Lithotripsy and Non-Invasive Lithotripsy. May 22, 1986.
11. Riehle R (ed): *Principles of Extracorporeal Shock Wave Lithotripsy.* Churchill Livingstone, New York, 1987.
12. Rous S (ed): *Stone Disease Diagnosis and Management.* Grune and Stratton, Orlando, 1987, p 314.

MEDSTONE 1050 ST LITHOTRIPTER

The Medstone 1050 ST lithotripter is an advanced dual-purpose and dual-imaging system. Using the same unit, both kidney stones and gallstones can be treated with either x-ray or real-time ultrasound imaging. It is a complete system that includes components for stone localization, patient handling and positioning, and shockwave generation. General anesthesia is not required.

The device is approved for the treatment of kidney stones and approved by the FDA for investigational use in the treatment of gallstones. Currently, there are seven Medstone investigational sites for gallstone treatment in the United States. The first gallstone disintegration in the United States was in January 1988 at Baylor University Medical Center in Dallas, using the Medstone 1050 ST lithotripter. The patients in the gallstone study are also receiving adjuvant Actigal (ursodiol) as part of their therapy.

The Medstone 1050 ST lithotripter was designed as a dry lithotripter from its inception. A spark-gap shockwave generated in a water column is focused through a membrane-covered port in the tabletop using computer-generated positioning. The patient maintains contact with the table membrane or in some instances a fluid-filled bag is used as a coupling medium. The shockwaves are gated to the ECG to prevent extrasystoles. The table top is a solid flat unit to ensure patient safety. Because of the flat table top, the unit can also be used for routine radiography and with the stirrups in place for urologic procedures such as retrograde pyelograms, placements of stents, and so on.

The spark-gap mechanism is a proven technology that has been improved upon by Medstone engineers. Consistent high-energy shockwaves are produced so that fewer shockwaves are needed and the retreatment rate is very low.

The computer system is sophisticated but simple to operate. Not only does it provide for precise localization of the stones, but also it monitors every critical part of the lithotripsy procedure to ensure safe treatment of the patients. The computer also produces a "chart ready" report immediately after treatment.

Because a majority of renal stones are calcified, localization is usually by x-ray though with noncalcified stones ultrasound can be used. For x-ray localization, two angled films are obtained and by the use of a "digipad" on the films the XYZ coordinates are computed for positioning of the patient's stone over the shockwave. During the procedure, progress in fragmentation is determined by overhead films. This has been found to be more accurate, particularly with low-density stones and also with heavier patients. This has allowed several patients weighing over 300 pounds to be successfully treated. Fluoroscopy is not used in current models because of the difficulties in visualizing large patients, low-density stones, and small fragments, as well as the increased radiation dosage to the patients and the personnel in the room. The radiation dosage is very low with the Medstone 1050 ST lithotripter (Table 1).

Real-time ultrasound can also be used during the treatment for monitoring of the stone fragmentation.

Following the use of extracorporeal shockwave lithotripsy for the treatment of kidney stones, it became apparent that this technology would be applied to the biliary tract.

A number of considerations increase the complexity of treatment in the biliary tract. Cholecystectomy has been the treatment of choice for approximately the last 100 years. It is safe, in most instances curative, and associated with a short hospital stay. Despite the widespread use of this procedure, shockwave therapy holds considerable appeal for many patients as it is not associated with an incision and the patient can resume normal activity the next day without the abdominal pain that surgery produces. Most gallstones contain cholesterol and occur as a result of a failure of the bile to keep cholesterol dissolved in a micellar solution due to an imbalance in the concentrations of cholesterol, bile acids, and phospholipids in the bile, as well as by factors which contribute to nucleation, gallstone growth, and impairment of gallbladder contraction. The administration of ursodeoxycholic acid, the 7-beta epimer of chenodeoxycholic acid, facilitates cholesterol stone resorption by desaturating the bile.

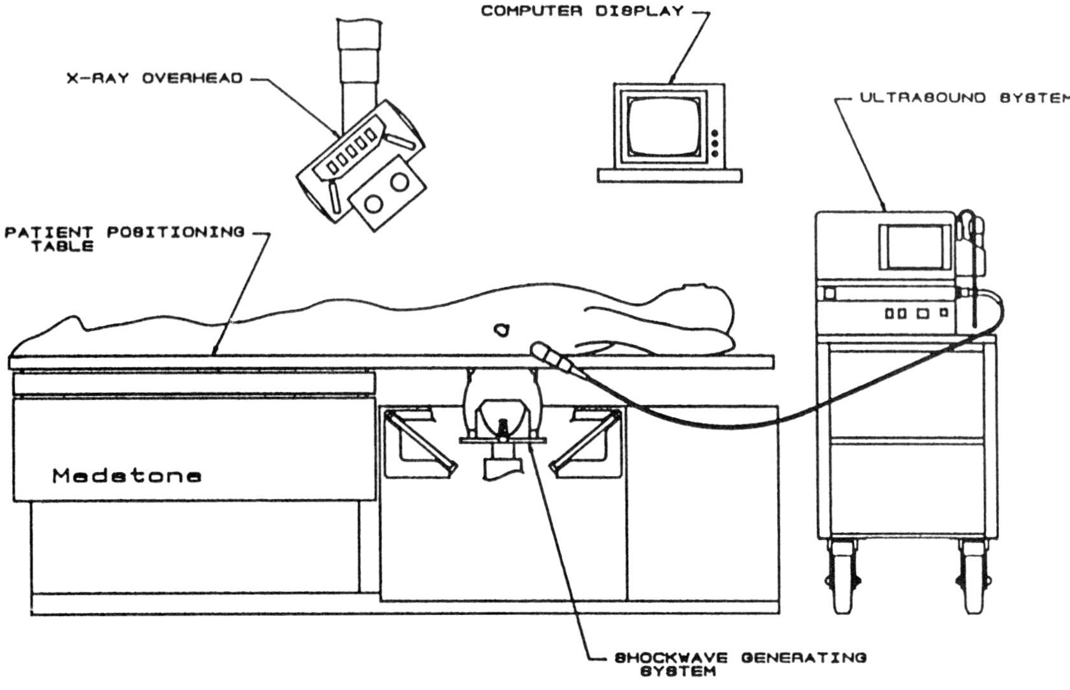

TABLE 1
Estimated Organ Dose from Lithotripsy Procedure Using Medstone 1050 ST

ORGAN	LITHOTRIPSY	KUB	LIMITED IVP	LITHOTRIPSY AS PERCENTAGE OF IVP
	(20 Films)	(1 Film)	(7 Films)	
Testicle	< 1 mR	11 mR	77 mR	< 1%
Ovary	55 mR	140 mR	980 mR	6%
Active Bone Marrow	52 mR	26 mR	182 mR	29%
Embryo	5 mR	189 mR	1323 mR	< 1%

It also produces a choleretic effect that may help to flush out small stone particles. While there is a low incidence of new stone formation after cholecystectomy, shockwave therapy alone would not be expected to change the lithogenic properties of bile or reduce the risk of future stones. It is therefore reasonable to suppose that a percentage of patients' gallstones will recur after lithotripsy unless the lithogenic state of the bile can be altered.

In the gallbladder study initiated at Baylor University Hospital, Dallas, in January 1988, there had been 30 patients treated as of early April 1988. The patients' ages ranged from 26 to 62 years, with a mean age of 43. Their weights ranged from 47 to 99 kg (103 to 218 lbs), with a mean weight of 72 kg (159 lbs). Twenty-five of the patients were women. Ten patients had solitary stones, and 20 had 2 or more stones. Sixteen of the patients had stones 10 mm or less, while 14 had larger stones. Twenty-nine of the 30 patients had their stones fragmented, for a fragmentation rate of 96.6 percent. No significant complications were encountered from the lithotripsy treatments.

For gallstones the real-time ultrasound system is used for positioning as well as monitoring the disintegration of the stones. The ultrasound localization is a unique system that is user-friendly. A freely moveable transducer localizes the gallstone, and through monitoring by overhead sensors the XYZ coordinates are computed. The patient is then positioned for treatment. Because of the freely moveable real-time ultrasound transducer used with the Medstone 1050 ST lithotripter, the not uncommon problem of the misalignment of articulated arm transducers is eliminated.

While lithotripsy for kidney stones has established itself as an effective and safe technique, biliary lithotripsy is in its early stages of development. This emerging modality may be expected to play an important role in the future treatment of calculi in the gallbladder and biliary ducts.

TECHNICAL DESCRIPTION OF THE SIEMENS LITHOSTAR FOR BILIARY LITHOTRIPSY

Laura Lee Murphy

Siemens Medical Systems has conducted studies using the Lithostar system to evaluate the applicability of shockwave lithotripsy on gallstones. These studies have led to the design and manufacture of an additional shock wave generator mounted over the Lithostar table on an articulated arm. This simple upgrade makes the Siemens Lithostar truly a multifunctional, multipurpose lithotripsy system.

The Lithostar is the only lithotripter that uses the electromagnetic principle for shockwave generation. In brief, the electromagnetic technology uses an electric current passed through a coil to produce a magnetic field. The resulting magnetic induction causes an aluminum-rubber membrane to deflect, propagating an acoustic wave through a column of degassed water. The wave is focused with an acoustic lens, generating a highly reproducible shockwave. This technology requires no consumables; the shockwave generators developed by Siemens have an average lifetime worldwide in excess of 200,000 shocks.

The Lithostar provides two undertable shockwave generators with fixed focal depth. Biplanar x-ray is used for localization and focusing. The intersection of the two x-ray planes, one anterior-posterior and one caudal-cranial, corresponds with the focal zone depth of the shockwave generators. Focusing is accomplished by placing the image of the stone in the cross hairs on the monitor for each plane.

The Lithostar allows x-ray imaging with the use of contrast for localization of biliary duct stones. Studies performed with the Lithostar on gallstones around the world led to the incorporation of a third shockwave generator and ultrasound localization into the Lithostar system. The combination of x-ray and ultrasound in one system maximizes the flexibility available for localization.

This third shockwave generator is housed in an overhead module which is easily mounted next to the overhead x-ray tubes. The same proven electromagnetic technology is used for shockwave generation.

The overhead module includes an in-line ultrasound probe for localization of typically radiolucent biliary calculi. The pressure and diameter of the shockwave generator are designed to allow treatment of biliary stones with little or no anesthesia. The overhead module has a diameter of 30 cm and pressures approximately double those of the undertable shockwave generators.

The in-line ultrasound probe can be extended to contact the patient in order to provide excellent images without decoupling the shockwave generator from the patient. Probe extension can be used at any time during the treatment to verify the progress seen with the real-time ultrasound capability.

The ultrasound probe can be rotated 90 degrees to obtain images in two planes. As with the basic Lithostar system, localization is easily achieved by placing the image of the stone in the cross hairs on the ultrasound monitor.

The acoustic lens can be displaced laterally within the housing, allowing for more accurate targeting without repositioning the patient. Fragments visualized with ultrasound can be targeted in this manner. In addition, stone movement can be followed during the procedure with this lateral variation.

Variable focal depth from approximately 4 cm inside the body to roughly 12 cm is achieved via movement of the acoustic lens. Stones can easily be brought into focus without repositioning the patient once coupling has occurred. A wide range of patient anatomies can be treated with this built-in flexibility.

The overhead module is easily manipulated with user-friendly controls. The simple keypad enables rapid technician training and provides a consistent set of commands for the user.

The overhead module is easily moved into a wide number of positions. This maneuverability facilitates optimum pa-

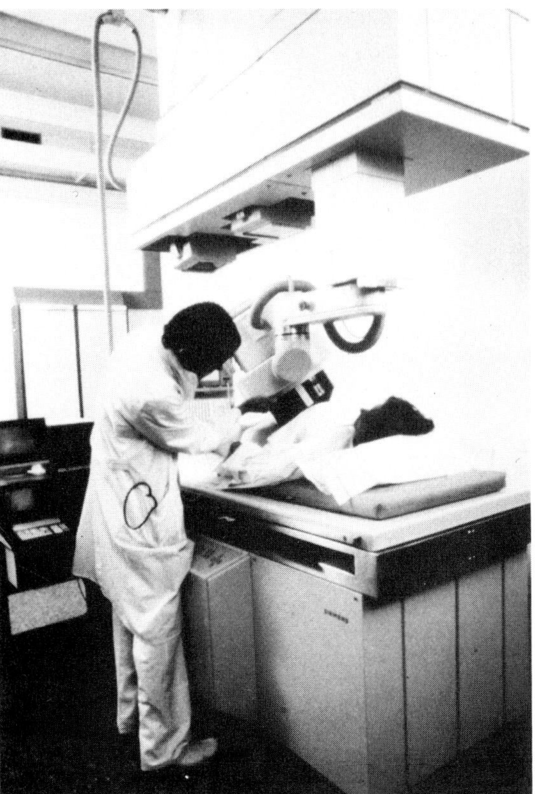

FIG 1.
Lithostar with overhead module in operation.

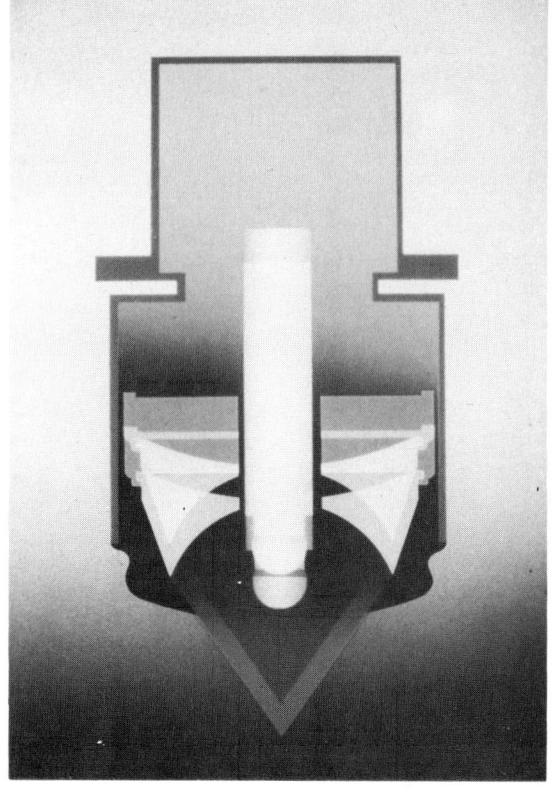

FIG 2.
Shock tube head showing in-line ultrasound probe with variable focal zone depth.

tient positioning so that the shockwave path avoids liver and lung tissue while targeting the gallstones. The patient is first placed in a left lateral position on the table and the shockwave generator is then coupled to the patient.

The overhead module can be parked out of the way so that other procedures, such as ERCP or renal lithotripsy, can be performed on the Lithostar table.

The Lithostar with the overhead module will be used at 10 investigational sites here in the United States to collect data necessary to submit a premarket approval application for biliary calculi. Research and clinical procedures on biliary stones are being performed in Europe and Canada. Data collected at these sites will be verified by the clinical trial sites in the United States.

EDAP LT.01

Robert A. W. Reeders
Executive Vice President
EDAP International Corp.

Overview

The Lithedap LT.01, a new generation lithotripter designed and manufactured by EDAP International of France, is revolutionary in its treatment of urinary lithiasis (kidney stones) and its potential for treating cholelithiasis (gallstones).

Extracorporeal shockwave lithotripsy (ESL) is a proven technique which enables remote disintegration of specific solid matters within the body (urinary stones, gallstones). The Lithedap LT.01 lithotripter device employs a piezoelectric emitter which generates elastic shockwaves of required amplitude and shape focused on the stone in such a manner that stress applied to the structure exceeds its elastic limit, disintegrating the stone and allowing for natural elimination by the body.

The system consists of a lithotripter head which is independent of the table, utilizing a flexible membrane coupling to the patient.

A standard urology table is ergonomically designed for multipurpose use and is fully adjustable for all positions.

Each of the 320 piezoelectric electric transducers is activated by its own generator; therefore, failure of any of these generators will not effect the others, resulting in more than 99 percent uptime.

Inherent to the Lithedap LT.01 is real-time monitoring and targeting.

Piezoelectric emitters produce pulses that are short (1 microsecond), directed at a small focal point, produce no electrical or mechanical interference, and therefore have no effect on the heart rate, lung tissue, or other vital organs. As piezoelectric technology uses a spherical disk with a mosaic of 320 piezoelectric crystals, the energy transmitter through each element is moderate which allows for durability and does not require periodic replacement of components. Electrohydraulic emitters generate massive amounts of energy through the use of electrodes which generally require replacement prior to each patient treatment. Therefore, the electrohydraulic method is more expensive than the EDAP LT.01 and requires far more maintenance by qualified technicians.

Because the piezoelectric emitter is able to transmit elastic waves of short duration and has an adjustble power setting, patients are now able to receive treatment without anesthesia or analgesia. Conventional lithotripters, which make use of a huge and archaic electrohydraulic emitter, transmit waves that are painful to the patient. The more intense shocks produced by this device requires anesthesia. Pain experienced by the patient is proportional to the firing rate; only the piezoelectric emitter allows adjustment of the power and frequency of waves produced (from 1 to 128 per second). The EDAP treatment involves a gradual erosion of the stone as opposed to an "explosion" caused by first-generation lithotripters. There is also significant noise reduction with the EDAP LT.01, which in turn reduces patient stress.

Because of the Lithedap LT.01's ability to focus shockwaves accurately and precisely, individual treatment time is reduced. Coupled with the decreased need for general or local anesthesia, treatment with the Lithedap LT.01 results in decreased costs and lower risk for both the hospital and patient.

The entire procedure is done on an outpatient basis without surgery, anesthesia, or hospitalization.

The new-generation EDAP technology, now under investigation, represents lower operating costs and a more reliable implementation for the treatment of cholelithiasis.

Energy is transmitted to the patient by utilizing a flexible membrane coupling.

The lithotripter operates 60 degrees in three planes so there is good patient access. It is the lithotripter that is adjusted while the patient remains in a comfortable supine or prone position.

Our European experience has confirmed the Lithedap LT.01 features in treating gallbladder stones; over 600 patients have already been treated worldwide with a high success rate.

EDAP International Corporation has obtained an investigational device exemption from the Federal Food and Drug Administration for gallstone lithotripsy testing at 10 sites.

Functional Description

The EDAP LT.01 Lithotripter, pictured in Figure 1, consists of the following major components:

- Treatment head and support
- Electronic generator
- Ultrasound scanner
- Control console
- Treatment table
- Power supply
- Optional peripheral equipment

TREATMENT HEAD AND SUPPORT

The treatment head, illustrated in Figure 2, is the major element of the LT.01 system and serves two purposes: it combines an ultrasound imaging probe for localization of the stone and a piezoelectric system for destruction of the stone, both of which are housed in a fluid-filled container.

The stone destruction system is based on the convergence on a single focal point of a series of ultrashort (less than 1 microsecond) shockwave pulses generated by 320 ceramic piezoelectric elements. This system is depicted in Figure 3. The piezoelectric elements are uniformly distributed across the surface of a segment of a spherical cup and around the ultrasound imaging transducer. In this way they are all focused on the same point, located at the center of the sphere. Each piezoelectric element is excited by a separate emitter module in the electronic generator. A shockwave is produced when all 320 piezoelectric elements are pulsed in synchrony and the resulting individual pressure waves are focused exactly at the center of the sphere that constitutes the focal point.

Each piezoelectric element used in the treatment head contains a titanade lead zirconate ceramic made by the French company Quartz et Silice. Each element is 20 mm in

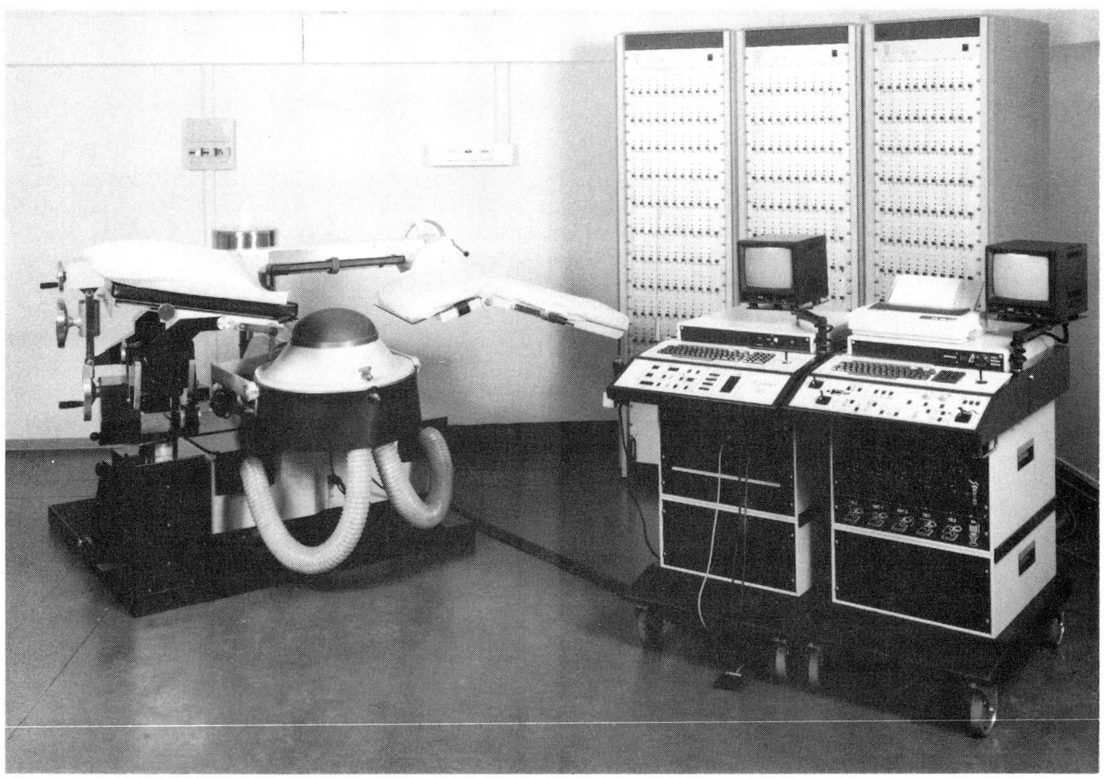

FIG 1.
The EDAP LT.01.

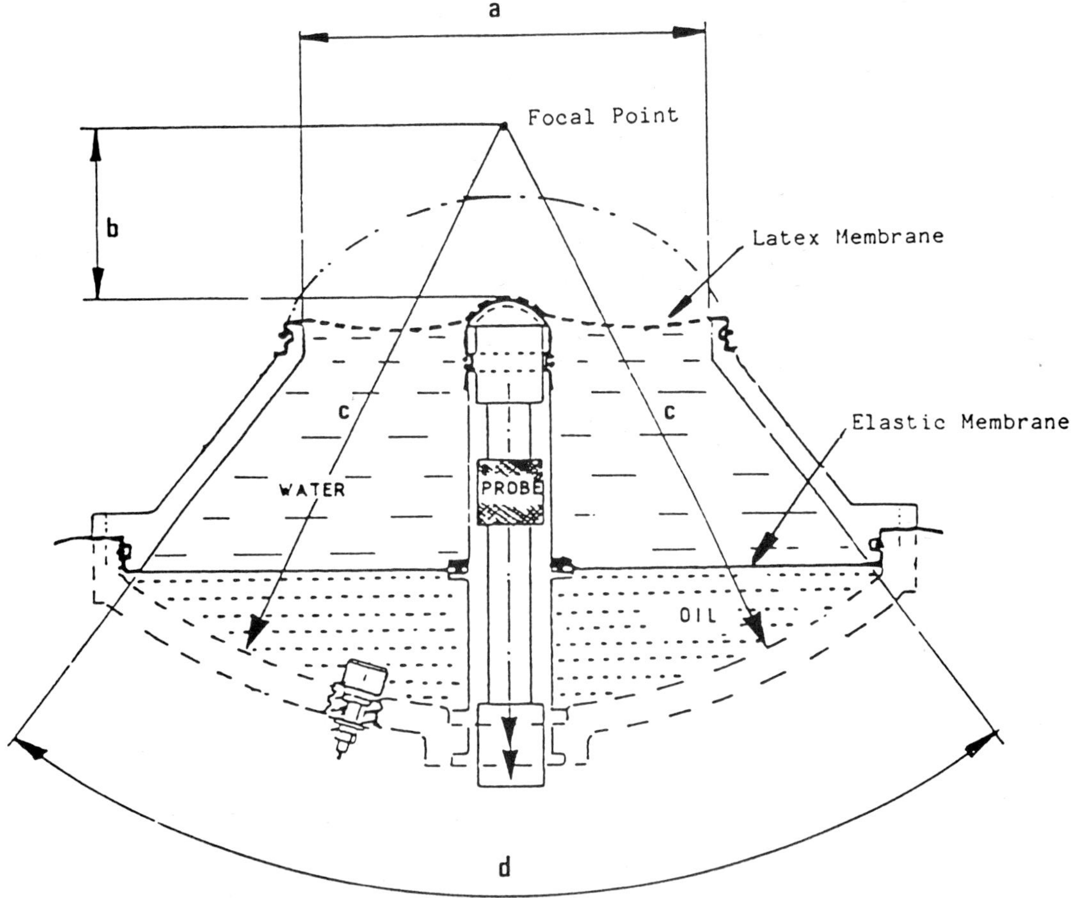

FIG 2.
Treatment head; a = diameter of treatment head; b = distance to focal point (fully inflated); c = radius of spherical cup; d = angle of emitting surface.

diameter and 5 mm thick and is highly damped to produce short pulses. The complete assembly is injection molded in plastic, and each element is removable.

There are 320 piezoelectric elements mounted on the surface of the spherical cup. Each of the piezoelectric elements has a surface area of 3.14 cm^2. Thus the total transmitting surface area is approximately 1005 cm^2 spread out over the area of the spherical cup.

The spherical segment of the cup with the piezoelectric elements is covered with insulating oil. An elastomer membrane separates the oil from a water chamber.

The water chamber is made of a light alloy cone placed over the spherical cup and closed at its upper part with a flexible latex membrane. The chamber has a variable height, which is adjusted by adding or removing water. The latex membrane is placed into contact with the lumbar fossa of the patient, making immersion in a tub unnecessary. An ultrasound conducting gel is placed on the membrane to ensure a good contact between the membrane and the patient's skin. By inflating or deflating the water chamber, the distance between the focus and the surface of the membrane can be varied from 0 to about 14.6 cm.

The pulse produced by the piezoelectric elements is very brief (approximately one microsecond), which reduces the risk of damage to biological tissues. An oscilloscopic illustration of the pressure pulse at the focus is given in Figure 4.

A real time 5 MHz sectorial ultrasound probe is fitted through a cylindrical sleeve at the center of the treatment head. The probe is connected to the ultrasound scanner (see description below). The probe is a rotating transducer and provides longitudinal and transverse images and all oblique views.

The ultrasound probe provides an image of the area around the focal point of the shockwaves, which is displayed on the ultrasound scanner monitor. The ultrasound scanner provides an electronic cursor that marks the position of the

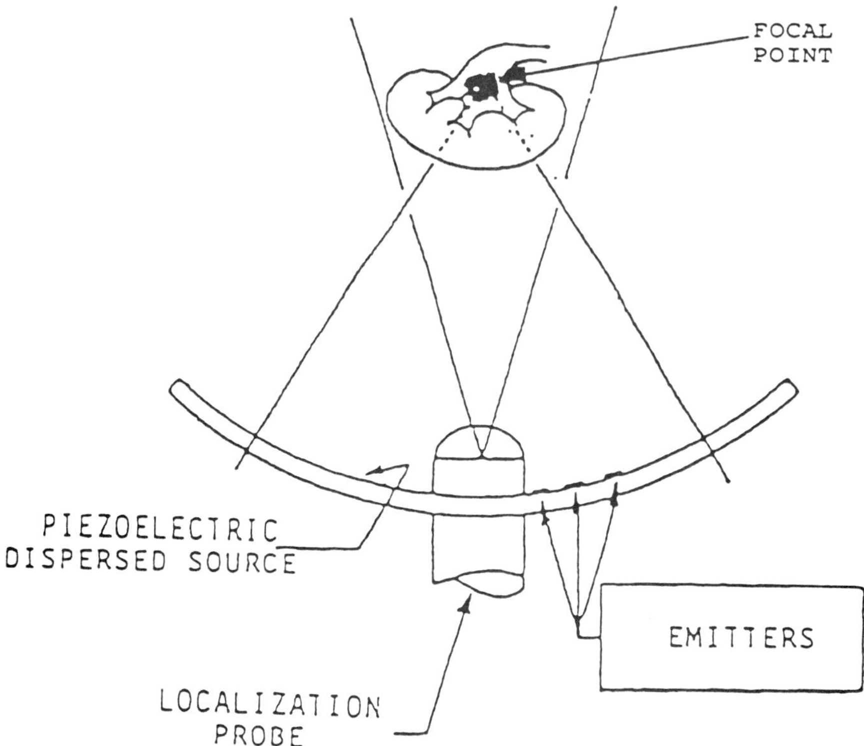

FIG 3.
Diagram of components of treatment head.

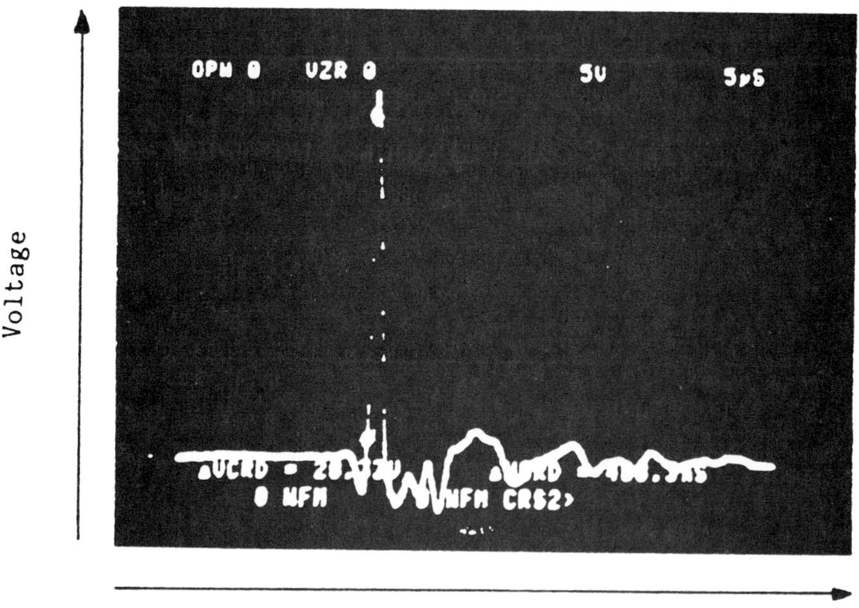

FIG 4.
Oscilloscope pattern of pressure pulse at the focal point (pulse duration = approximately 1 microsecond).

focal point on the scanner monitor so that the stone can be precisely positioned. Using the displayed image, the progress made in disintegration may be monitored in real time throughout the entire treatment.

The treatment head is mounted on a mobile support and is controlled electronically from the control console and can be moved in five different directions: three linear ones (X, Y, and Z) and two rotating ones in perpendicular planes. The movable support is placed under the treatment table and can be locked in place. In use, the treatment head is positioned so that it is in direct contact with the patient and the patient's stone is positioned in the treatment head focal using the ultrasound scanner.

A reservoir for water is also located on the movable treatment head support. The reservoir can be raised or lowered with an electric jack and is connected to the treatment head with a flexible tube. It supplies water to fill the treatment head.

Since the treatment head can be oriented in all directions, the best firing axis can be selected. The energy delivered can be adjusted by means of a potentiometer on the control console. The rate of firing can be varied from 1.25 to 160 shots per second. In most applications, firing rates below 5 or 10 shots per second are used to reduce the pain level and avoid the use of anesthetics.

The pressure wave generated by this treatment system has extremely steep sides, reaching its maximum within one microsecond (see Figure 4). In vivo, the maximum pressure at the focus is approximately 900 bars. The pressure pulse falls as rapidly as it rises and does not possess any significant negative components. The size of the focal point is approximately 5 mm by 23 mm.

ELECTRONIC GENERATOR

The electronic generator is the powering unit for the piezoelectric elements on the treatment head. The generator contains 320 emitter modules mounted in 32 racks and distributed in three cabinets (two cabinets have 11 emitter module racks and one cabinet has 10). The 320 emitter modules contain high-power semiconductors that excite the corresponding piezoelectric elements arranged in the spherical segment of the treatment head.

All of the piezoelectric elements are actuated simultaneously, using a single pilot board that supplies controlling signals to 320 emitter modules through a series of buffering stages. The pilot board generates the command signals, which control each module in the generator as well as the go-stop orders.

The frequency of firing is controlled from the electronic generator central rack. Firing frequencies can be selected from a front panel control and can have the following values: 1.25, 2.5, 5, 10, 20, 40, 80, or 160 Hz.

ULTRASOUND SCANNER

The ultrasound scanner, illustrated in Figure 5, is a mechanical sector scanner for localization of the calculus. The commercially available EDAP Sonedap 260 Universal Ultrasound Scanner has been adapted for this purpose.

Continuous real-time visualization of the area under treatment using the ultrasound scanner allows very precise positioning and monitoring of the position of the stone.

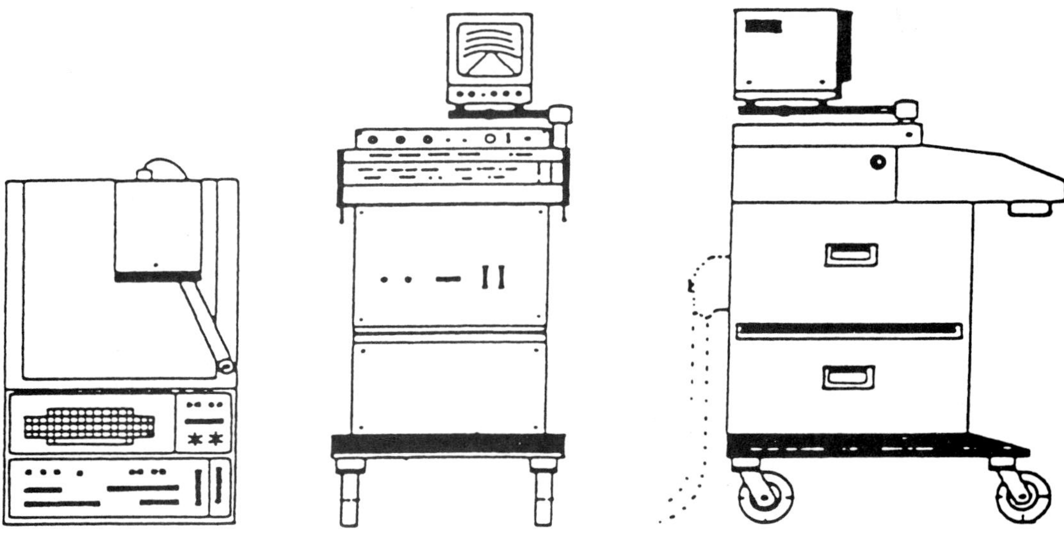

FIG 5.
Ultrasound scanner.

The ultrasound scanner is equipped with a circuit that detects the presence of the stone in the focal point and controls discharges according to this presence. This feature is used especially if the stone makes large movements due to the patient's breathing. When used, the circuit automatically fires the lithotripter only when an echo is detected in an area corresponding to the focus. The detection level is adjustable so that the echo presented by the stone can be selected from other echos.

PROBES

The LT.01 system is equipped with two probes that are wide in diameter so as to obtain optimal focalization. In both probes, the focusing is achieved through acoustic lenses mounted directly on the crystals. One of these probes is operated manually, and the other is an integral part of the treatment head.

The hand-operated probe is a standard mechanical sector probe operating at 4.8 MHz. The crystal diameter is 20 mm, the focus is in the range of 7 to 10 cm, and the maximum sweep angle is 90 degrees. The probe is used to verify the position of the calculus and the possibility of access prior to the installation of the patient of the treatment table. This prior localization serves for piloting the movement of the treatment head later.

The localization probe is a 5 MHz mechanical sector probe that operates at 3.3 MHz and is mounted in the center of the treatment head. It is coupled to the water bath through a water membrane to avoid any leakage of water. The treatment head, and therefore the localization probe, is movable in all directions by a remote control. The crystal diameter of the probe is 30 mm, and the focus is in the range of 120-150 mm. This long focus is necessary to take into account the water path between the probe and the patient's skin. The localizing probe is used for the precise, real-time imaging of the calculus prior to and during treatment.

CONTROL CONSOLE

The control console, illustrated in Figure 1, consolidates all system controls except those for the ultrasound scanner. The frame of the console is identical to that of the scanner and is placed to the right of it. The control console is composed of three major parts:

a) Control Panel. The control panel comprises all the controls. Significant controls include those for the selection of the motion of the treatment head and the different treatment modes. The LT-01 operator's manual provides a detailed description of the control panel functions and use.

All displacements of the treatment head are controlled by joysticks, and the coordinates of the position are displayed on the monitor of the control console. The treatment mode is determined by operator-adjustable controls which define the rate of shots and the amplitude of the shockwaves. All necessary information concerning the treatment is displayed on the monitor, for example, the maximum power, the mean power, the total energy produced, and the number of shots. Either manual or automatic firing modes can be selected. In automatic firing mode, the lithotripter fires only when the echo of the stone is detected within the focal point.

b) Computerized control system and monitor. An Acorn Microcomputer Model BBC Master is integrated into the control console and is used to display information relative to the position of the treatment head, record the patient's file, and drive a printer for reports. When the control panel is turned on, the program is loaded automatically and is ready to operate.

c) Manual control switches. These switches are located on the lower front of the control console and may be used to manually position the treatment head.

TREATMENT TABLE

The treatment table, illustrated in Figure 1, is a multiposition table which allows for the placement of patients in various positions useful in urology. The table allows a plain x-ray or fluoroscopic image to be performed by horizontal rotation. The table is also fitted with two leg pieces which are useful for endoscopic manipulations concomitant with extracorporeal lithotripsy, for example, flushing of ureteric stones.

PRODUCT SPECIFICATIONS

a) Shockwave generator

type	piezoelectric
diameter of water bladder	306 mm
water bladder height adjustments	0 to 14.6 cm
diameter of focal point	approximately 5 mm × 23 mm
focal point pressure	adjustable, approximately 0 to 900 bars
pulse rates	1.25, 2.5, 5, 10, 20, 40, 80, 160 Hz

b) Stone location method: Integral ultrasound imager with fixed and hand probes

c) Mechanical movements of treatment head

linear	
longitudinal	255 mm
transversal	270 mm
vertical	140 mm
rotation	
Y axis	± 30 degrees
X axis	± 30 degrees
Z axis (ultrasound probe only)	± 100 degrees

RICHARD WOLF: PIEZOLITH 2300

H. Wurster

The Wolf Company, well known in the endoscopic field and endoscopic stone treatment, started in 1978 to develop extracorporeal shockwave equipment for kidney stones.

Spark-gap generators were primarily used until 1980, when piezoceramic transmitters were constructed and tested. It was eventually demonstrated that the piezoelectric effect is useful in generating shockwaves that have enough energy to destroy stones.

Shockwave Generator

The piezoceramic elements, made of lead zirconate titanate, are fused together and polarized into the direction for operation.

If a voltage is applied to such elements, they may expand or contract, depending on the polarity. The degree of movement is proportional to the amount of the voltage. An array of such piezo elements forms the shockwave transducer.

There is an acoustic backing on each of the elements that has to be matched to the crystals and is very important for the proper function of such a system. If a high-voltage pulse is applied to the elements, the ceramic expands, and a positive pressure pulse is emitted and transmitted to the focal point.

The shockwave transducer is made of multiple small piezoceramic elements that in toto give a better performance. To get the energy needed, about 3,000 of these elements placed in a spherical array are necessary.

To get a high gain and a small focal point, the aperture of the transducer was made large. Figure 1 compares the piezo transducer to the spark gap in which the shockwave is generated directly by the spark discharge at Fl, reflected at the ellipsoid, and then refocused at F2.

In the piezo system, an ultrasonic wave is generated, which directly propagates to the focal point and on its way the shockwave front is established.

Due to the nonlinear relation between sound speed in water versus pressure, which starts at about 300 bars, the low-pressure parts of the pressure pulse are slower than the high-pressure parts of the pulse, which leads to a stepping up of the pulse shape.

Therefore, by propagation of the sound pulse, the rise time shortens the closer the pulse gets to the focal point. Due to accumulation of the positive pressure parts, there is a much larger increase in the positive than in the negative part of the pulse, which is very beneficial in terms of minimizing tissue destruction.

The Piezolith transducer has a focal point of about 3 mm in diameter and 11 mm in length (half pressure). Compared to focal points of low-aperture spark-gap systems, with 12 mm focal diameter, the energy ratio calculated at the same pressure output is 16. It has been shown clinically that the Piezolith causes no pain during its application, and the reason for this is the large aperture which allows distribution of the energy over a large skin surface area.

In addition, measurements show that the shockwave front forms some centimeters before the focal point, so that the wave entering the skin may not actually be a shockwave.

The pressures achieved with the 4 power settings are between 600 and 1,200 bars. The maximum pressure depends on the excitation of the piezoceramic crystal and of the efficiency of the piezoceramic itself.

For skin coupling to transmit the shockwave into the patient's body, water has proven to be the best transmission medium. It has to be degassed and the temperature adjusted to the patient's comfort. Air bubbles at the patient's skin surface should be wiped off so they do not disturb sound penetration.

The Location System

The location system is as important as the system for stone disintegration. The Piezolith 2300 uses real-time ultra-

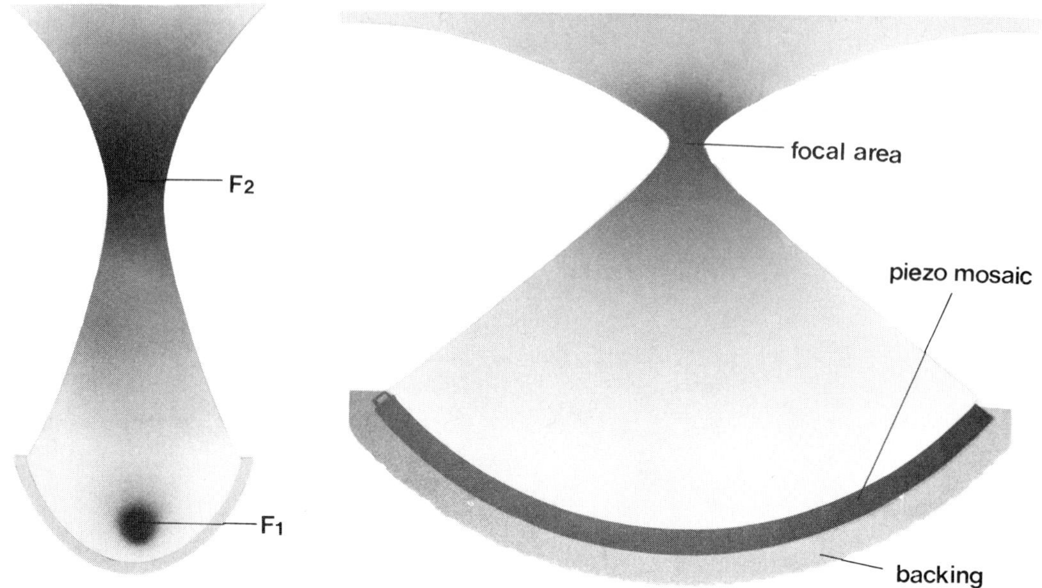

FIG 1.
A. Ellipsoid transducer; **B.** Piezoelectric transducer.

sound for location, which has proven very effective. It is important that the ultrasound scanner is oriented in line with the direction the shockwave is propagated. This is to confirm the ultrasonic shockwave pathway and to assure that there are no obstacles such as air bubbles, which will reflect the shockwaves, and bones, which reflect too much of the energy. These obstacles can be shown with ultrasound but cannot be seen using x-rays.

The system was initially designed with a single diagnostic ultrasound scanner mounted centrally in the piezomosaic array. However, it was found that in some cases stone localization was difficult because of ribs. Therefore, two ultrasound scanners are now used, each inclined 15° to the central axis. One displays the caudal and the other the cranial field. With this two-scanner method, the user can select that scanner which is more suitable for the ultrasonic image information. One scanner is used at a time, and the other is in park position. The scanners are integrated into the spherical transducer; they are adjustable in their height and can be rotated by 90° to move the scanning plane into transverse and longitudinal position (Fig 2).

The advantage of an ultrasonic location system versus x-ray, which was used in the early lithotripters, is that there is no radiation exposure to the patient during localization, and therefore continuous observation of the stone with ultrasound is possible. This is of critical importance because the small focal point of the shockwave generator and respiratory movements of the patient may allow the stone to move out of the focus. Shockwaves would then miss the stones and be absorbed by tissues. By continuous real-time ultrasound monitoring, shockwaves release can be interrupted for repositioning to produce an effective treatment with minimal tissue injury (Fig 3).

To get a good ultrasonic image, it is important that the diagnostic scanner head is touching the patient's skin. There is also no adverse effect of the shockwave on heart rhythm. Extrasystoles are not created, and therefore ECG-triggered release of the shockwave is not necessary.

The final well-known advantage of the ultrasound localization system is that all stones can be seen with ultrasound, even though they are radiolucent. Of course, most cholesterol stones are radiolucent. Therefore, ultrasound localization is the method of choice for gallstones.

Treatment

For gallbladder stones, the patient is placed in the prone position on the treatment table so that the body is partially within the water bath to guarantee good contact of the shockwaves. The spherical dish with integrated US-scanners is then moved in three directions—transverse, longitudinal, and vertical—to identify the gallstone. If the stone is seen, it is brought into the cross hair, which is electronically displayed on the monitor and represents the focal point of the spherical dish (Fig 4).

All the functions of the machine are controlled from the console, which is connected to the treatment table by a 2-meter-long connection hose.

If the stone is in the cross hair, the shockwaves are released either manually or continuously by pressing the bot-

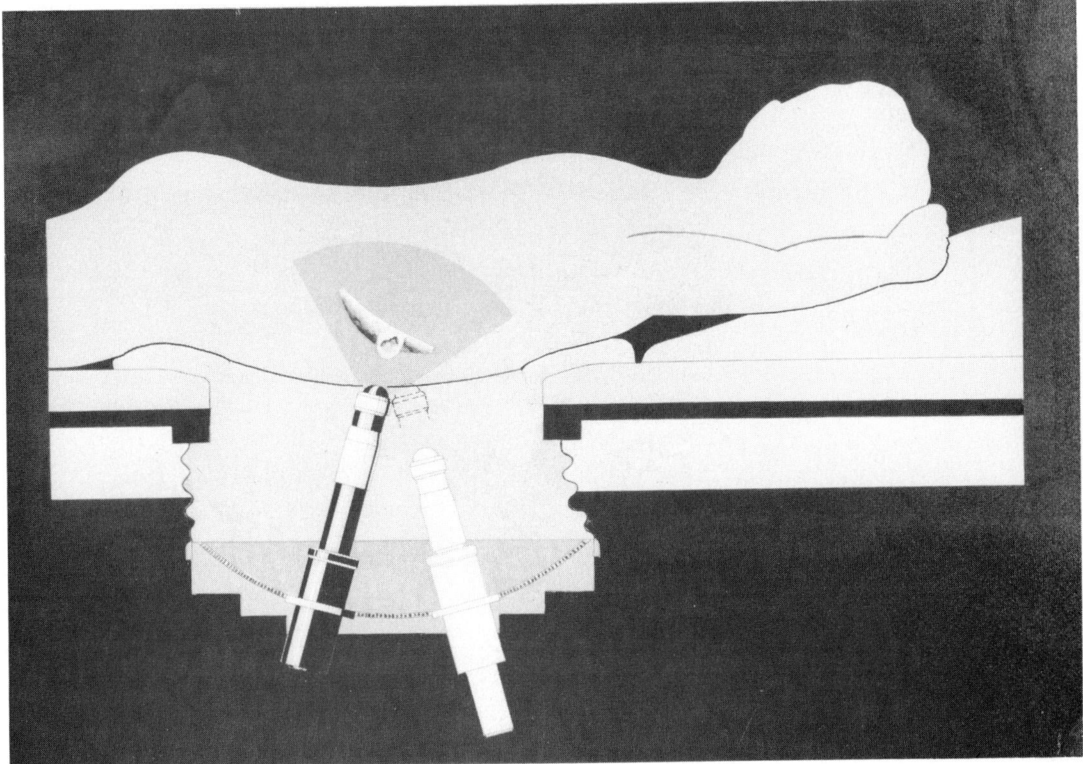

FIG 2.
Location system with dual ultrasound scanners.

tom. Shockwave administration should be given only under direct ultrasonic monitoring; to guarantee a safe and effective treatment, shockwaves should be released only when the stone is in the focal point within the cross hair.

During stone destruction, the acoustic shadow of the stone gets fainter and the echogenic arc of the stone gets wider. This is a sign that the stone is disintegrated and the treatment should be stopped. The stone actually erodes from the surface shock by shock like a woodpecker. The treatment is totally painfree, and no analgesia or sedation is needed. However, very anxious patients may wish some sedation.

Most of the patients fall asleep during treatment, for the warm water is very soothing. Since there is really no preparation of the patient before treatment, a treatment which cannot be completed fully in one session can be completed in a second session.

To disintegrate a 10 mm gallstone, about 1,500 to 2,500 shocks are needed. The number of shocks depends on the hardness of the stones, inasmuch as soft gallstones need more shocks for disintegration than harder kidney stones. This is due to differences in acoustical impedance.

The range of indications for use of the Piezolith is very wide. Without major modifications of the unit, it can be used to treat kidney stones and ureteral stones in the upper and lower part of the ureter excluding the pelvic ureter, which is obstructed by bone.

While gallbladder stones are very easy to find and treat with this unit, common bile duct stones can also be treated in the supine position if they can be seen with ultrasound and are not covered by the air-filled duodenum.

The Unit

The unit was designed to be very universal and mobile. Therefore, it consists of two parts, the treatment table and the operating console.

The treatment table contains all parts needed to do the shockwave treatment, especially the spherical piezoceramic shockwave transducer, which is movable in four directions: longitudinal, transversal, vertical, and cranial tilt.

The treatment system for the water is incorporated and provides for the water to be degassed and heated to body temperature.

There is a hydraulic system for sliding out the table plate

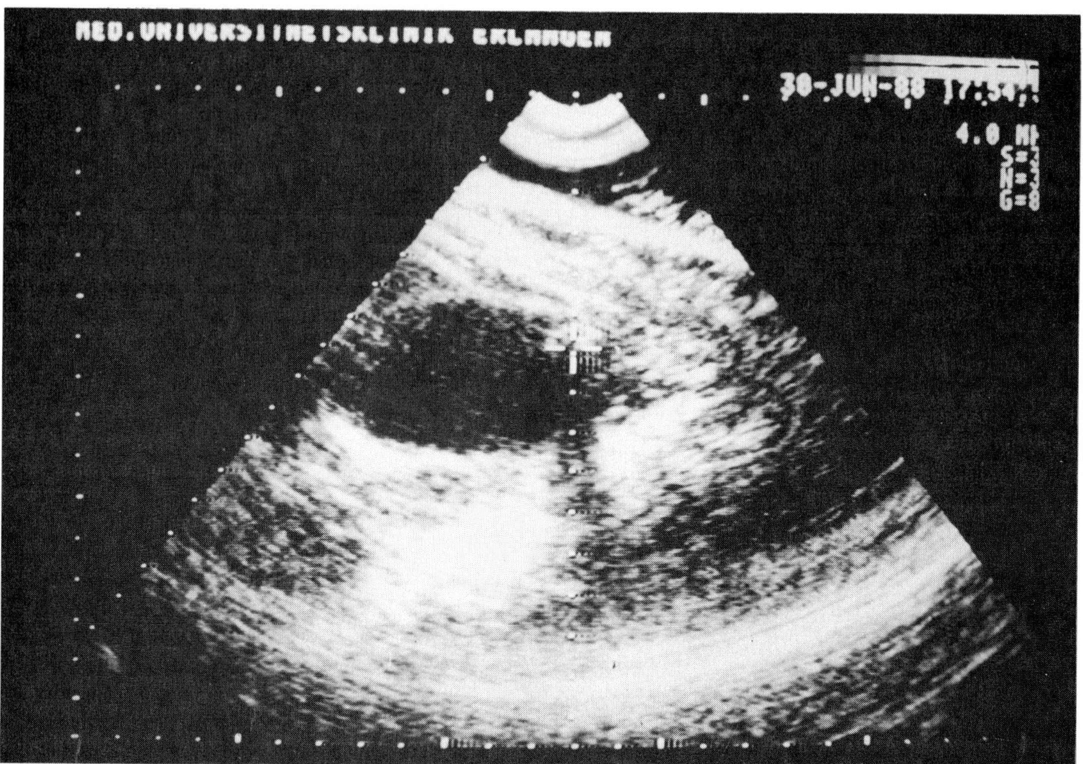

FIG 3.
Ultrasonic image of gallstone.

when the table is used for other urological treatments or if a fluoroscopic C-arm is needed to make x-rays of the area treated without moving the patient.

The console contains the ultrasonic unit, the monitor, and all the keyboards needed to operate the machine and control the ultrasonic unit, including input of patient data on the screen for documentation. The shockwave power can be set in four separate steps, and the shockwave repetition rate can also be selected in four steps from 0.5 to 2.5 per second. Digital readouts display the position of the spherical transducer, temperature of the water, number of shockwaves given, scanner height, and rotation position.

The unit is mobile, can be moved on casters, and thus needs no special site preparation. Facilities required include a wall outlet with power of 3.5 kW at 50 or 60 cycles and a water tap with cold or warm water as well as a sink for the used water. Most of the power is used for warming up the water. The lithotripter can be used in any room that provides these conveniences.

With regard to the operating personnel, one person could do the total treatment. Most times this person is the physician.

There are nearly no operating or maintenance costs. Due to the mobility of the unit, it can also be transported easily into a van from one hospital to another and then moved inside for treatments. This concept has worked well in Europe.

Results

Many of the Piezolith 2300 systems that have been in operation for kidney stones have also been used for gallstone treatment. Up to now more than 300 gallbladder patients have been treated and their gallbladder stones disintegrated. Due to the long dissolution time of the stone fragments, even with ursodeoxycholic acid, the stone-free success rate can not yet be given completely. It appears, however, that the short-term results show that they are comparable to those reported from Dornier in Munich. The results from Erlangen (Dr. Ell) and London (Prof. Dowling) will be presented in this volume.

Stones in the common bile duct have also been treated if endoscopic methods have failed. About 40 common bile duct stones have been treated successfully.

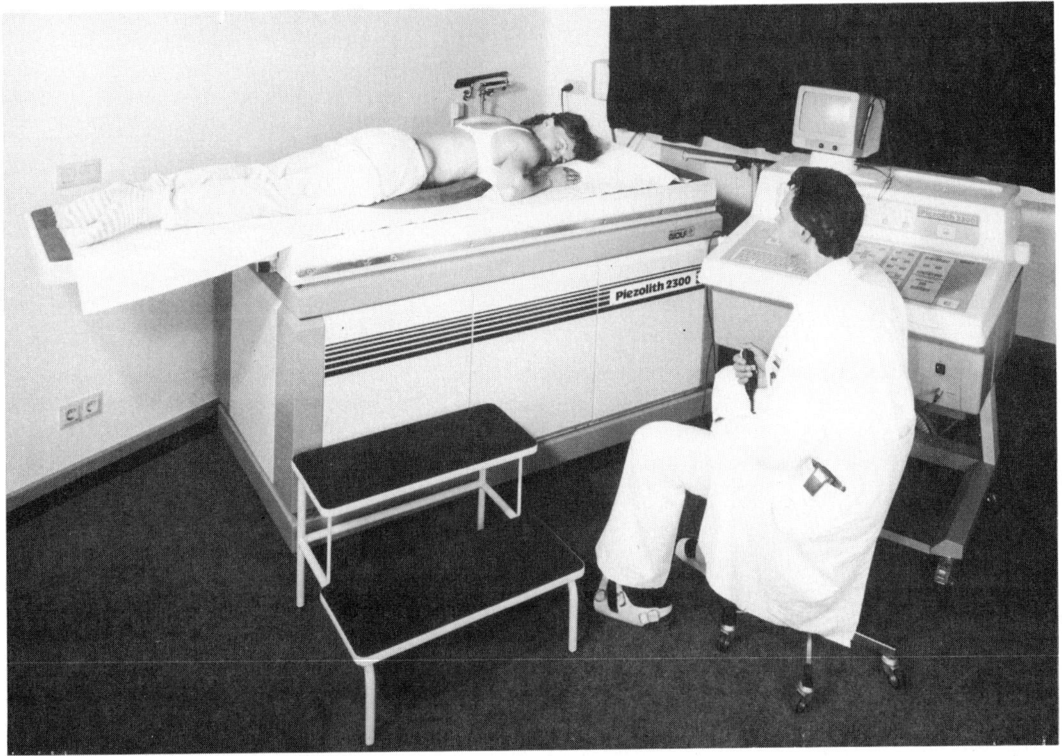

FIG 4.
Treatment of gallbladder stones with patient in the prone position on the Piezolith 2300.

REFERENCES

1. Riedlinger R, Ueberle F, Wurster H, Krauss W, Vallon P, Konrad G, Kopper B, Stoll HP, Goebbels R, Gebhardt T, Ziegler M: Die Nertrümmerung von Mierensteinen durch piezoelektrisch erzeugte Hochenergie-Schallpulse. Physikalische Grundlagen und experimentelle Untersuchungen, *Urologe A* 1986; 25:188–192.
2. Krass W, Vallon P, Wurster H: Der Piezolith—eine piezoelektrische Geräteeinheit zur extrakorporalen Zertrümmerung von Nierensteinen, in von Manfred Ziegler, ed: *Die extrakorporale und laserinduzierte Stosswellenlithotripsie bei Harn- und Gallensteinen: Grundlagen—Anwendung—Klinik* Springer, 1987.
3. Ziegler M, Mast G, Neisius D, Zwergel Th, Riedlinger R, Wurster H: Die schmerzfreie extrakorporale piezoelektrische Lithotripsie (EPL) von Harnsteinen, Dt. Ärzteblatt 84, A-2452 – A-2461, bzw. B-1704 – B-1712 (1987).
4. Coptcoat MJ, Miller RA, Wickham JEA, eds, Lithotripsy II, London, BDI publishing, 1987.
5. Hood KA, Dowling RH, Keightley A, Dick JA, Mallinson C: Piezo-ceramic lithotripsy of gallbladder stones: Initial experience in 31 patients. *Lancet*, June 11, 1988, pp 41–43.
6. Tolley DA, Reid J: Painless lithotripsy. *Lancet,* March 19, 1988, pp 650–651.
7. Bird NC, Johnson AG, Ross B: Lithotripsy of gallstones. *Lancet,* Dec. 19, 1987, pp 1468–1469.
8. Ell Ch, Kerzel W, Heyder N, Becker V, Hermanek P, Domschke W: Piezoelectric lithotripsy of gallstones. *Lancet,* Nov. 14, 1987, pp 1449–1450.
9. Ell Ch, Domschke W: Extrakorporale Lithotripsie von Gallensteinen. *Deutsche Medizinische Wochenschrift* 113 (1988): 317–318.
10. Marberger M, Türk Ch, Steinkogler I: Painless piezo-electric extracorporeal Lithotripsy. *AUA Journal of Urology,* Vol. 139, April 1988: 695–699.
11. Sackmann M, Delius M, Sauerbruch T, Holl J, Weber W, Ippisch E, Hagelauer U, Wess O, Hepp W, Brendel W, Paumgartner G: Shock-wave lithotripsy of gallbladder stones. *N Engl J Med,* 318(7):393–397.

DIASONICS: THERASONIC LITHOTRIPSY TREATMENT SYSTEM

J. Pell, A. Stein, and K.W. Marich

The THERASONIC Lithotripsy Treatment System combines the clinical advantages of ultrasonic shock wave technology with both x-ray *and* ultrasound imaging for accurate localization and real-time treatment monitoring. The system was designed for treatment of renal and biliary calculi. In addition, the modular design allows the SPA 1000 ultrasound and UroView x-ray systems to be used independently for other diagnostic and therapeutic procedures. This versatility, combined with dramatically reduced siting and operating costs, results in superior financial performance and should bring the opportunity for lithotripsy treatment within the reach of smaller medical centers.

SYSTEM COMPONENTS AND FUNCTIONS

The THERASONIC Lithotripsy Treatment System consists of three major components, providing a physician with the ability to localize stones using x-ray or ultrasound, position the patient over the shock wave apparatus, and disintegrate the stone under real-time ultrasound observation (Fig 1). The specifics of each component are described below:

THERASONIC CONTROL CONSOLE.—The THERASONIC Control Console is incorporated in the Diasonics SPA 1000 ultrasound system (Fig 2). The SPA 1000 is a complete, fully functional ultrasound system that can be used with the lithotripter or independently. When used with the lithotripter, the ultrasound console functions as the lithotripsy operator's console, displaying the localization image as well as providing real-time viewing of stone fragmentation.

UROVIEW X-RAY SYSTEM.—The UroView X-Ray System consists of the tomographic version of the Liebel-Flarsheim HUT III urology table with a Diasonics fluoroscopy system. The x-ray console, which comes with display screens, is programmed to calculate three-dimensional positioning from two x-ray projections and communicate the position information to the lithotripsy system controller.

THERASONIC Treatment Table

The THERASONIC Treatment Table is a moveable table that physically docks to the x-ray system and consists of the major subsystems listed below:

Piezoelectric Stonebreaker Assembly
Custom, Coaxial Ultrasound Probe
5-Axes Positioning System
System Controller Electronics
Power Supplies and Patient Table

PRINCIPLES OF OPERATION

ACOUSTIC PRESSURE WAVE GENERATOR AND FOCUSING ASSEMBLY

The pressure wave generator consists of a mosaic of piezoelectric elements mounted in a flat, 40-cm circular pattern and electrically driven in parallel by a high-energy pulse source.

The acoustic energy generated by the piezoelectric elements creates uniform planar pressure waves that are focused to a nominal spot size of 2.5 mm diameter by an acoustic lens mounted integral to the transducer array. The pressure wave is coupled to the body through a water cushion. The focal distance was chosen with the requirement of efficient stone breaking up to 12 cm from the skin surface. The pressure at the focal region bears a linear relationship to the excitation voltage and, therefore, is easily adjusted for a specific application.

SERVO POSITIONING AND REAL-TIME STONE VISUALIZATION

The five-axes positioner system positions the shock wave generator such that the shock wave path propagates along the best anatomical window with the focus on the urinary stone. The localization of the stone is aided by the real-time high-resolution image generated by the coaxially mounted

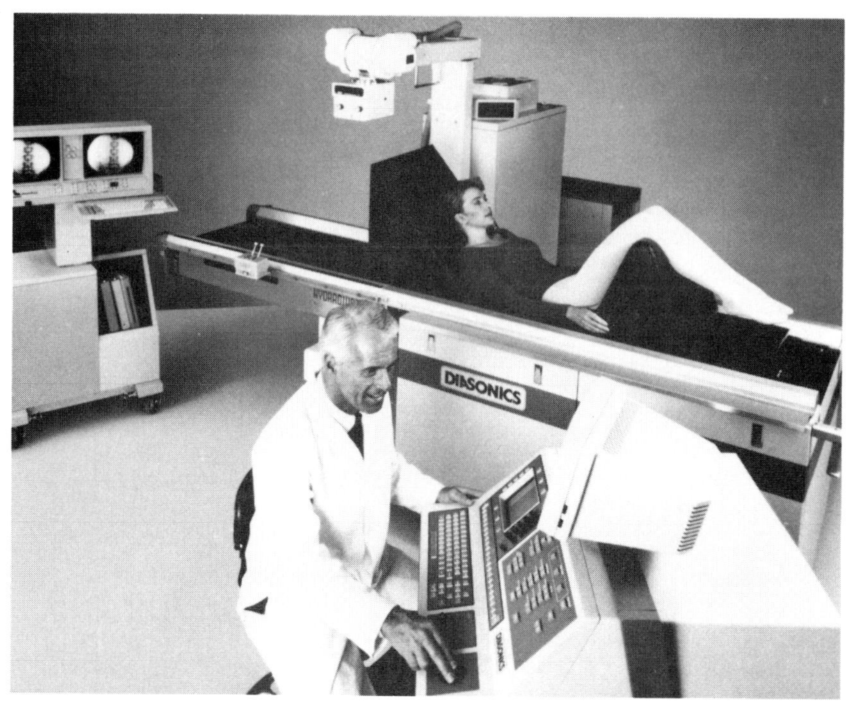
DIASONICS

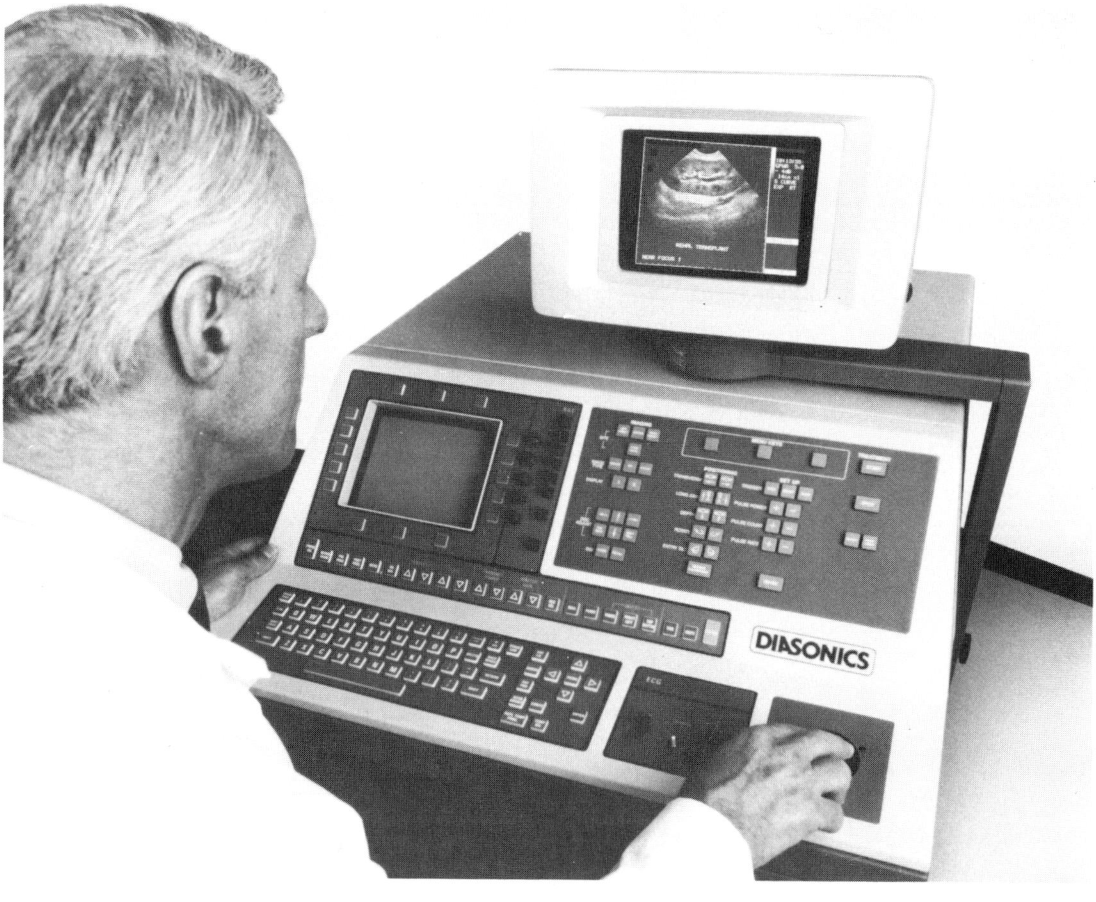

FIG 1.
THERASONIC Lithotripsy Treatment System combines the clinical advantages of ultrasonic shock wave generation technology with both x-ray and ultrasound imaging for accurate localization and real-time treatment monitoring.

sector scan ultrasound transducer (Fig 3). The imaging transducer is a 50-mm annular array, mechanically scanned over a 60-degree sector.

The real-time image is displayed on the ultrasound imaging system and a trackball-controlled cursor is used to position the shock wave focus. The system automatically moves the shock wave generator assembly to focus the shock wave at the point indicated by the operator.

The stone disintegration process is monitored in real time by the ultrasound imaging system and can be triggered to fire only when the stone is in the focus, thus minimizing the number of unnecessary shocks and reducing the overall duration of the procedure.

DEVICE OPERATION

The physician may choose, if appropriate, to acquire a flat film x-ray as a baseline. For x-ray localization, the UroView system will be used in tomographic mode. The operator simply defines the stone position in the two views acquired (Fig 4), and the system will calculate the stone position in three-dimensional space. This positional data will be transferred to system controller, and the patient is moved to the treatment table (Fig 5).

The physician can also use ultrasound independently for localization. However, if x-ray was used for preliminary localization, the stone will automatically appear centered on the ultrasound image.

By rotating the coaxial imaging transducer, the shock wave path can be visualized and evaluated for acoustic obstructions (Fig 6). In the event of an obstruction, the stonebreaker assembly can be tilted while maintaining the shock wave focus at the stone. The physician may then evaluate the path again with the imaging transducer to confirm a clear path for the shock wave. The lithotripsy procedure can then commence under real-time ultrasound visualization. The physician has control of the pulse pressure, repetition rate, and number of pulses.

FIG 2.
The THERASONIC lithotripsy control console is incorporated in the Diasonics SPA 1000 ultrasound system.

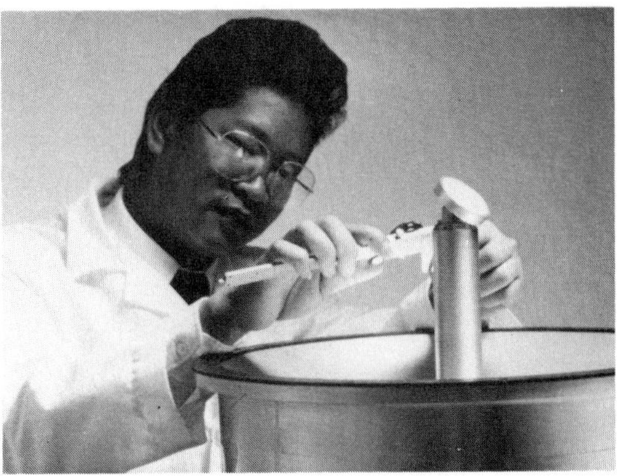

FIG 3.
A custom 3.0 MHz lithotripsy imaging probe is located coaxial with the shock wave transducer. The 50-mm annular array with multi-zone focusing provides excellent spatial resolution over an extended field of view.

SHOCK WAVE CHARACTERISTICS: LABORATORY TESTS

Figure 7 shows the waveform typically recorded at the focus of the lithotripter in degassed water. Relevant characteristics of the shock wave, including peak pressure, pulse rise time, pulse width, and beam profile are summarized in Figure 8.

The measurements to determine the shock wave characteristics of the lithotripter have been made with a custom-built, calibrated hydrophone and then confirmed with a commercial Marconi membrane hydrophone. The custom hydrophone consists of a layer of PVDF piezoelectric material, metalized on both sides and epoxy-bonded to a brass backing and is calibrated against the commercial Marconi hydrophone.

ADVANCED IMAGING TECHNIQUES

While ultrasound imaging is playing an important role in renal lithotripsy, it is anticipated that ultrasound will play the primary role in visualization of radiolucent biliary stones and in real-time monitoring of fragmentation during treatment.

Enhanced visualization of stone morphology and fragmentation is being investigated using Reflex Transmission Imaging (RTI), a proprietary ultrasound imaging technique being developed by SRI International (Menlo Park, CA) and licensed exclusively by Diasonics for lithotripsy applications. Reflex Transmission Imaging produces an orthographic image similar to a flat field x-ray that allows accurate visualization of calculi without the acoustic shadowing normally present in B-scan ultrasound (Figs 9, 10, and 11). Additionally, RTI can display changes in both acoustic at-

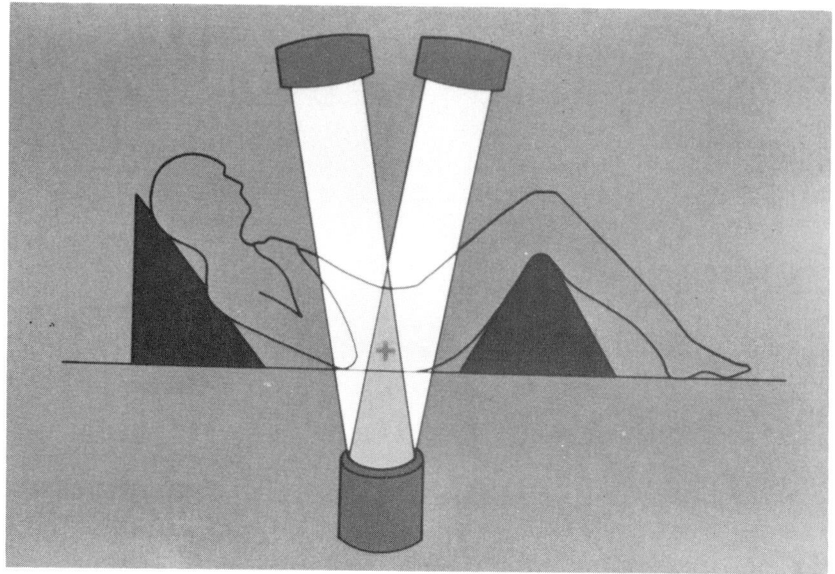

FIG 4.
The operator defines stone position with a cursor in the two views acquired, and the system automatically calculates the stone position in three-dimensional space.

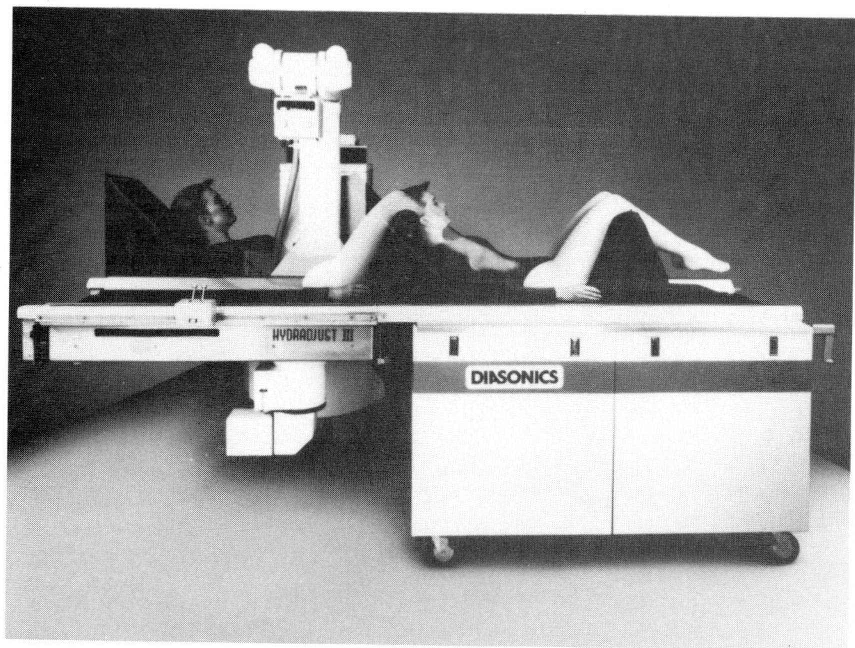

FIG 5.
After x-ray localization, the patient is easily moved to the treatment table. Coordinates from x-ray localization are automatically transferred to the system controller.

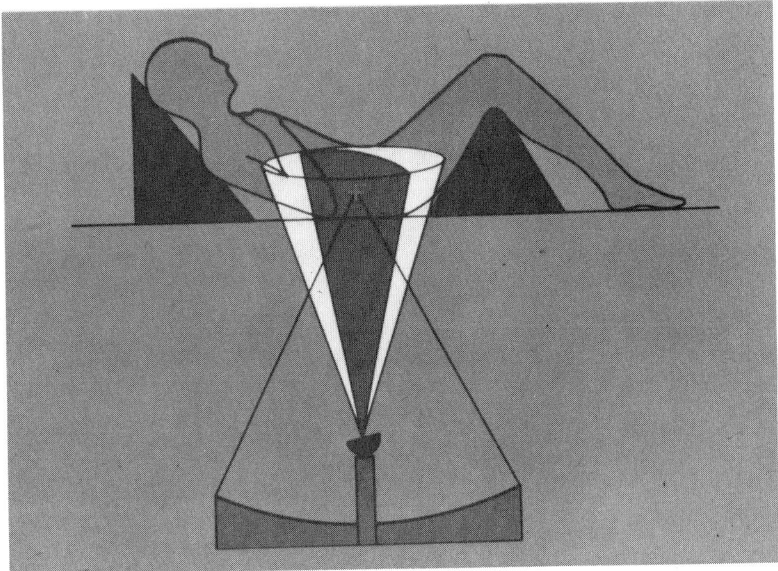

FIG 6.
The operator can rotate the ultrasound transducer in order to evaluate the shock wave treatment path for acoustic obstructions.

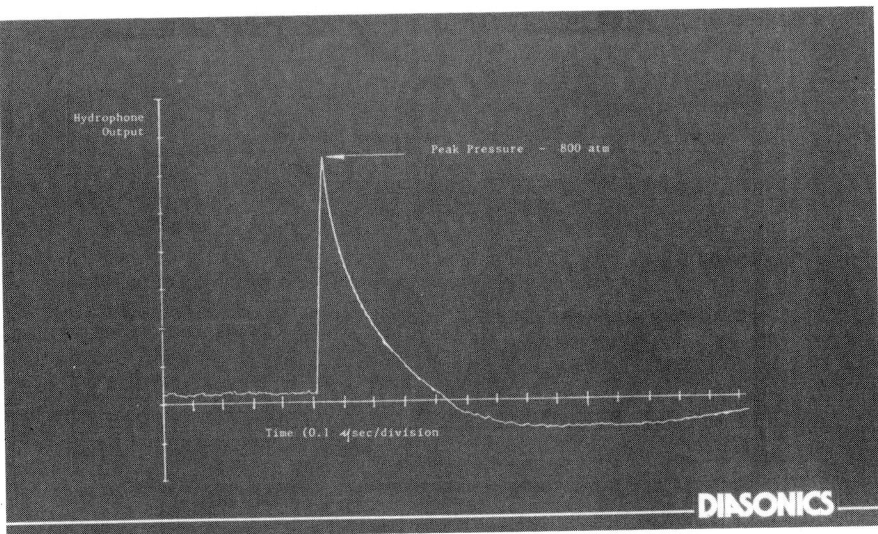

FIG 7.
Typical waveform at shock wave focus measured in degassed water.

Shock Wave Characteristics

Peak Pressure	
Positive	**800** Atmosphere
Negative	**100** Atmosphere
Rise Time (10%-90%)	**30** nanosec
Pulse Width (FWHM)	**115** nanosec
Beam Profile (-6b6)	
Lateral	**3** mm
Axial	**25** mm
Focal Pressure Gain	**150**

DIASONICS

FIG 8.
Summary of THERASONIC shock wave characteristics.

tenuation and reflectivity, which may be useful in monitoring the degree of stone fragmentation.

CONCLUSION

We believe that the design of this device with a small shock wave focal region, low total energy, the ability to localize with x-ray or ultrasound and to monitor stone fragmentation with real-time ultrasound will result in the effective disintegration of upper urinary and biliary stones with minimal anesthesia requirements and reduced peripheral tissue damage. In addition, the reduced size, versatility, and cost effectiveness of this system should bring the opportunity for lithotripsy treatment within the reach of smaller medical centers.

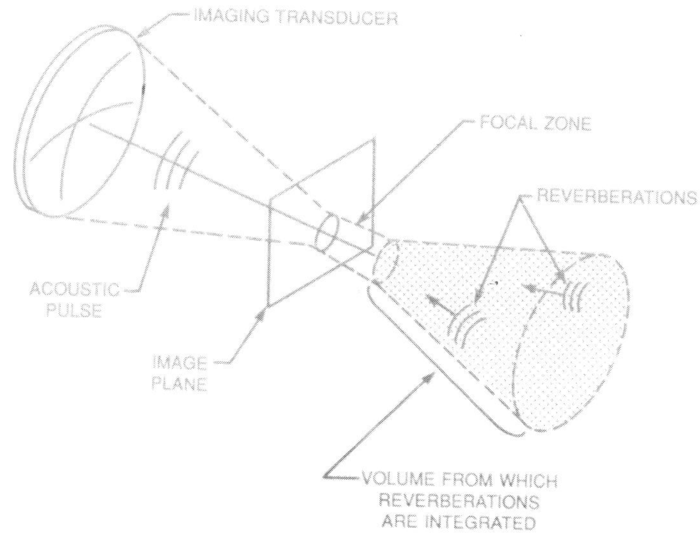

FIG 9.
Reflex Transmission Imaging (RTI) produces an orthographic image similar to a flat field x-ray and can accurately demonstrate stone morphology and acoustic attenuation.

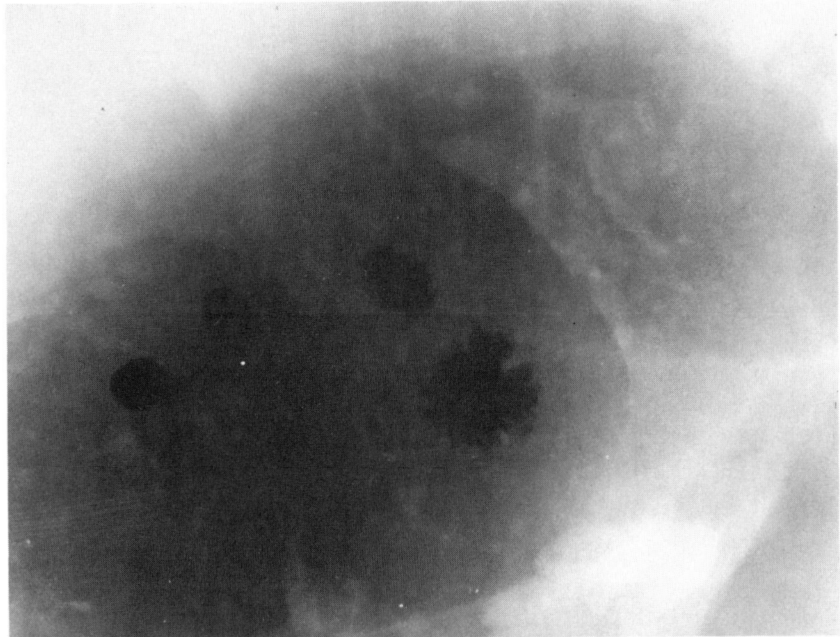

FIG 10.
X-ray image of four stones in a lamb kidney.

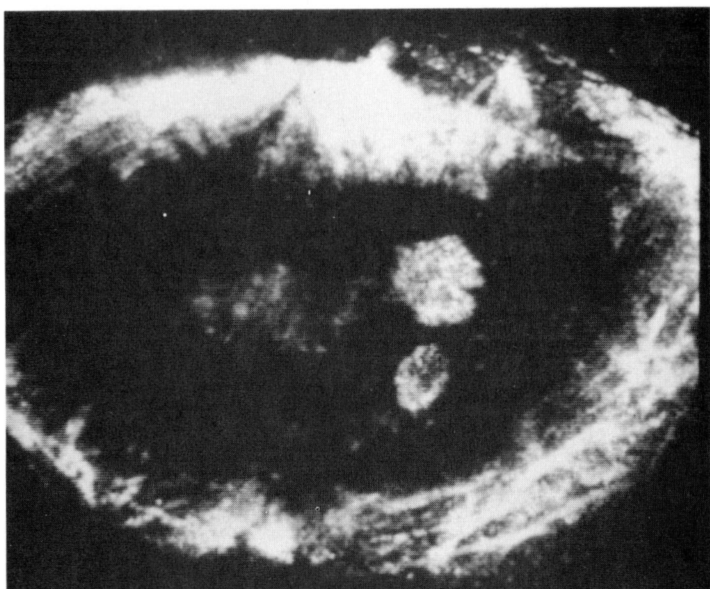

FIG 11.
RTI image demonstrates two stones in the acquired plane. The other two stones are in a deeper slice. Note the clear visualization of the stone without the shadowing normally present in conventional B-scan ultrasound.

Index

H